HUMAN ANATOMY AND PHYSIOLOGY

# POSTURE: TYPES, ASSESSMENT AND CONTROL

# HUMAN ANATOMY AND PHYSIOLOGY

Additional books in this series can be found on Nova's website under the Series tab.

Additional E-books in this series can be found on Nova's website under the E-books tab.

Human Anatomy and Physiology

# Posture: Types, Assessment and Control

Adrienne M. Wright
and
Samuel P. Rothenberg
Editors

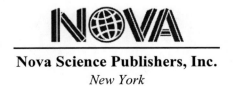

Nova Science Publishers, Inc.
*New York*

Copyright © 2011 by Nova Science Publishers, Inc.

**All rights reserved.** No part of this book may be reproduced, stored in a retrieval system or transmitted in any form or by any means: electronic, electrostatic, magnetic, tape, mechanical photocopying, recording or otherwise without the written permission of the Publisher.

For permission to use material from this book please contact us:
Telephone 631-231-7269; Fax 631-231-8175
Web Site: http://www.novapublishers.com

**NOTICE TO THE READER**

The Publisher has taken reasonable care in the preparation of this book, but makes no expressed or implied warranty of any kind and assumes no responsibility for any errors or omissions. No liability is assumed for incidental or consequential damages in connection with or arising out of information contained in this book. The Publisher shall not be liable for any special, consequential, or exemplary damages resulting, in whole or in part, from the readers' use of, or reliance upon, this material. Any parts of this book based on government reports are so indicated and copyright is claimed for those parts to the extent applicable to compilations of such works.

Independent verification should be sought for any data, advice or recommendations contained in this book. In addition, no responsibility is assumed by the publisher for any injury and/or damage to persons or property arising from any methods, products, instructions, ideas or otherwise contained in this publication.

This publication is designed to provide accurate and authoritative information with regard to the subject matter covered herein. It is sold with the clear understanding that the Publisher is not engaged in rendering legal or any other professional services. If legal or any other expert assistance is required, the services of a competent person should be sought. FROM A DECLARATION OF PARTICIPANTS JOINTLY ADOPTED BY A COMMITTEE OF THE AMERICAN BAR ASSOCIATION AND A COMMITTEE OF PUBLISHERS.

Additional color graphics may be available in the e-book version of this book.

**Library of Congress Cataloging-in-Publication Data**

Posture : types, assessment, and control / editors, Adrienne M. Wright and Samuel P. Rothenberg.
    p. ; cm.
 Includes bibliographical references and index.
 ISBN 978-1-61324-107-3 (hardcover)
 1. Posture. I. Wright, Adrienne M. II. Rothenberg, Samual P.
 [DNLM: 1. Posture. WE 103]
 RA781.5.P675 2011
 613.7'8--dc22
                            2011008478

*Published by Nova Science Publishers, Inc. †New York*

# CONTENTS

**Preface** vii

**Chapter 1** Postural Control: Changes with Ageing and Exercise 1
*Zachary Crowley, Pedro Bezerra and Shi Zhou*

**Chapter 2** Postural Control: From Prescription to Emergence 33
*R. Thouvarecq and D. Leroy*

**Chapter 3** Influence of Sport Training on Sagittal Spinal Curvatures 63
*P. A. López-Miñarro, J. M. Muyor,
F. Alacid, and P. L. Rodríguez*

**Chapter 4** Human Standing Posture: Mathematical Models,
their Biofidelity and Applications 99
*P. B. Pascolo, G. Pagnacco and R. Rossi*

**Chapter 5** The Relationship between Muscle-Tendon Unit Stiffness,
Joint Stability and Posture, The Risk of Injury, Performance,
Resonance and Energy Expenditure 137
*Aurélio Faria, Ronaldo Gabriel, João Abrantes,
Helena Moreira, Paola Wood, and Tanya Camacho*

**Chapter 6** H-Reflex Assessment as a Tool for Understanding
Motor Functions in Postural Control 155
*Yung-Sheng Chen and Shi Zhou*

**Chapter 7** Body Support and Driving Operation
of a Vehicle for Wheelchair Users 175
*Hiroshi Ikeda and Akihiro Mihoshi*

**Index** 191

# PREFACE

Standing is the static posture most commonly evaluated in balance assessments. This is because of its ubiquitous nature and because the act of precariously balancing two thirds of our body mass some distance from the ground imposes critical demands on the postural control system. In this new book, the authors present topical research in the study of posture, including the changes with aging and exercise of postural control; the influence of sport training on sagittal spinal curvatures; mathematical models, their biofidelity and applications in human standing posture; the relationship between muscle-tendon unit stiffness, joint stability and posture and H-reflex assessment in understanding motor functions in postural control.

Chapter 1 - Ageing is frequently accompanied by a decrease of neuromuscular capacities which is associated with increased risk of falls and morbidity. Postural control is one of the functional capacities that are fundamental to an independent lifestyle. Postural control is the ability to maintain the body's centre-of-gravity within the base of support during upright stance. The sensory inputs from visual, vestibular, and proprioceptive modalities are processed by a number of structures in the central nervous system, including the cerebellum, basal ganglia, and cortex, and integrated to produce appropriate motor responses that maintain upright stance and reduce postural sway. Both strength and power, as appropriate motor responses, are important factors in the control of balance and preventions of falls. Decreased muscle strength and power associated with ageing can cause adaptations in the strategies used by the nervous system in control of posture. For example, it has been reported that there is a change from an "ankle strategy" which relies on large moments at the ankle, to a "hip strategy" which relies on moments at the hip to rotate ankle and hip joints in opposite directions. The ability in control of posture can be assessed using either traditional posturography or stabilogram diffusion analysis. Traditional postural control variables are most often characterised with the measures based on the displacement of the centre-of-pressure (COP), while the stabilogram diffusion analysis generates a stabilogram diffusion function that summarises the mean square COP displacement as a function of the time interval between COP comparisons. However, further research is needed to identify the most appropriate postural measures for upright quiet stance. Evidence in the current literature indicates that appropriate exercise has a beneficial effect on the postural control. Amongst the training modalities that have been examined it appears that exercises that involve coordinative balance tasks, such as balance training and Tai Chi, are the most effective in delaying the age-related decline in postural control.

This chapter provides a review of current literature and our understanding on control of upright stance posture, with a focus on the effects of ageing on the factors that are essential for control of posture and the effects of exercise interventions for improving postural control.

Chapter 2 - Studies of postural control using the theoretical framework of complex systems have multiplied over the past 20 years, challenging the traditional cognitive approach to this topic. According to Abernethy and Sparrow (1992), these opposing perspectives, generally concerning "motor control", reflect a paradigmatic crisis as defined by Kuhn (1964). This chapter develops this point of view on the basis of four points. (i) We briefly recall the theoretical origins and fundamental principles of these two approaches to motor function: both arose from the cybernetics research conducted in the 40s and 50s but can be distinguished by their respective control determinants. The cognitive framework assumes that motor function arises from the execution of prescribed programs that are controlled by feedback (Schmidt, 1975). The complex systems framework is based on the assumptions that coordination emerges from the interaction of constraints (Newell, 1986) and is self-organizing (Haken, Kelso, Bunz, 85). (ii) We then show the consequences of these two perspectives in posture research, with major but not exclusive reference to the proposals of Nashner and McCollum (1985) and Massion et al. (1992) for the cognitive perspective, and those of Bardy, Marin, Stoffregen, and Bootsma (1999) for the complex systems perspective. In both cases, recent developments are also considered. (iii) The limits of each perspective are then discussed. (iv) Last, we show the difficulty of reconciling these two approaches to postural control research and discuss the strong possibility that we are headed for a (probably) long period of so-called "normal science", particularly in that these two paradigms will have to coexist.Many studies on motor control, particularly regarding posture, have been published without a clear statement of the authors' ontological position. In most cases, the authors have based their work on cognitivist theory but this has been implicit. At times, internal contradictions are observed, suggesting that the lack of positioning may have been due to an inadequate understanding of the available theoretical perspectives. This issue is not without importance. In 1992, Abernethy and Sparrow published an article titled "The rise and fall of dominant paradigms in motor behavior research" and showed that the field of motor control research was in a period of paradigmatic crisis, as defined by Kuhn (1962). Essentially, since the early 1980s, the nearly exclusive domination of the cognitivist approach in motor behavior studies has been repeatedly contested by proposals based on complexity theory. In this chapter, we briefly review the ontological foundations of these two approaches and the insight into posture that each approach has contributed. We then examine the issue of whether these two approaches have points in common, at least in the field of posture research.

Both cognitivism and complexity theories were inspired by the Macy conference series held between 1946 and 1956 (see Dupuy, 1994, for a review), but they express radically different points of view regarding motor control1. Conversely, the study of motor behavior cannot proceed without a theoretical context]. In the cognitivist approach, the production and control of movement are assumed to be prescribed by a higher information-processing system. In turn, this system receives information from the environment and the musculoskeletal system through the sensory systems. Working from this perspective, Schmidt (1975) presented a model in the 1970s that was to become the reference. According to

---

[1] The research questions and fields of application of both cognitivist and complexity theories extend well beyond motor behavior research, a mere epiphenomenon in this debate (see, for example, Varela, 1993).

Schmidt (1975, 1988), the production and regulation of movement are not based on a single mental schema stored in memory, but on two schemas. Depending on the initial conditions and the goal, the recall schema containing the general rules for movement (the basis of the program) to be carried out permits movement initiation. This Generalized Motor Program (GMP) is applied to a set of similar movements that control certain segments. Once parameterized (segments, force, speed direction), the program issues a series of instructions (composed of invariants and parameters) that will be applied to the musculoskeletal system in the form of muscle contractions (and relaxation) that in turn will provoke feedback from the proprioceptive system (essentially via the neuromuscular spindles), the vestibular system, and so on. The muscle contractions have an effect on the environment, which is then captured by the external receptors (mainly vision). The recognition schema is evoked at the same time as the recall schema. This schema contains information on the expected proprioceptive and exteroceptive feedback. The comparison of these two types of information (proprioceptive and exteroceptive, the "subjective reinforcement")—that is, that which is perceived and that which is expected—then allows for movement correction, if there is sufficient time. Within this framework, representations have a major role and the main research focus is on the information processing that will result in prescriptions and the regulation of muscle activity.

In contrast, complex systems theories do not accord an important role to representations. Instead of a hypothesized higher information-processing system, complexity theories focus on notions of self-organization and emergence. In research on perception and action, three approaches can be distinguished, not contradictory but instead focused on slightly different topics. The first grew out of Gibson's work (1958, 1979) and is focused on the subject-environment relationship. This approach provides an alternative to the notion of action guided by the actor's internal representations and emphasizes perception-action coupling and the theory of affordances. Dynamical systems theory (Turvey, 1990), which built on the works of Bernstein (1967) and Von Holst (1969), has been more concerned with how motor coordination emerges from organismic, task and environmental constraints (Newell, 1986). Last, the synergetic approach (Haken, 1985) applies a model validated in other fields to the study of motor coordination (Kelso and Schoner, 1988). These three approaches share the same ontology and, although proposals for their integration have been made (Warren, 2006), this remains far from evident (Michaels, 1998). These two paradigms have provided the general theoretical framework for much of the research on postural control.

Chapter 3 - Sagittal spinal curvatures are geometric parameters which influence mechanical properties of spinal tissues. Sagittal alignment influences postural loading and load balance of the intervertebral disc.

Sagittal spinal curvatures may adapt gradually when training intensively for long periods. Theoretically, intensive training could lead to adaptations in the spine and might be an important factor associated with changes in the degree of spinal curvatures.

The spinal curvatures of an intensively trained athlete may differ in sagittal configuration from one sport to another. There have been studies on the sagittal spinal curvatures in female rhythmic gymnasts, young ballet dancers, soccer players, runners, Greco-Roman and free style wrestlers, cyclists, rowers, paddlers, skiers... Other studies have analyzed heterogeneous samples of athletes of differing in sports participation. All these studies revealed that specific and repetitive movements and postures of each sport influence spinal curvatures. These differences have been associated to specific spine positions during the training and competition activities. Furthermore, several studies have found some differences between athletes participating in different sports and with respect to control groups of age-matched sedentary subjects.

Sagittal alignment influences postural loading and load balance of the intervertebral disc in healthy subjects. Alterations in spinal curvatures may influence the development of low-back pain, which is a common injury among athletes. Greater spinal angles produce larger shear forces, larger contributions from passive components and greater intradiscal pressures on the thoracic and lumbar tissues. This is of special concern in young athletes, because an increased thoracic angle and/or kyphotic lumbar postures impose great demands on the immature spine, altering the spine's exposure to mechanical loadings during growth. Moreover, prolonged static and cyclic loading has been related to creep deformation in the lumbar viscoelastic tissues. These changes seem to be associated with microdamage to the collagen structure since it was shown to elicit spasms in spinal muscles.

Because the specific positions and movements of the sport training may influence the spine posture, the aim of this chapter is to analyze the influence of sport training in the thoracic and lumbar spinal curvatures of young and adult athletes.

Chapter 4 - In the last decades, several mathematical models of increased complexity have been developed with the goal of better understanding human standing posture and the mechanisms that control it. The sophistication and biofidelity of the models has increased from simple one-link inverted pendulum to full three-dimensional multi-link models. Although models have and continue to provide invaluable insights, they are still at this time too simple to allow the modeling of many pathological conditions and therefore much more work is needed in this field.

Chapter 5 - The predominant role that the musculoskeletal system and, more specifically, the muscle tendon unit play in human motion performance and rehabilitation has been questioned in recent investigations. An attempt to deepen the understanding of how the muscle-tendon unit may contribute to improve human motion performance and rehabilitation has been undertaken by various researchers however this understanding is still limited. The biomechanical properties of the muscle tendon unit and their association to joint stability and posture, the risk of injury, performance, resonance and energy expenditure as well as possible differences between sexes needs to be a source of constant enquiry to ensure a better understanding of this topic and thereby assisting in the application of this knowledge into the fields of sport performance, clinical decision making and rehabilitation. With the purpose to provide an update of the muscle-tendon unit stiffness literature this review includes relevant information for the assessment and comprehension of this biomechanical property and its relationship with joint stability and posture, the risk of injury, performance, resonance and energy expenditure. More specifically the following topics are reviewed: (1) Definition of stiffness and methods used in stiffness evaluation; (2) Stiffness, stability and posture; (3) Stiffness, resonance and energy expenditure; (4) Stiffness and performance; (4) Stiffness and the risk of injury. Finally some directions for future work are proposed. This review will contribute to increase the knowledge of the musculoskeletal system and provide a stronger basis for the development of future works and intervention programs in the fields of sport performance, clinical decision making and rehabilitation.

Chapter 6 - The Hoffmann reflex (H-reflex) has been extensively used to investigate spinal reflexive function in clinical and human movement studies. The H-reflex is induced by applying an electrical stimulation on a peripheral nerve branch and recording EMG from a muscle innervated by this nerve. The response of the α-motoneuron pool to the stimulation, as indicated by the peak-to-peak amplitude of H-reflex, reflects inhibitory and excitatory modulation of the spinal motoneuron pool during a motor task. Recently, the H-reflex modulation in relation to postural control has been addressed in a number of laboratory-based investigations. There has been evidence that the modulation of H-reflex is task-dependent. Specificity of the H-reflex in adaptation to exercise intervention has also been revealed. This chapter provides a discussion on the H-reflex modulation during a variety of postural tasks and its adaptation to exercise training. The soleus (SOL) H-reflex is the focus because this muscle plays a critical role in maintaining an upright standing posture and the studies on SOL H-reflex modulation may help us to understand the neural mechanisms in postural control.

Chapter 7 - Driving a vehicle is an important means to realizing participation in society for disabled people who want to become independent, however, the maintenance of laws in Japan concerning the driving environment is insufficiently established when compared to the support and welfare for disabled drivers in other advanced countries. A better and safer driving environment will be created if public opinion is taken into account positively, in a similar way to stations and other public areas. In this chapter, in order to determine the driving safety of wheelchair drivers, both a questionnaire survey and an experiment to measure the steering angle and acceleration-velocity during driving were conducted. As a result, it is shown that the driving environment for wheelchair drivers does not grant enough modifications for safe driving, and there are differences between physically unimpaired drivers and wheelchair drivers in the tendency for hazardous driving behavior. When driving at faster speeds, the methods of keeping body balance are shown to be different on right and left curves, and also a difficulty in maintaining a stable position during operation of the vehicle is indicated. Especially at the end of a curve, where there is greater acceleration velocity, the body balance is easily disrupted in terms of driving posture, and a reduction of both stability and usability of driving operation of the steering wheel and the acceleration lever is shown.

In: Posture: Types, Assessment and Control
Editors: A. Wright and S. Rothenberg, pp. 1-32

ISBN 978-1-61324-107-3
© 2011 Nova Science Publishers, Inc.

*Chapter 1*

# POSTURAL CONTROL: CHANGES WITH AGEING AND EXERCISE

## *Zachary Crowley,*[1] *Pedro Bezerra*[2] *and Shi Zhou*[*1]

[1]School of Health and Human Science, Southern Cross University, Australia
[2]Instituto Politecnico Viana do Castelo, Portugal

### ABSTRACT

Ageing is frequently accompanied by a decrease of neuromuscular capacities which is associated with increased risk of falls and morbidity. Postural control is one of the functional capacities that are fundamental to an independent lifestyle. Postural control is the ability to maintain the body's centre-of-gravity within the base of support during upright stance. The sensory inputs from visual, vestibular, and proprioceptive modalities are processed by a number of structures in the central nervous system, including the cerebellum, basal ganglia, and cortex, and integrated to produce appropriate motor responses that maintain upright stance and reduce postural sway. Both strength and power, as appropriate motor responses, are important factors in the control of balance and preventions of falls. Decreased muscle strength and power associated with ageing can cause adaptations in the strategies used by the nervous system in control of posture. For example, it has been reported that there is a change from an "ankle strategy" which relies on large moments at the ankle, to a "hip strategy" which relies on moments at the hip to rotate ankle and hip joints in opposite directions. The ability in control of posture can be assessed using either traditional posturography or stabilogram diffusion analysis. Traditional postural control variables are most often characterised with the measures based on the displacement of the centre-of-pressure (COP), while the stabilogram diffusion analysis generates a stabilogram diffusion function that summarises the mean square COP displacement as a function of the time interval between COP comparisons. However, further research is needed to identify the most appropriate postural measures for upright quiet stance. Evidence in the current literature indicates that appropriate exercise has a beneficial effect on the postural control. Amongst the training modalities that have been examined it appears that exercises that involve coordinative balance tasks,

---

[*] Corresponding Author: Professor Shi Zhou, School of Health and Human Sciences, Southern Cross University, Lismore, NSW 2480, Australia, Tel: + 61 2 66203991, Fax: + 61 2 66269583, E-mail: shi.zhou@scu.edu.au.

such as balance training and Tai Chi, are the most effective in delaying the age-related decline in postural control.

This chapter provides a review of current literature and our understanding on control of upright stance posture, with a focus on the effects of ageing on the factors that are essential for control of posture and the effects of exercise interventions for improving postural control.

## 1. BIOMECHANICS OF UPRIGHT STANCE

The ability in maintaining an upright standing position is of fundamental importance to daily life. The upright stance is a naturally unstable position that requires continuous adjustments of muscle contractions to maintain joint positions from the neck to the ankle (Maurer and Peterka, 2005). It requires maintenance of body's centre of gravity (COG) within the supporting base, ie. between the feet (King, Judge, and Wolfson, 1994; Laughton et al., 2003; Ryushi et al., 2000). The COG is usually located within the body at approximately the level of the second sacral segment. Despite this relatively large distance from the base of support (BOS) the body is able to provide suitable responses to changes in the location of the COG. The movement of the COG during an unconstrained standing can be measured by the trajectory of the Centre of Pressure (COP) when an individual stands on a force platform. The movements of COP are derived from the location of the vertical ground reaction forces on the surface of a force platform under the feet (Prieto, Myklebust, Hoffmann, Lovett, and Myklebust, 1996; Santos, Delisle, Lariviere, Plamondon, and Imbeau, 2008; Winter, 1995). These COP trajectories have, for many years, been used to infer biomechanical mechanisms of postural control (Lord and Sturnieks, 2005; Melzer, Benjuya, and Kaplanski, 2004; Prieto, et al., 1996) and some of the commonly used COP assessment methods are described in Section 2 of this chapter.

In the static erect posture the vertical projection of the COG is often termed the line of gravity (LOG) and this line has important implications in the maintenance of posture. Any shift in the location of the COG e.g. anterior translation, will cause movement of the LOG in the same direction i.e. anteriorly. However, during static erect posture the LOG must fall within the border of the supporting feet to maintain equilibrium (Nashner, 1990).

When the LOG passes directly through the axis of rotation of a joint no net gravitational torque is produced. However, during quiet upright bipedal stance this optimal alignment of joints or "optimal posture" does not exist. Often when maintaining postural control the LOG passes either anteriorly or posteriorly to the axis of rotation of all joints involved which will cause gravitational torque around the joints. This torque will cause rotation around the joint which will consequently require a counterbalancing torque, through muscular contractions, to maintain the upright posture. Also the gravitational moment magnitude increases as the distance between the LOG and joint axis increases (Levangie and Norkin, 2001).

When analysing upright stance in the sagittal plane it can be seen that the LOG falls either anteriorly or posteriorly to the ankle, knee, and hip joint axes. For the ankle joint the LOG usually passes anteriorly to the lateral malleolus which is the ankle axis of rotation (Danis, Krebs, Gill-Body, and Sahrmann, 1998). This anterior LOG positioning causes a gravitational dorsiflexion moment. To counteract this dorsiflexion moment there is a need to activate posterior muscles such as the soleus and gastrocnemius (Izquierdo, Aguado,

Gonzalez, Lopez, and Hakkinen, 1999). The activation of posterior lower limb muscles has been establish on several occasions (Borg, Finell, Hakala, and Herrala, 2007; Runge, Shupert, Horak, and Zajac, 1999) with some authors stating that the strength of these muscles is the main modulator for ankle movement during postural control (Horak, Earhart, and Dietz, 2001).

Like the ankle joint, during upright stance the LOG does not pass through the joint axes of the knee and hip joints. The knee joint is usually close to full extension during quiet posture, however the LOG passes just anterior to the knee joint axis which creates a gravitational moment causing extension at the knee joint (Danis, et al., 1998). Posterior knee joint capsule tension and associated ligaments are usually sufficient to counterbalance the gravitational moment at the knee, therefore little muscle activity is needed. A small amount of activity, however, has been identified that a small amount of activation occurs in posterior thigh muscles (Levangie and Norkin, 2001) which would help to counteract the extension moment due to gravity. It has also been hypothesised that activity of the soleus may augment the gravitational extension moment at the knee through its posterior pull on the tibia as it acts at the ankle joint (Levangie and Norkin, 2001). The LOG acting at the hip passes through the greater trochanter, which is slightly posterior to the axis of rotation. This posteriorly located gravitational line creates an extension moment at the hip which causes posterior rotation of the pelvis on the femoral head (Kagaya, Sharma, Kobetic, and Marsolais, 1998). This is supported by research that has shown activity within the hip flexors during standing (Basmajian, 1978).

While all the above examples were discussed in relation to a near optimal posture, in reality there is always movement of the body segments to counter the destabilisation torque due to gravity. The LOG will often pass on the opposite side of the joint axis and would therefore require activation of the opposing muscles, compared to what was explained above. For example, if an individual adopted a flexed knee posture or the movement of the COG was posterior then the LOG would pass posterior to the knee joint and create a flexion moment. To stabilise the knee and maintain erect posture, activation of the quadriceps muscles would then be required (Levangie and Norkin, 2001).

## 2. ASSESSMENTS OF POSTURE CONTROL

Static posturography is a method in which the performance of the postural control system in a static position and environment is characterised. When an individual attempts to stand still, the COP under their feet moves relative to a global coordinate system. A plot of the time-varying coordinates of the COP is known as a stabilogram (Collins, De Luca, Burrows, and Lipsitz, 1995). Many researchers have measured the anterior-posterior (AP) and medial-lateral (ML) displacements of the COP in an attempt to evaluate and interpret the behaviour of the postural control system. The measurement of posture control is often conducted using either traditional posturography or stabilogram diffusion analysis, which are methods of computing the COP behaviours. Traditional postural control variables are most often characterised with the measures based on the displacement of the COP measured with a force platform (also known as summary statistics) (Prieto, et al., 1996). The stabilogram diffusion analysis generates a stabilogram diffusion function that summarises the mean square COP displacement as a function of the time interval between COP comparisons and is based on the assumption that erect posture is, in part, a stochastic process (Collins and De Luca, 1993).

## 2.1. Stabilogram Traditional Parameters

The COP is the location of the vertical reaction vector on the surface of the force platform on which the subject stands. The COP reflects the orientation of the body segments (joint angles), as well as the movements of the body to keep the COP within the base of support. The anterior-posterior, medial-lateral displacement of the COP can be measured with the force platform. The COP parameters can be measured in 1) Time-Domain "distance" measures, 2) Time-Domain "area" measures, and 3) Time-Domain "hybrid" measures (Prieto, et al., 1996). Several authors in the literature have used combinations of these COP measurements to characterise the behaviour of the postural control system (Doyle, Hsiao-Wecksler, Ragan, and Rosengren, 2008; Raymakers, Samson, and Verhaar, 2005; Santos, et al., 2008; Vieira, de Oliveira, and Nadal, 2009) with a large majority of these parameters being drawn from the work of Prieto et al. (1996).

The COP coordinate time series, AP and ML, are commonly used to compute measures of postural steadiness, and characterise the static performance of the postural control system. These two time series also define the COP path relative to the origin of the force plate. The resultant distance (RD) time series is the vector distance from the mean COP to each pair of points in the AP and ML time series (Prieto, et al., 1996). The following procedures are for the composite measures computed using both the AP and ML time series, and those based on the AP time series. Every measurement defined for the AP time series is similarly defined for the ML time series (Prieto, et al., 1996).

Time-domain distance measures estimate a parameter associated with either the displacement of the COP from the central point of the stabilogram, or the velocity of the COP. The mean distance (Mdist) is the mean of the RD time series, and represents the average distance from the mean COP, while the mean distance-AP is the mean absolute value of the AP time series and represents the average AP distance from the mean COP (Prieto, et al., 1996). The root-mean-squared (RMS) distance from the mean COP is the RMS value of the RD time series and can also be calculated for just the RMS distance-AP and ML time series (Prieto, et al., 1996). The mean velocity (Mvel) is the average velocity of the COP and is also calculated for all three time series (RD, AP, and ML). In effect, this normalises the total excursions to the analysis interval. The COP time series are filtered to the frequency range of interest to minimise the quantisation noise that may inadvertently inflate measures such as mean velocity and total excursions (Prieto, et al., 1996).

Time-domain area measures and time-domain hybrid measures have also been used in the past but generally not to the same degree. These measures are methods that are statistically based estimates of the area enclosed by the stabilogram or are measures that model the stabilogram with a combination of distance measures respectively. Examples of Time-domain area measures include the 95% confidence circle area (Area-CC) (Santos, et al., 2008) and the 95% confidence ellipse area (Area-CE) (Doyle, et al., 2008) while the sway-area (Area-SW) (Raymakers, et al., 2005) and mean frequency (MFreq) (Prieto, et al., 1996) are examples of time-domain hybrid measures. Although this is not an exhaustive list of the parameter used in traditional stabilogram analysis, there still is a need for future investigations to elucidate which measures best represent changes in the postural control system, e.g. due to ageing.

## 2.2. Stabilogram Diffusion Parameters

The statistical-biomechanics method of assessing the COP trajectories named stabilogram-diffusion analysis (SDA) was developed by Collins and De Luca (1993). This analysis is based on the assumption that the movement of the COP represents the combined output of co-existing deterministic and stochastic mechanisms. The COP displacement analysis is calculated by computing the square of the displacements between all pairs of points separated by a specific time interval and averaged over the number of time intervals making up a COP time series. These analyses reveal that over short-term intervals of time during undisturbed stance the COP behaves as a positively correlated random walk whereby the COP tends to drift away from a relative equilibrium point. This is interpreted as an indication that the postural control system uses open-loop control mechanisms which operates without sensory feedback (descending commands which set the steady-state activity levels of the postural muscles) (Laughton, et al., 2003). In long-term intervals of time, it resembles a negatively correlated random walk whereby the COP tends to return to a relative equilibrium point, indicating that the postural control system now uses closed-loop control mechanisms. It is inferred that this period is one in which the postural control system operates with sensory feedback (from visual, vestibular and somatosensory systems) (Collins and De Luca, 1993; Collins, et al., 1995; Laughton, et al., 2003). This perspective has the advantage that it leads to the extraction of repeatable COP parameters which can be directly related to the steady-state behaviour and functional interaction of the neuromuscular mechanisms underlying the maintenance of upright stance (Collins, et al., 1995).

Stabilogram-diffusion analysis involves the extraction of three sets of posturographic parameters: diffusion coefficients, scaling exponents, and critical point coordinates (Collins, et al., 1995). The diffusion coefficient is an average measure of the stochastic activity of a random walker, i.e. it is directly related to its jump frequency and/or amplitude, and can be thought of as an indicator of the relative stability of the system (Doyle, et al., 2008). The short-term and long-term COP diffusion coefficients characterise the stochastic activity of the open-loop and closed-loop postural control mechanisms, respectively (Collins, et al., 1995). Diffusion coefficients are calculated from the slopes of the resultant linear-linear plots of mean square COP displacement versus the change in time (Collins, et al., 1995). The long-term and ML diffusion coefficients are usually lower than the respective short-term and AP diffusion coefficients which reflects the increased level of stochastic activity over the short-term time series and AP direction comparatively to long-term time series and ML direction, respectively (Collins and De Luca, 1993).

Quantification of the correlation between the step increments that make up an experimental time series is the second posturographic parameter used in SDA and is termed "scaling exponents" (Collins, et al., 1995). Scaling exponents are calculated from the slopes of the resultant log-log plots of mean square COP displacement versus the change in time. This measure can be thought of as providing an indication whether the motion of the COP is more or less likely to continue moving in the same direction that it is currently moving (Doyle, et al., 2008). Scaling exponents may assume a value in the range of 0 to 1. If the scaling exponents are equal to 0.5, then the increments in COP displacements are statistically independent. If the scaling exponent value is greater than 0.5, then past and future increments are positively correlated, i.e. future displacement increments tend to move in the same direction as the current displacement value (persistent behaviour). If scaling exponents are less than 0.5, then the stochastic activity is negatively correlated, i.e. increasing/decreasing trends in the past imply decreasing/increasing trends in the future (anti-persistent behaviour) (Collins, et al., 1995; Peterka, 2000). From a physiological standpoint, SDA scaling exponents quantify the correlated behaviour of the respective postural control mechanisms, i.e., short-term scaling exponents characterise the drift-like dynamics of the open-loop postural control mechanisms, whereas the long-term scaling exponents characterise the antidrift-like dynamics of the closed-loop postural control mechanisms (Collins, et al., 1995).

The critical point coordinates approximate the transition region that separates the short-term and long-term regions. The estimation of the critical point coordinates is determined as the intersection point of the straight lines is fitted to the two regions of the linear-linear version of the resultant stabilogram-diffusion plot. The transition points occur at relatively small time intervals (0.33 to 1.67 s) and small means square displacement (1.10 mm2 to 29.37 mm2) (Collins and De Luca, 1993; Collins, et al., 1995). These coordinates approximate the temporal and spatial characteristics of the region over which the physiological postural control system switches from open-loop control to closed-loop control.

Several studies have utilised the SDA technique since the work of Collins and De Luca was first published with some authors using the technique to examine the age-related changes in postural control (Baratto, Morasso, Re, and Spada, 2002; Collins, et al., 1995; Dozza et al., 2005; Laughton, et al., 2003). The SDA approach has the advantage that it can be directly related to the steady-state behaviour and functional interaction of the neuromuscular mechanisms underlying the maintenance of upright position. Thus, this statistical-biomechanics approach seems be useful to formulate and test hypothesis concerning the relative contribution of different sensorimotor subsystems (visual, vestibular and proprioceptive) and strategies to control posture (Collins and De Luca, 1993, 1995; Collins, et al., 1995; Doyle, et al., 2008; Newell, Slobounov, Slobounova, and Molenaar, 1997; Peterka, 2000).

## 3. PHYSIOLOGY OF POSTURAL CONTROL

Any detected angular deviation from upright stance applies neural strategies, at supraspinal and spinal levels, involving the interaction between the sensory and motor system to create continuous corrective torque to compensate for disturbances. Postural control involves integration of sensory information from the vestibular, visual and tactile-proprioceptive receptors which stimulate motor responses to maintain balance via several parts of the brain including the cerebellum, brainstem, basal ganglia and sensory-motor cortex (Lord, Clark, and Webster, 1991b; Lord, Ward, Williams, and Anstey, 1994). Once the postural system has integrated all sensory information the CNS sends out appropriate motor responses to effector muscles in an effort to maintain the posture. These corrective movements imply the ability to choose appropriate motor responses based on past experience, to modify these responses on the basis of the continuous sensory input and to produce the needed muscular contraction to stabilise posture (Era et al., 1996).

Proprioception, vision, and vestibular inputs are the main sources of sensory information to guide and control posture and movement. This information is provided via kinaesthetic receptors located in the muscles, tendons, joints, skin, the eyes, and vestibular receptors and provide essential feedback for the maintenance of postural control (Lord, Clark, and Webster, 1991c). The peripheral sensations appear to be the most important sensory input in the maintenance of the postural control (Era, et al., 1996; Melzer, et al., 2004) and consists of two main sensory organs, the muscle spindle and the Golgi tendon organ. The vestibular and visual systems seem to contribute to the postural control system more when there is a reduced sensory feedback from proprioceptive inputs especially in some pathological conditions and ageing (Era, et al., 1996).

Muscle spindles are distributed throughout the belly of muscles and report the absolute amount of stretch and the rate of change of stretch in a particular muscle (Mynark and Koceja, 2001). The response to muscle length change, known as stretch reflex, plays an important role in counteracting the pull of gravity in upright posture (Barr and Kiernan, 1993). The tendon receptors, known as Golgi tendon organs, are sensitive to the amount of tension developed on a tendon and send the impulses to the spinal cord. This proprioceptive information is important in maintaining balance and adjusting posture during standing and has an increased role when both visual and vestibular information are poor or reduced (J. Winter, Allen, and Proske, 2005). The vestibular apparatus is centrally involved in body balance and has close reflex connections with the visual system (Horak, et al., 2001; Horak, Shupert, Dietz, and Horstmann, 1994). A diminutive vestibular reflex has an impact on the maintenance of posture when both proprioceptive and visual information are unavailable or ambiguous (Bacsi and Colebatch, 2005; Horak, et al., 2001; Horak, Nashner, and Diener, 1990; Nashner, Black, and Wall, 1982).

In the motor system, the main factors associated with decreased postural control include the decline in muscle strength and power, and the reduced capacity to respond appropriately to disturbances in postural activity (Dean, Kuo, and Alexander, 2004; Grasso, Zago, and Lacquaniti, 2000). The hip and lower limb muscle groups (knee extensors, knee flexors, ankle planarflexors, and ankle dorsiflexors) should be examined closely because of their influence in controlling posture (Laughton, et al., 2003). The dynamic interaction between the agonists and antagonists in maintaining posture has received limited attention, however it has been suggested that an increase in strength of lower limb muscle groups may be a factor that could improve not only postural control but the stability of muscle contractions (Collins, et al., 1995; Laughton, et al., 2003). This is especially important as the hamstrings are the antagonists of the quadriceps muscle and *vice versa* in the thigh, while in the lower leg the same principle applies to the plantarflexors (eg. gastrocnemius) and dorsiflexors (eg. tibialis anterior) during postural control. Several studies have demonstrated that a reduced quadriceps and ankle dorsiflexion strength greatly increases body sway in a situation of reduced sensation and visual input (King, et al., 1994; Laughton, et al., 2003; Maki, Holliday, and Topper, 1994), highlighting the importance of lower limb strength as a limiting factor in the control of upright stance.

## 3.1. Effects of Ageing on Postural Control

Ageing is a natural process that brings with it many biological, physiological, and psychological changes. These changes often affect the individual's quality of living; nevertheless the fact remains that the ageing body can accomplish most, if not all, of the functions of its youth. However, these functions are often diminished with ageing, the main differences being that movements are less precise, take significantly longer time to produce, and require much more motivation (Porth and Matfin, 2009). But as in youth, physiological function can be maintained to a degree through continued use and exercise (Carter, Kannus, and Khan, 2001).

In chronological terms, the older adult population is characteristically defined as individuals 65 years and older. Still there is considerable heterogeneity among this age group and as a result older adults are often sub grouped into young-old (65 – 74 years), middle-old (75 – 84 years), and old-old (85+ years) categories. This further grouping of older individuals reflects more accurately the changes in physiological function (Porth and Matfin, 2009).

Physiological changes often seen with ageing reflect a general decline in body system functions. These declines result in a diminution of various systems such as the muscular and neurologic systems resulting in a reduction of physical capabilities. The ageing muscular system experiences a decrease in muscular strength which is directly related to both a reduction in the size of existing muscle fibres (muscular atrophy) as well as a loss of muscle fibres. Accompanying this strength loss is a decline in reaction time which is often associated with type II muscle fibre loss while type I fibres are said to remain relatively stable throughout life (Timiras, 2003c). The progressive ageing-related decline in musculoskeletal strength cannot be stopped in entirety, however, it is said that it can be slowed with the introduction of appropriate exercise interventions (Carter, et al., 2001; Sherrington et al., 2008). Neurological structural changes also occur with the ageing process that may interfere with day-to-day routines including a loss of neurons in both the brain and spinal cord. Another change in the nervous system with ageing is neuronal dendrite atrophy which results in impaired synaptic connections and diminished electrochemical reactions leading to the slowing of many neuronal processes (Timiras, 2003a). Sensorimotor changes with ageing include a decline in motor strength, slowed reaction time, diminished reflexes (especially in the ankles), and proprioceptive changes. These changes have functional consequences such as a compromised balance and postural control, and slowed and more deliberate movements (Porth and Matfin, 2009; Timiras, 2003b).

Morphological and physiological alterations associated with ageing often cause degradation in the human's ability to maintain upright stance (Abrahamová and Hlavačka, 2008; Horak, Shupert, and Mirka, 1989; Woollacott, 1993). It is often found that with ageing there is a decline in the capacity of postural control with an associated increase in the incidences of falls and a decrease in mobility (Laughton, et al., 2003). This ageing process often results in a decrease in stability of the open-loop postural control mechanisms (Laughton, et al., 2003) and also a greater delay in the closed-loop postural control (Amiridis, Hatzitaki, and Arabatzi, 2003; Prieto, et al., 1996) Both the delay in the onset of the closed-loop postural control and the larger instability of the open-loop postural control causes an increase in the short-term postural sway through endorsing a higher level of stochastic activity (Amiridis, et al., 2003; Kuo and Zajac, 1993b). It is possible that these age-related changes in the open-loop postural control mechanisms are due to a postural control strategy adopted by elderly individuals whereby they increase the level of muscle activity across their lower-limb joints (Laughton, et al., 2003). Moreover, compared with healthy young adults, older adults exhibit significantly increased levels of antagonist muscle co-activation in response to postural perturbations (Amiridis, et al., 2003; Benjuya, Melzer, and Kaplanski, 2004). This co-activation of antagonistic muscles has been said to improve joint impedance and more specifically joint stiffness, which in turn contributes to the overall stability of the system (van Soest, Haenen, and Rozendaal, 2003).

It is also common in the postural control literature to find that, when using measures of COP traditional summary statistics, the elderly exhibit greater measured COP velocities, distances, and amplitude and/or frequencies. For example, Abrahamová and Hlavačka (2008) found that under four sensory organisation test (SOT) conditions (combination of eyes open and closed on either hard or foam surface), the older group (60-82 years) exhibited significantly greater anterioposterior (AP) COP amplitude, velocity, and root mean square values when compared to a young group (20-40 years). In another study, Du Pasquier et al. (2003) found that velocity measures were best at reflecting postural stability impairment with ageing. They also found that closure of the eyes increased sway but to a much greater degree in the older individuals compared to the younger group. All of the above authors attributed the decreased functionality of the postural control system to physiological changes in sensory and motor systems that are often seen with ageing.

## 3.2. Sensory Inputs and Ageing

Effective maintenance of postural control not only relies on appropriate application of muscle forces to maintain body position but also requires sensory inputs. These sensory inputs allow the nervous system to decide on the *when* and *how* of the restorative forces in an effort to maintain upright stance (Woollacott, 1993). When sensory inputs are altered or absent, as is the often experienced with natural ageing, the control system must interpret and respond to incomplete data. This partial reduction or complete lack of sensory feedback often causes alterations in a person's stability and postural control (Du Pasquier, et al., 2003; Fransson, Kristinsdottir, Hafstrom, Magnusson, and Johansson, 2004). These variations in sensory feedback can either be environmental, as in weightlessness, or physiological such as visual, vestibular, or proprioceptive abnormalities. All three of these physiological factors have been proven to diminish with ageing and have been implicated in alterations in postural control (Baloh, Ying, and Jacobson, 2003; Du Pasquier, et al., 2003; Lord and Menz, 2000).

### 3.2.1. Vision

Visual inputs provide important information to the CNS regarding the motion and position of the head in relation to the surrounding environment. Visual inputs not only provide the postural system with motion information but it also provides a reference for verticality and further information such as colour, form, and depth which all contribute to sensory feedback and orientation with reference to the external environment. This visual information can have significant effects on the maintenance of upright posture. For example, Hafström et al. (2002) found that sway increased when visual motion feedback was deprived or visual field was restricted. In other studies, similar results have been found in that visual environmental motion induces postural adjustments (Guerraz, Gianna, Burchill, Gresty, and

Bronstein, 2001; Mergner, Schweigart, Maurer, and Blümle, 2005) as well as illusions of self-motion (Guerraz and Bronstein, 2008).

In another study, Collins and De Luca (1995) investigated the effects of eyes-open and eyes-closed on both open-loop and closed-loop postural control mechanisms in a group of healthy young adults. The authors interpreted the results as that the visual system is integrated into the postural control system in one of two ways: either causes a decrease in the mediolateral and anteroposterior stochastic activity of the open-loop control mechanism, or causes an increase in the stochastic activity and uncorrelated behaviour of the closed-loop control mechanism in the anteroposterior direction. It was hypothesised that in both schemes visual input serves to decrease the stiffness of the musculoskeletal system. However these alterations in postural control strategies in relation to visual inputs can differ when comparing young to older adults.

With ageing, there are multiple structural changes in the eye which cause functional constraints affecting the ability to maintain adequate postural control. There is typically a loss of visual field, a reduction in light transmission to the retina (causing an increase in visual threshold), a decline in visual acuity (caused by an increase in lens' stiffness, colour opacity, increased incidents of cataracts, and macular degeneration), and reduction in visual contrast sensitivity (which causes problems in contour and depth perception) (Harwood, 2001; Shumway-Cook and Woollacott, 2007). Many previous studies have demonstrated that age-related changes in visual information have undesirable effects on functional skills including postural control (Lord and Menz, 2000; Matheson, Darlington, and Smith, 1999; Teasdale, Stelmach, and Breunig, 1991; Teasdale, Stelmach, Breunig, and Meeuwsen, 1991). For example, Anand et al. (2003a) investigated postural stability changes in elderly while influenced by cataract simulation and refractive blur. They found that cataract simulation and refractive blur caused significant increases in COP-root mean square and concluded that changes in contrast sensitivity rather than resolution changes are responsible for increasing postural instability.

As humans age, the resulting reduction or alteration in the amount and quality of visual sensory information available to the motor cortex (Prieto, et al., 1996) is often associated with the deterioration in postural control (Kristinsdottir, Fransson, and Magnusson, 2001; Peterka, 2000). It is a common finding that the elderly exhibit significantly faster centre-of-pressure (COP) velocities, COP distances, and COP excursions in comparison with younger adults with the trend being exacerbated when eyes are closed (Kuo and Zajac, 1993a). A study by Lord and Ward (1994) found that under challenging conditions (standing on foam with eyes open or closed), vision, along with muscle strength and reaction time, played a significant role in postural maintenance. It was concluded that up until age 65, balance control was significantly influenced by vision and that increasing sway areas in the oldest age groups (Over 65 years) were, in part, attributable to visual deficits effecting peripheral inputs.

### 3.2.2. Vestibular Apparatus

Although we are not conscious of the vestibular sensation, as we are with other senses, vestibular inputs are important for the coordination of many motor functions. The vestibular organs are located in the inner ear and have a connection to the CNS. They contribute to the reflex activity necessary for effective posture and movement and provide information about the position and movement of the head with respect to gravity and inertial forces (Horak, 2010; Shumway-Cook and Woollacott, 2007). In humans, the sense of equilibrium is facilitated by hair cells that line the vestibular apparatus of the inner ear. These hair cells are tonically active and synapse, via primary sensory neurons, to the vestibular nerve, in the vestibular nuclei of the medulla or run without synapsing to the cerebellum, which is the primary site of equilibrium processing (Silverthorn, 2010). This vestibular sensory information has been shown on several occasions to be integral in the maintenance of upright posture. For example, in a study by Bacsi and Colebatch (2005), it was confirmed that vestibulospinal reflexes were acutely facilitated as body sway increased and vestibular reflexes appeared to have a specific role in the maintenance of upright stance, especially under conditions where postural information was absent or attenuated.

Acute unilateral or bilateral loss of vestibular function has been shown to have devastating effects on postural control. This is particularly evident with ageing where there is a loss of 40% of the vestibular hair and nerve cells by 70 years of age (Rosenhall and Rubin, 1975) which often leads to deteriorations in vestibular function (Ray and Monahan, 2002). The extent of this disturbance, however, is often dependant on the ability of the nervous system to compensate for the loss of this important sensory input (Horak, 2010). This is due to the vestibular system functioning as a reference system for other sensory modalities (vision and somatosensory). For example, Horak et al. (1990) found that sensory deficits resulted in postural response alterations. Vestibular loss gave rise to a normal ankle strategy and a lack of hip strategy, even when required for the task of maintaining posture on a shortened surface.

Although about one third of older adults suffer from disturbed vestibular reflexes, many studies have not found any effects on postural control (Lord, et al., 1991b; Lord and Ward, 1994; Lord, et al., 1994). The proposed reason for this lack of effect on postural control is that older people with adequate peripheral sensation and/or vision can compensate for reduced vestibular function (Lord and Sturnieks, 2005). However, individuals with vestibular dysfunction experience conditions such as vertigo and nystagmus, suggesting that vestibular disorders influence postural control and that further research is required to better understand the vestibular contributions to the control of balance (Lord and Sturnieks, 2005).

### *3.2.3. Proprioception*

Proprioception is the afferent information that contributes to conscious sensation (muscle sense) and segmental posture (joint stability). The sensory organs that are most commonly referred to as proprioceptors include muscle spindles, Golgi tendon organs, and joint receptors (Shumway-Cook and Woollacott, 2007; Silverthorn, 2010). Muscle spindles relay information about the muscles length and rate of stretch and are distributed throughout the belly of the muscle, while Golgi tendon organs are found in muscle tendons and transmit information regarding muscle tension or force. Muscle spindles provide sensory information by means of primary endings connected to the spinal cord via type Ia afferent fibres and secondary endings connected to the central nervous system via type II afferent fibres. The Golgi tendon organs send their impulses to the spinal cord via the Ib afferents fibres. Joint receptors are the third type of proprioceptor and are found in the capsules and ligaments around joints of the body. These receptors are stimulated by mechanical distortion that is experienced when the relative position of bones linked by flexible joints is changed (Porth and Matfin, 2009; Silverthorn, 2010).

Proprioceptors provide the CNS with position and motion information which provides the body with a reference to the supporting surface and is arguably the most important contributor to postural stability (Lord and Sturnieks, 2005). Proprioceptive information from the ankle, regarding joint position in normal healthy individuals, has been said to be of principal importance in controlling standing balance (Fitzpatrick and McCloskey, 1994). Other studies of young individuals have found that lateral ligament anesthesia of the ankle (McKeon, Booi, Branam, Johnson, and Mattacola, 2010) and changes in support surface conditions (Fransson, Gomez, Patel, and Johansson, 2007; Isableu and Vuillerme, 2006) have significant effects on postural control.

Many previous studies have repeatedly found that with ageing, there are proprioceptive deficits including decreases in both cutaneous vibratory and joint sensation. These and other proprioceptive losses increase the threshold to movement detection and decrease postural stability (Hay, Bard, Fleury, and Teasdale, 1996; Kristinsdottir, et al., 2001; Speers, Kuo, and Horak, 2002). Age-related differences have been demonstrated when proprioceptive information was perturbed by means of tendon vibration of tibialis anterior and soleus muscles; and the differences were even greater when proprioceptive inputs needed to be reintegrated after the perturbation was removed (Teasdale and Simoneau, 2001). Doumas and Krampe (2010) investigated adaptations and reintegration of proprioceptive information in young and older adults when undertaking postural tasks. Their results indicated that AP sway path length increased when inaccurate proprioception was introduced. These increases were, however, comparable in both the young and older groups. What was different between the two age groups was the reintegration phase on restoration of a stable platform. In this stage, there was a sizable increase in AP path length which was greater in magnitude and duration for older adults. In another study, Kristinsdottir et al. (2001) found that vibration sensation was the major determinant for postural control with those older adults that lacked intact vibration sensation exhibiting an increased high frequency sway compared with younger adults and those older with intact sensation. They concluded that the status of sensory receptors of the lower limbs were of the utmost importance for postural control in older people.

## 3.3. Motor Outputs and Ageing

The maintenance of upright postural control is not only reliant on effective sensory input but also the application of appropriate motor outputs. Both strength and power of lower limbs have been indicated as important factors in the control of balance, gait and preventions of falls, and have traditionally been the focus of many papers in the ageing and postural control literature (Barrett and Lichtwark, 2008; Izquierdo, Aguado, et al., 1999; Perry, Carville, Smith, Rutherford, and Newham, 2007). More recently however, there has been growing interest into the possible role that steady muscular contractions (usually termed steadiness) has on the control of posture (Kouzaki and Shinohara, 2010).

### *3.3.1. Muscular Strength*

Muscular strength, or the amount of force a muscle produces, is a major contributor to the maintenance of posture. With ageing there is a decline in the strength of nearly all muscles of the body. However, in relation to lower limbs, strength declines at steady rates of approximately 1–2% per year (Vandervoort, 2002) and it has been found that 20% to 40% of muscular strength is lost from the third to eighth decade (Doherty, 2003). Though, it is often seen that the major decrease in strength occurs after the fifth decade (Doherty, Vandervoort, and Brown, 1993; Izquierdo et al., 1999; Petrella, Kim, Tuggle, Hall, and Bamman, 2005) which often results in modifications in functional tasks such as the control of posture.

It seems that muscle strength, as a musculoskeletal characteristic of postural control, is important in generating basic acceleration vectors to control posture. In both cross sectional and longitudinal studies, lower extremity muscle weakness has been identified as a risk factor contributing to falls in the older populations (Lord, Clark, and Webster, 1991a). This has been shown to be especially true when considering muscles on the posterior side of the lower limbs. Kou and Zajac (1993a) conducted a biomechanical analysis of muscle strength based on a musculoskeletal model of the lower limb and reported that a 1% increase in knee flexors strength may result in approximately 0.9% increase in the maximum acceleration vector, while a similar increase in other muscles such as gluteus may have no such effect. It was also concluded that knee flexion muscle strength is thought to have increased participation in both hip and ankle strategies to control posture. However, research has not examined whether the loss in knee flexors' force has any impact on balance.

In a study by Lord et al. (1991b) it was shown that poor performance in two clinical measures of postural stability was associated with reduced quadriceps and ankle dorsiflexion strength. This suggests that in situations where there is a reduction in ankle proprioceptive inputs older subjects are more reliant on motor outputs such as muscular strength. In a similar study by Daubney and Culham (1999) it was found that the difference between fallers and non-fallers was in the muscular strength of the knee extensors and ankle dorsiflexors, which provides further evidence that the force generating capacity of lower limb muscles is important in the maintenance of postural control.

### *3.3.2. Power*

Muscular power can be defined as the amount of work that is performed per unit of time and has been linked to the ability to control posture by many authors (Izquierdo, Aguado, et al., 1999; Katayama et al., 2004; Perry, et al., 2007; Robinovitch, Heller, Lui, and Cortez, 2002). Generally, muscle power has been shown to decline at a faster rate than isometric muscle strength with age, at a rate of approximately 3.5% per annum, compared to the rate of strength decline of approximately 1.5% per annum (Thomas, Tomlinson, Hong, and Hui, 2006). It has also been shown that power output can decrease by 50% or more from the third to the eighth decade (Izquierdo, Ibanez, et al., 1999; Kostka, 2005; Runge, Rittweger, Russo, Schiessl, and Felsenberg, 2004).

Izquierdo et al. (1999) examined the maximal and explosive force production capacity and balance performance in men of different ages. They found that the rate of force development was lower in older men compared with middle aged and was as much as 64% lower than young men. In both middle age and older groups the rate of force development (RFD) was significantly correlated with individual balance measures. It was concluded that ageing may lead to impaired postural control with a decrease in the speed of postural adjustments and that the decreased ability to develop force rapidly in older people seems to be associated with a lower capacity for neuromuscular responses in controlling posture.

Power output has also been implicated in the postural differences between fallers and non-fallers. Perry et al. (2007) examined the difference between young and older people and between older fallers and non-fallers to determine if the history of falling is associated with strength and power output. Younger individuals were much stronger and more powerful compared to older people while there were significant differences between fallers and non-fallers. The fallers exhibited only 85% of the strength and 79% of the power of non-fallers. It was concluded by the authors that power output appears to be the most relevant measure of fall risk and its importance to postural control should be further studied.

Finally in a study by Bezerra et al. (2009) in which they assessed RFD of the knee extensors and flexors in static knee extension and flexion and analysed the relationship with traditional COP and stabilogram parameters. Three groups of healthy volunteers, aged 18-30 (YG), 40-50 (MG) and 60-77 (OG) years, with 10 males and 10 females in each group, participated in the study. Results showed significantly lower RFD between OG compared with YG and MG in knee extensors and flexors. Both MG and YG were significantly better than OG in COP mean distance in AP direction and COP mean velocity in AP and ML directions. Moderate negative correlations were found between COP mean velocity in ML and the strength of the knee extensors and flexors in all posture testing conditions. It was concluded that higher RFD in the thigh musculature may contribute to better postural control performance. It was suggested that RFD be further examined for its validity as an indicator in postural control, particularly in the knee flexors.

### *3.3.3. Steadiness of Force Production*

The ability to control force, termed steadiness (ST), can be understood as the magnitude of fluctuation in force when performing either isometric or anisometric (concentric and eccentric) steady contractions (Enoka, 1997). Muscle steadiness has been examined in several muscle groups and it has been reported that the upper limbs demonstrate a better control of force than do the muscle groups of the lower limbs (Christou, Zelent, and Carlton, 2003; Tracy and Enoka, 2002). These findings have led to suggestions by some authors that individuals who experience an impaired ST within lower limb muscle groups may also have difficulties in the performance of daily activities (Kouzaki and Shinohara, 2010).

Available research has reported that the muscle steadiness is better maintained in young adults than older adults (Burnett, Laidlaw, and Enoka, 2000; Christou and Carlton, 2001; Enoka, Burnett, Graves, Kornatz, and Laidlaw, 1999; Laidlaw, Bilodeau, and Enoka, 2000) and both isometric and anisometric muscle steadiness may be limiting factors for older adults in performing daily tasks (Seynnes et al., 2005) such as repeated rising from a chair (Manini, Cook, Ordway, Ploutz-Snyder, and Ploutz-Snyder, 2005) or postural control (Kouzaki and Shinohara, 2010). This line of thoughts seems logical because the maintenance of upright bipedal stance is another motor task requiring the capacity to control forces of the lower limb because of the continuous need to neutralise destabilising forces (Wolfson, Whipple, Derby, Amerman, and Nashner, 1994). Despite this assumption, the potential association between the performance of daily activities and force fluctuations during isolated voluntary steady contractions has not been clearly shown.

Of the limited research that has been completed there have been some promising results. Kouzaki and Shinohara (2010) investigated the functional significance of force fluctuations during voluntary contractions of the plantar flexors and postural sway during quiet stance. They found a positive correlation between the coefficient of variation (CV) of COP measures and CV of force during plantar flexion in both young and older adults. This correlation was only seen at contraction intensities of ≤5% maximal voluntary contraction which corresponds to commonly seen muscle activity levels during quiet stance. In another study in our laboratory (Bezerra, Zhou, Crowley, and Baglin, 2010) it was found that in older adults moderate correlations existed between COP mean distance and root means square in anterior-posterior direction and steadiness at low contraction intensities of the plantar flexors, dorsiflexors, and knee extensors. Therefore further research should be conducted to verify whether ST of all four muscle groups of the lower limbs is important in postural control.

### 3.3.4. Strength Ratio between Agonists and Antagonists

It has been emphasised in the literature that the Hamstring to Quadriceps Ratio (HQR) is of integral importance in the maintenance of knee joint stability and the prevention of knee injuries such as ACL ruptures or hamstring muscle tears (Gabbe, Finch, Bennell, and Wajswelner, 2005; Mjolsnes, Arnason, Osthagen, Raastad, and Bahr, 2004; Verrall, Slavotinek, Barnes, Fon, and Spriggins, 2001). Previously it has been found that the HQR appears not to be affected by age in young individuals (12 to 17 years) (Highgenboten, Jackson, and Meske, 1988; Rosene, Fogarty, and Mahaffey, 2001) and no differences in HQR have been reported across sport, gender or side of the body (Bahr and Holme, 2003; Gabbe, et al., 2005; Verrall, et al., 2001). However, in adult athletes age does have an influence on the HQR and hence injury (Baratta et al., 1988; Mesfar and Shirazi-Adl, 2006). However, very little investigation has been conducted on the age-related changes of the HQR in older populations and the possible complications that may cause in the everyday functioning of these individuals.

Just as the HQR has been proven to provide stability to the knee joint, the DPR also has a potential functional role. It is common in the literature to highlight that strength on the lower limb musculature is a limiting factor in the maintenance of postural control especially when considering the muscles acting at the ankle joint (Daubney and Culham, 1999; Kuo and Zajac, 1993a; Lord, et al., 1991a, 1991b). Considering that there is a dynamic interaction between the ankle plantarflexors and dorsiflexors during functional task such as postural control, it is surprising that there has not been more in depth examination of the influence of these strength ratios in relation to posture and falls.

From the above information, it seems plausible that the balance between agonist/antagonist muscle strength may play a key role in knee and ankle stability and therefore functional tasks such as postural control. These roles seem to increase when the ankle joint is in the neutral position and when the knee joint angle approaches those angles commonly used in daily tasks such as posture. Therefore, the age-related decline in knee flexors and plantar flexors' strength may contribute to a lack of knee and ankle stability respectively and eventually may compromise posture in an older population. To date, little research has investigated the HQR or DPR and their age-related changes in relation to postural stability. Whether the HQR and DPR are correlated with the ability to control posture, and whether and how this relationship is affected by ageing and/or training, has not been extensively examined.

However, of the few studies that have investigated the role of strength ratios of lower limb agonist/antagonist muscle pairs in postural control, there have been some interesting findings. In our laboratory it was found that there are significant age-related declines in quadriceps and hamstrings maximal voluntary contraction strength and HQR. An additional finding was that the HQR exhibited significant negative correlations with most stabilogram parameters. The authors concluded that a higher HQR may be associated with better postural control performance and suggested that the HQR should be further examined for its validity as a meaningful indicator in postural control, particularly in relation to ageing (Bezerra, Zhou, and Crowley, 2008).

## 3.4. Postural Strategies and Ageing

When standing in an upright position the COG is said to be continuously repositioned via a flexible inverted pendulum about the ankles (Amiridis, et al., 2003) and is dependent on the effective control of the torques at the ankle, knee and hip joints (Edwards, 2007). This COG fluctuation causes a COP drift away from the relative equilibrium point during the maintenance of stance (Collins, et al., 1995). Such slow movements of the body are detected by the sensory system and integrated by the CNS and reflex pathways. These signals generate the commands necessary to drive the muscles involved around the lower limb joint, so that these muscles restore body balance (Fujisawa et al., 2005; Morasso and Schieppati, 1999). These postural control movements are often categorised into two discrete control strategies: either "ankle strategy" or "hip strategy" (Fujisawa, et al., 2005). However, other strategies have been hypothesised that highlight the role of knee joint dynamics and also the use of muscle coactivation around the joints of the lower limb (Benjuya, et al., 2004). The strategy selected by individuals is based on sensory information, area of support, musculoskeletal characteristics, degree of freedom, task constraints, and particularly the age of the individual.

### *3.4.1. Ankle Strategy*

The ankle strategy was defined first by Nashner and McCollum (1985) who characterised the human postural control system as a single-segment inverted pendulum. This strategy was said to occur when there was early activation of ankle joint muscles and then activation radiated in sequence to the thigh and then trunk muscles. Therefore, it is thought that the nervous system controls postural movement through activation of the ankle joint muscle groups, while keeping the knee and hip joints in a fixed position (Fujisawa, et al., 2005; Kuo and Zajac, 1993b). Keeping the knee fixed is not equivalent to keeping the knee muscles inactivated as torque is still needed from both the agonists and antagonists to maintain the constraint (Kuo and Zajac, 1993b). Under this strategy, the aim is to keep the trunk parallel to the legs without changing the angle of the hip and knee joints, while at the same time the hip moment is regulated approximately proportional to the ankle moment (Fujisawa, et al., 2005). This strategy is mainly used in situations in which the perturbations to equilibrium are small, when the inclination angle is small, the area of support is large, and the support surface is firm (Fujisawa, et al., 2005; Kuo and Zajac, 1993b). The ankle strategy is also most commonly seen in young adults in comparison with older adults, who generally adopt a postural strategy termed hip strategy (Xu, Hong, Li, and Chan, 2004).

### *3.4.2. Hip Strategy*

The hip strategy has been categorised as the early activation of ventral trunk and thigh muscles, i.e. top down activation, and is related with the motion of the body as a double-segment inverted pendulum with counterphase motions at the hip and ankle joints (Colobert, Crétual, Allard, and Delamarche, 2006; Runge, et al., 1999). This strategy is more complex than the ankle strategy because the moments around the two joints are not simply proportional and require at least two independent sensory inputs. When a large disturbing force is applied to body segments, or the area of support is not wide enough to receive a sufficient amount of the ankle moment, the inclination angles of the body become so large that the ankle strategy may not be able to restore body balance. Therefore, near the body limits of stability, the nervous system regulates the joint moments using the hip strategy (Fujisawa, et al., 2005;

Kuo and Zajac, 1993b; Runge, et al., 1999; Saffer, Kiemel, and Jeka, 2008). This strategy has been reported to be highly effective in the maintenance of postural control and an efficient means of stabilising body posture especially in older individuals (Amiridis, et al., 2003).

The hip strategy is most often associated with older adults in comparison with young adults who utilise the ankle strategy more regularly (Xu, et al., 2004). This over-reliance on hip strategy in older adults has been linked to degeneration in neural, muscular, and skeletal mechanisms leading to increased susceptibility to falls (Amiridis, et al., 2003; Tsang and Hui-Chan, 2003). Possible explanations for the greater hip strategy dependence seen in the elderly include inadequate torque production by ankle muscles (Amiridis, et al., 2003; Widmaier, Raff, and Strang, 2004) and insufficient proprioceptive contribution from the distal lower limb and foot as a result of peripheral neuropathies (Anand, et al., 2003a; Anand, Buckley, Scally, and Elliott, 2003b).

### *3.4.3. Agonist/Antagonist Coactivation*

The concept of coactivation (also known as co-contraction) of agonist/antagonist pairs around the joint of the lower extremity has only recently gained much attention (Benjuya, et al., 2004). It has been found in past investigations that coactivation level is dependent on several factors. These factors include age, joint angle, and the muscle groups being investigated of which all may have an influence on the postural control strategy adopted (Hortobagyi and Devita, 2006; Melzer, et al., 2004).

Ageing may also have an influence on the coactivation level. Healthy young individuals produce the net torque at a joint by optimally scaling the activation of the prime movers and the concurrent activity of the antagonist muscles. In contrast, old adults generate the desired torque with a different neural strategy that involves a near complete activation of the agonist combined with a disproportionately heightened coactivation of the antagonist muscles. Changes in spinal reflex circuitry are the traditionally accepted mechanism that influences coactivation. However, recent imaging, EEG, microstimulation, and magnetic brain stimulation studies make the hypothesis tenable that, in conjunction with modulations of spinal circuits, cortical and possibly subcortical mechanisms also are responsible for the age associated changes in coactivation (Hortobagyi and Devita, 2006). It has been shown that during postural task and tasks that involve stepping the level of coactivation at the ankle joint is significantly increased in the elderly (Benjuya, et al., 2004; Hortobagyi and DeVita, 2000; Melzer, Benjuya, and Kaplanski, 2001). This association is further enhanced when older adults have restricted visual feedback, narrow base of support, or are required to undertake dual cognitive tasks while maintaining posture (Benjuya, et al., 2004; Melzer, et al., 2001). It has previously been speculated that the elderly adopt this coactivation strategy in an effort to stiffen the ankle joint which helps to reduce excessive movements thus decreasing postural sway (Melzer, et al., 2001). Due to this adopted strategy it may be hypothesised that the relative strength ratios of these agonist/antagonist muscles may play a role in the degree of coactivation during postural tasks.

## 4. EFFECTS OF EXERCISE INTERVENTION ON POSTURAL CONTROL

The regression of the physiological process and functional performance with ageing has evident impacts on the quality of life of older individuals. Loss of strength, decreasing aerobic capacity and increased risk of falls are well-known consequences associated with the ageing process (Lord, et al., 1991c; Lord and Ward, 1994). As the aged population continues to grow, the development and implementation of cost-efficient and effective exercise interventions for the improvement of postural control and prevention of falls is of utmost importance. Research concerning exercise habits and lifestyle choices in older adults has produced strong evidence that exercise and other forms of physical activity can produce health benefits (American College of Sports Medicine, 2006). Also, training studies involving resistance exercises (Ferri et al., 2003; Hess and Woollacott, 2005), Tai Chi (Choi, Moon, and Song, 2005), electromyostimulation (Amiridis, Arabatzi, Violaris, Stavropoulos, and Hatzitaki, 2005), balance exercises (Nagy et al., 2007), and walking exercises (Melzer, Benjuya, and Kaplanski, 2003) have shown that older adults respond positively to exercise and often produce enhancements in functional abilities and health variables.

## 4.1. Resistance Exercise

A decline in muscular strength occurs with ageing and is often associated with the observable decline in functional performance. This lack of capacity by the muscle effectors to respond appropriately is frequently linked to disturbances in postural control (Lord, et al., 1994). It has been shown that systematic strength training can lead to considerable increases in lower limb performance. For example, appropriate strength training may have a positive influence in maximal strength (Ferri, et al., 2003; Hakkinen and Hakkinen, 1995), muscle size (Hakkinen et al., 1998; Kryger and Andersen, 2007), muscle architecture (Blazevich, Cannavan, Coleman, and Horne, 2007), and the control of muscular contraction force (Manini, Clark, Tracy, Burke, and Ploutz-Snyder, 2005; Tracy, Byrnes, and Enoka, 2004).

Another function that is often observed to improve with resistance training is postural stability (Hess and Woollacott, 2005; Ryushi, et al., 2000). Ryushi et al. (2000) conducted a 10 week resistance training schedule that was focused on strength development of the quadriceps muscle group. It was found that the quadriceps strength and the percentage limits-of-stability to the rear were increased, and the percentage change in the path length was decreased significantly with strength training.

The authors concluded that strength gains in the quadriceps is thought to possibly enable accurate movement of the COG farther towards the rear, suggesting that strength gains have a positive influence on a person's perception of their postural control.

Similar findings were shown by Hess and Woollacott (2005) when they also conducted 10 weeks of high intensity strength training of the quadriceps, hamstrings, tibialis anterior, and triceps surae.

After training, there were considerable improvements in strength, Berg Balance Scale, Timed Up and Go, and the Activities-Specific Balance Confidence Scale in the experimental group. These findings showed that strength training can effectively strengthen lower extremity muscles in balance impaired older individuals which, in turn, results in significant improvements in functional balance ability and decrease falls risk.

## 4.2. Tai Chi Exercise

Postural equilibrium requires proprioceptive acuity. Proprioception is the afferent information that contributes to conscious sensation (muscle sense), total posture (postural equilibrium), and segmental posture (joint stability). It is well established in the literature that proprioception is impaired with age (Fong and Ng, 2006; Tsang and Hui-Chan, 2003; Xu, et al., 2004) and it has previously been postulated that this decrement in proprioceptive acuity makes it difficult for older individuals to detect changes in body position (Gauchard, Jeandel, Tessier, and Perrin, 1999). Indeed, some studies have shown that diminished proprioception is a major contributing factor to falls in older populations (Li, Xu, and Hong, 2008). Exercise has been shown to have beneficial effects on improving a number of sensorimotor systems that contribute to stability (Lord, et al., 1994). Of the exercise modes available, it appears that proprioceptive exercises such as Tai Chi have a more beneficial effect on the proprioceptive capacity post training compared with bioenergetic activities such as resistance exercise or walking (Gauchard, et al., 1999).

Tai Chi is a traditional Chinese exercise and has been used for centuries. It was originally developed as a form of martial arts, however now it has become popular among many older populations as a form of exercise to improve health and physical wellbeing. The basic exercise involved in Tai Chi is a series of individual movements that are linked together in a continuous manner and that flow smoothly from one movement to another. These elements incorporate the elements of postural muscle strengthening, balance, and postural alignment (Wolf, Barnhart, Ellison, and Coogler, 1997). The simple, soft, and fluid movements of Tai Chi are ideal for older people regardless of previous exercise experience. Tai Chi is performed in a semi-squat posture that can place a large load on the muscles of the lower extremities. The movements demand guided motions of the hip, knee, and ankle joints in various directions, requiring concentric, eccentric, and isometric contractions of the hip, knee, and ankle muscles (Xu, Hong, and Li, 2008). Tai Chi has been demonstrated to cause significant improvements in the neuromuscular and somatosensory systems which have particular importance in the performance of postural control and hence has become important in the areas of falls prevention and healthy ageing (Li, Hong, and Chan, 2001; Wong and Lan, 2008; Wu, 2002).

Several studies have examined the effects of Tai Chi interventions on balance control and the prevention of falls. In one such study, Voukelatos et al. (2007) examined the effectiveness of a 16 week Tai Chi program with the aim of improving balance and reducing falls in a group of adults with age 60 years and older. It was concluded in that study that participation in Tai Chi for one hour per week over 16 weeks can prevent falls and improve balance in relatively healthy community-dwelling older populations. In other studies, there have been shown significant improvements in postural control and falls risks when undertaking shorter Tai Chi interventions such as 4 to 8 weeks (Tsang and Hui-Chan, 2004) or 12 weeks (Choi, et al., 2005). The positive effect of Tai Chi on postural control and falls prevention has also been studied for older practitioners of Tai Chi who have practiced for one or more years. In a majority of these studies, positive health outcomes directly or indirectly related to improved posture and falls prevention have been establish. For example, long term Tai Chi practice (minimum of 1.5 hours per week for at least 3 years) was found to improve knee muscle strength, body sway in perturbed one-legged stance, and balance confidence (Tsang and Hui-Chan, 2005). In other studies that investigated the long term effects of Tai Chi practice in older adult population, it has been found that Tai Chi improves standing balance under reduced or conflicting sensory conditions (Tsang, Wong, Fu, and Hui-Chan, 2004), improves isokinetic knee extensor strength and reduces postural sway (Wu, Zhao, Zhou, and Wei, 2002), and improves balance control, flexibility, and cardiovascular fitness (Hong, Li, and Robinson, 2000).

## 4.3. Other Types of Exercise and Interventions

Several other exercise modes have been examined in the past in relation to their effect on postural control in older populations. Of these exercise modes, most are easily implemented, cost effective, and simple enough to be conducted at home.

### *4.3.1. Electromyostimulation*

Electromyostimulation (EMS) is a mode of training that induces a muscular contraction by the application of an external electrical stimulus on the muscle. The artificial stimulus evokes an action potential independent and different from normal voluntary contractions. Research has suggested that EMS recruits different types of muscle fibres in a reverse order relative to normal voluntary contractions (Feiereisen, Duchateau, and Hainaut, 1997; Heyters, Carpentier, Duchateau, and Hainaut, 1994; Knaflitz, Merletti, and De Luca, 1990).

EMS has been considered an important tool in physiotherapy and rehabilitation (Kramer, Lindsay, Magee, Mendryk, and Wall, 1984; Trimble and Enoka, 1991) and is increasingly used by post-injury and post-operation individuals (Bax, Staes, and Verhagen, 2005). However, EMS has only recently been considered as a training methodology to improve strength and postural control in older adults (Amiridis, et al., 2005; Bezerra, Zhou, Crowley, Brooks, and Hooper, 2009; Paillard et al., 2010). Little is known about whether EMS training is effective in improving postural control. Of the little research that has been conducted, it was found by Amiridis et al. (2005) that after 4 weeks of EMS training (40 mins per session, 4 sessions per week) there was a decrease in postural sway, greater ankle muscle EMG activity, greater stability of the ankle joint, and significant changes in the mean position of all three joints of the lower limb. Therefore further research should be conducted to clarify whether lower limb EMS training has a beneficial impact on postural control in older adults.

### *4.3.2. Balance Training*

Balance training is another coordinative exercise that has previously been utilised as a possible exercise intervention for the improvement of postural control. The inclusion of balance training in exercise programs appears to be important for older age groups and tailored balance training has been shown to improve postural stability (Judge, 2003; Judge, Whiple, and Wolfson, 1994). These exercise programmes, including low intensity strength and balance training, have improved the balance and reduced the fall rates compared with the controls. These finding are similar to that of Nagy et al. (2007) who found that 8 weeks of balance training produced a significant improvement in postural control.

Inclusion of balance training has previously shown to be effective in substantially reducing fall rates and improving postural control in older persons. In a systematic review and meta-analysis of effective exercise for the prevention of falls (Sherrington, et al., 2008), it was found that exercise could prevent falls and improve balance in older individuals and that greater relative effects were seen in programs that included exercises that challenged balance. The effect of exercise on postural control has been further highlighted in the publication, Frailty and Injuries: Co-operative Studies of Intervention Techniques (Province et al., 1995) which, on prospective meta-analysis of individual participant data from eight trials, found a pooled estimate of a 17% lower falls risk from exercise programs that included balance training.

### *4.3.3. Home-Based Exercise*

Home-based exercise (HBE) and community-based group exercise were first prescribed in the late 1980's to the early 1990's (King , et al., 1992). One potential advantage is the ability to incorporate the exercise sessions into the participants' own lifestyle, leading to higher amounts of incidental exercise and increased feeling of control over the exercise program (Ball, Crawford, and Owen, 2000; Daly, et al., 2005). Furthermore, HBE may foster long-term adherence through greater convenience and flexibility (King, et al., 1992), reducing the cost of transport and avoidance of the high cost of membership to fitness training providers (Daly, et al., 2005; Jette, et al., 1996). Most of the HBE training programs use body weight as the resistance and elastic bands as equipment, since the elastic-bands have been considered a valid alternative to machine-based resistance training (Yamauchi, et al., 2005).

## 5. SUMMARY

The human's ability to maintain upright posture is of the utmost importance and is essential to the everyday functioning of most people. To maintain this upright position the human body has to integrate several sensory modalities and produce appropriate motor responses to counteract internal and external perturbations. With ageing, however, there are many physiological degenerative processes that take place which reduce the effective control of posture. An effect of this diminished ability to maintain posture is often associated with falls and injuries. In an effort to reduce the incidents of falls and uncover those most at risk of postural control abnormalities, it is important to continue to develop appropriate postural control assessment techniques and the best intervention for improving balance control. The evidence in the current literature indicates that appropriate exercise has a beneficial effect on the postural control. Amongst the training modalities that have been examined it appears that exercises that involve coordinative balance tasks, such as balance training and Tai Chi, are the most effective in delaying the age-related decline in postural control.

## REFERENCES

Abrahamová, D., and Hlavačka, F. (2008). Age-related changes of human balance during quiet stance. *Physiological Research, 57*(6), 957-964.
American College of Sports Medicine. (2006). *ACSM's Guidelines for exercise testing and prescription* (7th ed.). Baltimore: Lippincott Williams and Wilkins.

Amiridis, I. G., Arabatzi, F., Violaris, P., Stavropoulos, E., and Hatzitaki, V. (2005). Static balance improvement in elderly after dorsiflexors electrostimulation training. *European Journal of Applied Physiology, 94*(4), 424-433.

Amiridis, I. G., Hatzitaki, V., and Arabatzi, F. (2003). Age-induced modifications of static postural control in humans. *Neuroscience Letters, 350*(3), 137-140.

Anand, V., Buckley, J. G., Scally, A., and Elliott, D. B. (2003a). Postural stability changes in the elderly with cataract simulation and refractive blur. *Investigative Ophthalmology and Visual Science, 44*(11), 4670-4675.

Anand, V., Buckley, J. G., Scally, A., and Elliott, D. B. (2003b). Postural stability in the elderly during sensory perturbations and dual tasking: the influence of refractive blur. *Investigative Ophthalmology and Visual Science, 44*(7), 2885-2891.

Bacsi, A. M., and Colebatch, J. G. (2005). Evidence for reflex and perceptual vestibular contributions to postural control. *Experimental Brain Research, 160*(1), 22-28.

Bahr, R., and Holme, I. (2003). Risk factors for sports injuries--a methodological approach. *British Journal of Sports Medicine, 37*(5), 384-392.

Ball, K., Crawford, D., & Owen, N. (2000). Too fat to exercise? Obesity as a barrier to physical activity. *Australian & New Zealand Journal of Public Health, 24*(3), 331-333.

Baloh, R. W., Ying, S. H., and Jacobson, K. M. (2003). A longitudinal study of gait and balance dysfunction in normal older people. *Archives of Neurology, 60*(6), 835-839.

Baratta, R., Solomonow, M., Zhou, B. H., Letson, D., Chuinard, R., and D'Ambrosia, R. (1988). Muscular coactivation. The role of the antagonist musculature in maintaining knee stability. *The American Journal of Sports Medicine, 16*(2), 113-122.

Baratto, L., Morasso, P. G., Re, C., and Spada, G. (2002). A new look at posturographic analysis in the clinical context: sway-density versus other parameterization techniques. *Motor Control, 6*(3), 246-270.

Barr, M. L., and Kiernan, J. A. (1993). *The Human Nervous System: an Anatomical Viewpoint* (6th ed.). Philadelphia: J. B. Lippincott Company.

Barrett, R. S., and Lichtwark, G. A. (2008). Effect of altering neural, muscular and tendinous factors associated with aging on balance recovery using the ankle strategy: a simulation study. *Journal of Theoretical Biology, 254*(3), 546-554.

Basmajian, J. V. (1978). *Muscles Alive* (4th ed.). Baltimore: Williams and Wilkins.

Bax, L., Staes, F., and Verhagen, A. (2005). Does Neuromuscular Electrical Stimulation Strengthen the Quadriceps Femoris?: A Systematic Review of Randomised Controlled Trials. *Sports Medicine, 35*(3), 191-212.

Benjuya, N., Melzer, I., and Kaplanski, J. (2004). Aging-induced shifts from a reliance on sensory input to muscle cocontraction during balanced standing. *Journals of Gerontology Series A-Biological Sciences and Medical Sciences, 59*(2), 166-171.

Bezerra, P., Zhou, S., and Crowley, Z. (2008). *Age-related changes in quadriceps to hamstrings strength ratio and its relation to postural stability.* Paper presented at the Australian Association for Exercise and Sports Science conference, Melbourne, Australia.

Bezerra, P., Zhou, S., Crowley, Z., and Baglin, R. (2009). *Age-related changes in knee extensors and flexors rate of force development and its relation to postural stability.* Paper presented at the 14th Congress of the European College of Sport Science, Oslo, Norway.

Bezerra, P., Zhou, S., Crowley, Z., and Baglin, R. (2010). *The relationship between lower limbs muscles steadiness and posture maintenance in older adults.* Paper presented at the 15th annual Congress of European College of Sport Science, Antalya, Turkey.

Bezerra, P., Zhou, S., Crowley, Z., Brooks, L., and Hooper, A. (2009). Effects of unilateral electromyostimulation superimposed on voluntary training on strength and cross-sectional area. *Muscle and Nerve, 40*(3), 430-437.

Blazevich, A. J., Cannavan, D., Coleman, D. R., and Horne, S. (2007). Influence of concentric and eccentric resistance training on architectural adaptation in human quadriceps muscles. *Journal of Applied Physiology, 103*(5), 1565-1575.

Borg, F., Finell, M., Hakala, I., and Herrala, M. (2007). Analyzing gastrocnemius EMG-activity and sway data from quiet and perturbed standing. *Journal of Electromyography and Kinesiology, 17*(5), 622-634.

Burnett, R. A., Laidlaw, D. H., and Enoka, R. M. (2000). Coactivation of the antagonist muscle does not covary with steadiness in old adults. *Journal of Applied Physiology, 89*(1), 61-71.

Carter, N. D., Kannus, P., and Khan, K. M. (2001). Exercise in the prevention of falls in older people: a systematic literature review examining the rationale and the evidence. *Sports Medicine, 31*(6), 427-438.

Choi, J. H., Moon, J.-S., and Song, R. (2005). Effects of Sun-style Tai Chi exercise on physical fitness and fall prevention in fall-prone older adults. *Journal of Advanced Nursing, 51*(2), 150-157.

Christou, E. A., and Carlton, L. G. (2001). Old adults exhibit greater motor output variability than young adults only during rapid discrete isometric contractions. *Journals of Gerontology Series A-Biological Sciences and Medical Sciences, 56*(12), B524-532.

Christou, E. A., Zelent, M., and Carlton, L. G. (2003). Force control is greater in the upper compared with the lower extremity. *Journal of Motor Behavior, 35*(4), 322-324.

Collins, J. J., and De Luca, C. J. (1993). Open-loop and closed-loop control of posture: a random-walk analysis of center-of-pressure trajectories. *Experimental Brain Research, 95*(2), 308-318.

Collins, J. J., and De Luca, C. J. (1995). The effects of visual input on open-loop and closed-loop postural control mechanisms. *Experimental Brain Research, 103*(1), 151-163.

Collins, J. J., De Luca, C. J., Burrows, A., and Lipsitz, L. A. (1995). Age-related changes in open-loop and closed-loop postural control mechanisms. *Experimental Brain Research, 104*(3), 480-492.

Colobert, B., Crétual, A., Allard, P., and Delamarche, P. (2006). Force-plate based computation of ankle and hip strategies from double-inverted pendulum model. *Clinical Biomechanics, 21*(4), 427-434.

Daly, R. M., Dunstan, D. W., Owen, N., Jolley, D., Shaw, J. E., & Zimmet, P. Z. (2005). Does high-intensity resistance training maintain bone mass during moderate weight loss in older overweight adults with type 2 diabetes? *Osteoporosis International, 16*(12), 1703-1712.

Danis, C. G., Krebs, D. E., Gill-Body, K. M., and Sahrmann, S. (1998). Relationship between standing posture and stability. *Physical Therapy, 78*(5), 502-517.

Daubney, M. E., and Culham, E. G. (1999). Lower-extremity muscle force and balance performance in adults aged 65 years and older. *Physical Therapy, 79*(12), 1177-1185.

Dean, J. C., Kuo, A. D., and Alexander, N. B. (2004). Age-related changes in maximal hip strength and movement speed. *Journals of Gerontology Series A-Biological Sciences and Medical Sciences, 59*(3), 286-292.

Doherty, T. J. (2003). Invited review: Aging and sarcopenia. *Journal of Applied Physiology, 95*(4), 1717-1727.

Doherty, T. J., Vandervoort, A. A., and Brown, W. F. (1993). Effects of ageing on the motor unit: a brief review. *Canadian Journal of Applied Physiology, 18*(4), 331-358.

Doumas, M., and Krampe, R. T. (2010). Adaptation and reintegration of proprioceptive information in young and older adults' postural control. *Journal of Neurophysiology, 104*(4), 1969-1977.

Doyle, R. J., Hsiao-Wecksler, E. T., Ragan, B. G., and Rosengren, K. S. (2008). Generalizability of center of pressure measures of quiet standing. *Gait and Posture, 25*(2), 166-171.

Dozza, M., Chiari, L., Chan, B., Rocchi, L., Horak, F. B., and Cappello, A. (2005). Influence of a portable audio-biofeedback device on structural properties of postural sway. *Journal of Neuroengineering And Rehabilitation, 2*, 13-13.

Du Pasquier, R. A., Blanc, Y., Sinnreich, M., Landis, T., Burkhard, P., and Vingerhoets, F. J. G. (2003). The effect of aging on postural stability: a cross sectional and longitudinal study. *Neurophysiologie Clinique, 33*(5), 213-218.

Edwards, W. T. (2007). Effect of joint stiffness on standing stability. *Gait and Posture, 25*(3), 432-439.

Enoka, R. M. (1997). Neural strategies in the control of muscle force. *Muscle and Nerve Supplement, 5*, S66-69.

Enoka, R. M., Burnett, R. A., Graves, A. E., Kornatz, K. W., and Laidlaw, D. H. (1999). Task- and age-dependent variations in steadiness. *Progress in Brain Research, 123*, 389-395.

Era, P., Schroll, M., Ytting, H., Gause-Nilsson, I., Heikkinen, E., and Steen, B. (1996). Postural balance and its sensory-motor correlates in 75-year-old men and women: a cross-national comparative study. *Journals of Gerontology Series A-Biological Sciences and Medical Sciences, 51*(2), M53-63.

Feiereisen, P., Duchateau, J., and Hainaut, K. (1997). Motor unit recruitment order during voluntary and electrically induced contractions in the tibialis anterior. *Experimental Brain Research, 114*(1), 117-123.

Ferri, A., Scaglioni, G., Pousson, M., Capodaglio, P., Van Hoecke, J., and Narici, M. V. (2003). Strength and power changes of the human plantar flexors and knee extensors in response to resistance training in old age. *Acta Physiologica Scandinavica, 177*(1), 69-78.

Fitzpatrick, R., and McCloskey, D. I. (1994). Proprioceptive, visual and vestibular thresholds for the perception of sway during standing in humans. *Journal of Physiology, 478 (Part 1)*, 173-186.

Fong, S.-M., and Ng, G. Y. (2006). The effects on sensorimotor performance and balance with Tai Chi training. *Archives of Physical Medicine and Rehabilitation, 87*(1), 82-87.

Fransson, P. A., Gomez, S., Patel, M., and Johansson, L. (2007). Changes in multi-segmented body movements and EMG activity while standing on firm and foam support surfaces. *European Journal of Applied Physiology, 101*(1), 81-89.

Fransson, P. A., Kristinsdottir, E. K., Hafstrom, A., Magnusson, M., and Johansson, R. (2004). Balance control and adaptation during vibratory perturbations in middle-aged and elderly adults. *European Journal of Applied Physiology, 91*, 595-603.

Fujisawa, N., Masuda, T., Inaoka, Y., Fukuoka, H., Ishida, A., and Minamitani, H. (2005). Human standing posture control system depending on adopted strategies. *Medical and Biological Engineering and Computing, 43*(1), 107-114.

Gabbe, B. J., Finch, C. F., Bennell, K. L., and Wajswelner, H. (2005). Risk factors for hamstring injuries in community level Australian football. *British Journal of Sports Medicine, 39*(2), 106-110.

Gauchard, G. C., Jeandel, C., Tessier, A., and Perrin, P. P. (1999). Beneficial effect of proprioceptive physical activities on balance control in elderly human subjects. *Neuroscience Letters, 273*, 81-84.

Grasso, R., Zago, M., and Lacquaniti, F. (2000). Interactions between posture and locomotion: motor patterns in humans walking with bent posture versus erect posture. *Journal of Neurophysiology, 83*(1), 288-300.

Guerraz, M., and Bronstein, A. M. (2008). Mechanisms underlying visually induced body sway. *Neuroscience Letters, 443*(1), 12-16.

Guerraz, M., Gianna, C. C., Burchill, P. M., Gresty, M. A., and Bronstein, A. M. (2001). Effect of visual surrounding motion on body sway in a three-dimensional environment. *Perception and Psychophysics, 63*(1), 47-58.

Hafström, A., Fransson, P.-A., Karlberg, M., Ledin, T., and Magnusson, M. (2002). Visual influence on postural control, with and without visual motion feedback. *Acta Oto-Laryngologica, 122*(4), 392-397.

Hakkinen, K., and Hakkinen, A. (1995). Neuromuscular adaptations during intensive strength training in middle-aged and elderly males and females. *Electromyography and Clinical Neurophysiology, 35*(3), 137-147.

Hakkinen, K., Newton, R. U., Gordon, S. E., McCormick, M., Volek, J. S., Nindl, B. C., et al. (1998). Changes in muscle morphology, electromyographic activity, and force production characteristics during progressive strength training in young and older men. *Journals of Gerontology Series A-Biological Sciences and Medical Sciences, 53*(6), B415-423.

Harwood, R. H. (2001). Visual problems and falls. *Age And Ageing, 30 Suppl 4*, 13-18.

Hay, L., Bard, C., Fleury, M., and Teasdale, N. (1996). Availability of visual and proprioceptive afferent messages and postural control. *Experimental Brain Research, 108*, 129-139.

Hess, J. A., and Woollacott, M. (2005). Effect of high-intensity strength-training on functional measures of balance ability in balance-impaired older adults. *Journal of Manipulative Physiological Therapeutics, 28*(8), 582-590.

Heyters, M., Carpentier, A., Duchateau, J., and Hainaut, K. (1994). Twitch analysis as an approach to motor unit activation during electrical stimulation. *Canadian Journal of Applied Physiology, 19*(4), 451-461.

Highgenboten, C. L., Jackson, A. W., and Meske, N. B. (1988). Concentric and eccentric torque comparisons for knee extension and flexion in young adult males and females using the Kinetic Communicator. *American Journal of Sports Medicine, 16*(3), 234-237.

Hong, Y., Li, J. X., and Robinson, P. D. (2000). Balance control, flexibility, and cardiorespiratory fitness among older Tai Chi practitioners. *British Journal of Sports Medicine, 34*(1), 29-34.

Horak, F. B. (2010). Postural compensation for vestibular loss and implications for rehabilitation. *Restorative Neurology And Neuroscience, 28*(1), 57-68.

Horak, F. B., Earhart, G. M., and Dietz, V. (2001). Postural responses to combinations of head and body displacements: vestibular-somatosensory interactions. *Experimental Brain Research, 141*(3), 410-414.

Horak, F. B., Nashner, L. M., and Diener, H. C. (1990). Postural strategies associated with somatosensory and vestibular loss. *Experimental Brain Research, 82*(1), 167-177.

Horak, F. B., Shupert, C. L., Dietz, V., and Horstmann, G. (1994). Vestibular and somatosensory contributions to responses to head and body displacements in stance. *Experimental Brain Research, 100*(1), 93-106.

Horak, F. B., Shupert, C. L., and Mirka, A. (1989). Components of postural dyscontrol in the elderly: a review. *Neurobiology of Aging, 10*(6), 727-738.

Hortobagyi, T., and DeVita, P. (2000). Muscle pre- and coactivity during downward stepping are associated with leg stiffness in aging. *Journal Of Electromyography And Kinesiology, 10*(2), 117-126.

Hortobagyi, T., and Devita, P. (2006). Mechanisms responsible for the age-associated increase in coactivation of antagonist muscles. *Exercise and Sport Sciences Reviews, 34*(1), 29-35.

Isableu, B., and Vuillerme, N. (2006). Differential integration of kinaesthetic signals to postural control. *Experimental Brain Research, 174*, 763-768.

Izquierdo, M., Aguado, X., Gonzalez, R., Lopez, J. L., and Hakkinen, K. (1999). Maximal and explosive force production capacity and balance performance in men of different ages. *European Journal of Applied Physiology and Occupational Physiology, 79*(3), 260-267.

Izquierdo, M., Ibanez, J., Gorostiaga, E., Garrues, M., Zuniga, A., Anton, A., et al. (1999). Maximal strength and power characteristics in isometric and dynamic actions of the upper and lower extremities in middle-aged and older men. *Acta Physiologica Scandinavica, 167*(1), 57-68.

Jette, A. M., Harris, B. A., Sleeper, L., Lachman, M. E., Heislein, D., Giorgetti, M., et al. (1996). A home-based exercise program for nondisabled older adults. *Journal of the American Geriatrics Society, 44*(6), 644-649.

Judge, J. (2003). Balance training to maintain mobility and prevent disability. *American Journal of Preventive Medicine, 25*, 150-156.

Judge, J., Whiple, R., and Wolfson, L. (1994). Effects of resistive and balance exercises on isokinetic strength in older persons. *Journal of American Geriatrics Society, 42*, 937-946.

Kagaya, H., Sharma, M., Kobetic, R., and Marsolais, E. B. (1998). Ankle, knee, and hip moments during standing with and without joint contractures: simulation study for functional electrical stimulation. *American Journal of Physical Medicine and Rehabilitation / Association of Academic Physiatrists, 77*(1), 49-54.

Katayama, Y., Senda, M., Hamada, M., Kataoka, M., Shintani, M., and Inoue, H. (2004). Relationship between postural balance and knee and toe muscle power in young women. *Acta Medica Okayama, 58*(4), 189-195.

King, A. C., Blair, S. N., Bild, D. E., Dishman, R. K., Dubbert, P. M., Marcus, B. H., et al. (1992). Determinants of physical activity and interventions in adults. *Medicine and Science in Sports and Exercise, 24*(6 Suppl), S221-S236.

King, M. B., Judge, J. O., and Wolfson, L. (1994). Functional base of support decreases with age. *Journal of Gerontology, 49*(6), M258-263.

Knaflitz, M., Merletti, R., and De Luca, C. J. (1990). Inference of motor unit recruitment order in voluntary and electrically elicited contractions. *Journal of Applied Physiology, 68*(4), 1657-1667.

Kostka, T. (2005). Quadriceps maximal power and optimal shortening velocity in 335 men aged 23-88 years. *European Journal of Applied Physiology, 95*(2-3), 140-145.

Kouzaki, M., and Shinohara, M. (2010). Steadiness in plantar flexor muscles and its relation to postural sway in young and elderly adults. *Muscle and Nerve, 42*(1), 78-87.

Kramer, J., Lindsay, D., Magee, D., Mendryk, S., and Wall, T. (1984). Comparison of Voluntary and Electrical Stimulation Contraction Torques. *The Journal of Orthopaedic and Sports Physical Therapy*(5), 324-331.

Kristinsdottir, E. K., Fransson, P. A., and Magnusson, M. (2001). Changes in postural control in healthy elderly subjects are related to vibration sensation, vision and vestibular asymmetry. *Acta Oto-Laryngologica, 121*(6), 700-706.

Kryger, A. I., and Andersen, J. L. (2007). Resistance training in the oldest old: consequences for muscle strength, fiber types, fiber size, and MHC isoforms. *Scandinavian Journal of Medicine and Science In Sports, 17*(4), 422-430.

Kuo, A. D., and Zajac, F. E. (1993a). A biomechanical analysis of muscle strength as a limiting factor in standing posture. *Journal of Biomechanics, 26 Suppl 1*, 137-150.

Kuo, A. D., and Zajac, F. E. (1993b). Human standing posture: multi-joint movement strategies based on biomechanical constraints. *Progress in Brain Research, 97*, 349-358.

Laidlaw, D. H., Bilodeau, M., and Enoka, R. M. (2000). Steadiness is reduced and motor unit discharge is more variable in old adults. *Muscle and Nerve, 23*(4), 600-612.

Laughton, C. A., Slavin, M., Katdare, K., Nolan, L., Bean, J. F., Kerrigan, D. C., et al. (2003). Aging, muscle activity, and balance control: physiologic changes associated with balance impairment. *Gait and Posture, 18*(2), 101-108.

Levangie, P. K., and Norkin, C. C. (2001). *Joint structure and function: A comprehensive analysis* (3rd ed.). Sydney: MacLennan and Petty.

Li, J. X., Hong, Y., and Chan, K. M. (2001). Tai Chi: physiological characteristics and beneficial effects on health. *British Journal of Sports Medicine, 35*(3), 148-156.

Li, J. X., Xu, D. Q., and Hong, Y. (2008). Tai Chi exercise and proprioception behavior in old people. *Medicine and Sport Science, 52*, 77-86.

Lord, S. R., Clark, R. D., and Webster, I. W. (1991a). Physiological factors associated with falls in the elderly population. *Journal of the American Geriatrics Society, 39*, 1194-1200.

Lord, S. R., Clark, R. D., and Webster, I. W. (1991b). Postural stability and associated physiological factors in a population of aged persons. *Journal of Gerontology, 46*(3), M69-76.

Lord, S. R., Clark, R. D., and Webster, I. W. (1991c). Visual acuity and contrast sensitivity in relation to falls in an elderly population. *Age and Ageing, 20*(3), 175-181.

Lord, S. R., and Menz, H. B. (2000). Visual contributions to postural stability in older adults. *Gerontology, 46*(6), 306-310.

Lord, S. R., and Sturnieks, D. L. (2005). The physiology of falling: assessment and prevention strategies for older people. *Journal of Science And Medicine In Sport, 8*(1), 35-42.

Lord, S. R., and Ward, J. A. (1994). Age-associated differences in sensori-motor function and balance in community dwelling women. *Age and Ageing, 23*(6), 452-460.

Lord, S. R., Ward, J. A., Williams, P., and Anstey, K. J. (1994). Physiological factors associated with falls in older community-dwelling women. *Journal of the American Geriatrics Society, 42*(10), 1110-1117.

Maki, B. E., Holliday, P. J., and Topper, A. K. (1994). A prospective study of postural balance and risk of falling in an ambulatory and independent elderly population. *Journal of Gerontology, 49*(2), M72-84.

Manini, T. M., Clark, B. C., Tracy, B. L., Burke, J., and Ploutz-Snyder, L. L. (2005). Resistance and functional training reduces knee extensor position fluctuations in functionally limited older adults. *European Journal of Applied Physiology, 95*(5-6), 436-446.

Manini, T. M., Cook, S. B., Ordway, N. R., Ploutz-Snyder, R. J., and Ploutz-Snyder, L. L. (2005). Knee extensor isometric unsteadiness does not predict functional limitation in older adults. *American Journal of Physical Medicine and Rehabilitation, 84*(2), 112-121.

Matheson, A. J., Darlington, C. L., and Smith, P. F. (1999). Further evidence for age-related deficits in human postural function. *Journal of Vestibular Research: Equilibrium and Orientation, 9*(4), 261-264.

Maurer, C., and Peterka, R. J. (2005). A new interpretation of spontaneous sway measures based on a simple model of human postural control. *Journal of Neurophysiology, 93*(1), 189-200.

McKeon, P. O., Booi, M. J., Branam, B., Johnson, D. L., and Mattacola, C. G. (2010). Lateral ankle ligament anesthesia significantly alters single limb postural control. *Gait and Posture, 32*(3), 374-377.

Melzer, I., Benjuya, N., and Kaplanski, J. (2001). Age-related changes of postural control: effect of cognitive tasks. *Gerontology, 47*(4), 189-194.

Melzer, I., Benjuya, N., and Kaplanski, J. (2003). Effects of regular walking on postural stability in the elderly. *Gerontology, 49*(4), 240-245.

Melzer, I., Benjuya, N., and Kaplanski, J. (2004). Postural stability in the elderly: a comparison between fallers and non-fallers. *Age and Ageing, 33*(6), 602-607.

Mergner, T., Schweigart, G., Maurer, C., and Blümle, A. (2005). Human postural responses to motion of real and virtual visual environments under different support base conditions. *Experimental Brain Research, 167*(4), 535-556.

Mesfar, W., and Shirazi-Adl, A. (2006). Knee joint mechanics under quadricepsâ€"hamstrings muscle forces are influenced by tibial restraint. *Clinical Biomechanics, 21*(8), 841-848.

Mjolsnes, R., Arnason, A., Osthagen, T., Raastad, T., and Bahr, R. (2004). A 10-week randomized trial comparing eccentric vs. concentric hamstring strength training in well-trained soccer players. *Scandinavian Journal of Medicine and Science in Sports, 14*(5), 311-317.

Morasso, P. G., and Schieppati, M. (1999). Can muscle stiffness alone stabilize upright standing? *Journal of Neurophysiology, 82*(3), 1622-1626.

Mynark, R. G., and Koceja, D. M. (2001). Effects of Age on the Spinal Stretch Reflex. *Journal of Applied Biomechanics, 17*(3), 188-203.

Nagy, E., Feher-Kiss, A., Barnai, M. r., DomjÃ¡n-Preszner, A., Angyan, L., and Horvath, G. n. (2007). Postural control in elderly subjects participating in balance training. *European Journal of Applied Physiology, 100*(1), 97-104.

Nashner, L. (1990). *Sensory, neuromuscular and biomechanical contribution to human balance.* Paper presented at the APTA Forum, Alexandria, Va.

Nashner, L., Black, F. O., and Wall, C., 3rd. (1982). Adaptation to altered support and visual conditions during stance: patients with vestibular deficits. *The Journal Of Neuroscience, 2*(5), 536-544.

Nashner, L., and McCollum, G. (1985). The organization of human postural movements: a formal basis and experimental synthesis. *Behavioral and Brain Sciences, 8*, 135-172.

Newell, K. M., Slobounov, S. M., Slobounova, E. S., and Molenaar, P. C. (1997). Stochastic processes in postural center-of-pressure profiles. *Experimental Brain Research, 113*(1), 158-164.

Paillard, T., Margnes, E., Maitre, J., Chaubet, V., François, Y., Jully, J. L., et al. (2010). Electrical stimulation superimposed onto voluntary muscular contraction reduces deterioration of both postural control and quadriceps femoris muscle strength. *Neuroscience, 165*, 1471-1475.

Perry, M. C., Carville, S. F., Smith, C. H., Rutherford, O. M., and Newham, D. J. (2007). Strength, power output and symmetry of leg muscles: effect of age and history of falling. *European Journal of Applied Physiology, 100*, 553-561.

Peterka, R. J. (2000). Postural control model interpretation of stabilogram diffusion analysis. *Biological Cybernetics, 82*(4), 335-343.

Petrella, J. K., Kim, J.-s., Tuggle, S. C., Hall, S. R., and Bamman, M. M. (2005). Age differences in knee extension power, contractile velocity, and fatigability. *Journal of Applied Physiology, 98*(1), 211-220.

Porth, C. M., and Matfin, G. (2009). *Pathophysiology - concepts of altered health sates* (8th ed.): Lippincott Williams andWilkins.

Prieto, T. E., Myklebust, J. B., Hoffmann, R. G., Lovett, E. G., and Myklebust, B. M. (1996). Measures of postural steadiness: differences between healthy young and elderly adults. *IEEE Transactions on Biomedical Engineering, 43*(9), 956-966.

Province, M. A., Hadley, E. C., Hornbrook, M. C., Lipsitz, L. A., Miller, J. P., Mulrow, C. D., et al. (1995). The effects of exercise on falls in elderly patients. A preplanned meta-analysis of the FICSIT Trials. Frailty and Injuries: Cooperative Studies of Intervention Techniques. *JAMA: The Journal of The American Medical Association, 273*(17), 1341-1347.

Ray, C. A., and Monahan, K. D. (2002). Aging attenuates the vestibulosympathetic reflex in humans. *Circulation, 105*(8), 956-961.

Raymakers, J. A., Samson, M. M., and Verhaar, H. J. J. (2005). The assessment of body sway and the choice of the stability parameter(s). *Gait and Posture, 21*(1), 48-58.

Robinovitch, S. N., Heller, B., Lui, A., and Cortez, J. (2002). Effect of strength and speed of torque development on balance recovery with the ankle strategy. *Journal of Neurophysiology, 88*(2), 613-620.

Rosene, J. M., Fogarty, T. D., and Mahaffey, B. L. (2001). Isokinetic hamstrings:quadriceps ratios in intercollegiate athletes. *Journal of athletic, training* (Dallas) 36(4), 378-383
Total No. of Pages 376.

Rosenhall, U., and Rubin, W. (1975). Degenerative changes in the human vestibular sensory epithelia. *Acta Otolaryngol, 79*, 67-81.

Runge, C. F., Shupert, C. L., Horak, F. B., and Zajac, F. E. (1999). Ankle and hip postural strategies defined by joint torques. *Gait and Posture, 10*, 161-170.

Runge, M., Rittweger, J., Russo, C. R., Schiessl, H., and Felsenberg, D. (2004). Is muscle power output a key factor in the age-related decline in physical performance? A comparison of muscle cross section, chair-rising test and jumping power. *Clinical Physiology and Functional Imaging, 24*(6), 335-340.

Ryushi, T., Kumagai, K., Hayase, H., Abe, T., Shibuya, K., and Ono, A. (2000). Effect of resistive knee extension training on postural control measures in middle aged and elderly persons. *Journal of Physiological Anthropology and Applied Human Science, 19*(3), 143-149.

Saffer, M., Kiemel, T., and Jeka, J. (2008). Coherence analysis of muscle activity during quiet stance. *Experimental Brain Research, 185*(2), 215-226.

Santos, B. R., Delisle, A., Lariviere, C., Plamondon, A., and Imbeau, D. (2008). Reliability of centre of pressure summary measures of postural steadiness in healthy young adults. *Gait and Posture, 27*(3), 408-415.

Seynnes, O., Hue, O. A., Garrandes, F., Colson, S. S., Bernard, P. L., Legros, P., et al. (2005). Force steadiness in the lower extremities as an independent predictor of functional performance in older women. *Journal of Aging and Physical Activity, 13*(4), 395-408.

Sherrington, C., Whitney, J. C., Lord, S. R., Herbert, R. D., Cumming, R. G., and Close, J. C. T. (2008). Effective exercise for the prevention of falls: a systematic review and meta-analysis. *Journal of the American Geriatrics Society, 56*(12), 2234-2243.

Shumway-Cook, A., and Woollacott, M. H. (2007). *Motor Control: translating research into clinical practice* (3rd ed.). Sydney: Lippincott, Williams and Wilkins.

Silverthorn, D. U. (2010). *Human Physiology: An intergrated approach.* (5th ed.). Sydney: Pearsons.

Speers, R. A., Kuo, A. D., and Horak, F. B. (2002). Contributions of altered sensation and feedback responses to changes in coordination of postural control due to aging. *Gait and Posture, 16*(1), 20-30.

Teasdale, N., and Simoneau, M. (2001). Attentional demands for postural control: the effects of aging and sensory reintergration. *Gait and Posture, 14*, 203-210.

Teasdale, N., Stelmach, G., and Breunig, A. (1991). Postural sway characteristic of the elderly under normal and altered visual and support surface conditions. *Journal of Gerontology, 46*, 238-244.

Teasdale, N., Stelmach, G., Breunig, A., and Meeuwsen, H. (1991). Age differences in visual sensory intergration. *Experimental Brain Research, 85*, 691-696.

Thomas, G. N., Tomlinson, B., Hong, A. W. L., and Hui, S. S. C. (2006). Age-related anthropometric remodelling resulting in increased and redistributed adiposity is associated with increases in the prevalence of cardiovascular risk factors in Chinese subjects. *Diabetes/Metabolism Research Reviews, 22*(1), 72-78.

Timiras, P. S. (2003a). Aging of the nervous system: Structural and biochemical changes. In P. S. Timiras (Ed.), *Physiological basis of aging and geriatrics* (3rd ed., pp. 99-117). Boca Raton, FL: CRC Press.

Timiras, P. S. (2003b). The nervous system: Functional changes. In P. S. Timiras (Ed.), *Physiological basis of aging and geriatrics* (3rd ed., pp. 119-140). Boca Raton, FL: CRC Press.

Timiras, P. S. (2003c). The skeleton, joints, and skeletal and cardiac muscles. In P. S. Timiras (Ed.), *Physiological basis of aging and geriatrics* (3rd ed., pp. 375-395). Boca Raton, FL: CRC Press.

Tracy, B. L., Byrnes, W. C., and Enoka, R. M. (2004). Strength training reduces force fluctuations during anisometric contractions of the quadriceps femoris muscles in old adults. *Journal of Applied Physiology, 96*(4), 1530-1540.

Tracy, B. L., and Enoka, R. M. (2002). Older adults are less steady during submaximal isometric contractions with the knee extensor muscles. *Journal of Applied Physiology, 92*(3), 1004-1012.

Trimble, M. H., and Enoka, R. M. (1991). Mechanisms underlying the training effects associated with neuromuscular electrical stimulation. *Physical Therapy, 71*(4), 273-280.

Tsang, W. W. N., and Hui-Chan, C. W. Y. (2003). Effects of tai chi on joint proprioception and stability limits in elderly subjects. *Medicine And Science in Sports And Exercise, 35*(12), 1962-1971.

Tsang, W. W. N., and Hui-Chan, C. W. Y. (2004). Effect of 4- and 8-wk intensive Tai Chi Training on balance control in the elderly. *Medicine And Science In Sports And Exercise, 36*(4), 648-657.

Tsang, W. W. N., and Hui-Chan, C. W. Y. (2005). Comparison of muscle torque, balance, and confidence in older tai chi and healthy adults. *Medicine And Science In Sports And Exercise, 37*(2), 280-289.

Tsang, W. W. N., Wong, V. S., Fu, S. N., and Hui-Chan, C. W. (2004). Tai Chi improves standing balance control under reduced or conflicting sensory conditions. *Archives of Physical Medicine And Rehabilitation, 85*(1), 129-137.

van Soest, A. J., Haenen, W. P., and Rozendaal, L. A. (2003). Stability of bipedal stance: the contribution of cocontraction and spindle feedback. *Biological Cybernetics, 88*(4), 293-301.

Vandervoort, A. A. (2002). Aging of the human neuromuscular system. *Muscle and Nerve, 25*, 17-25.

Verrall, G. M., Slavotinek, J. P., Barnes, P. G., Fon, G. T., and Spriggins, A. J. (2001). Clinical risk factors for hamstring muscle strain injury: a prospective study with correlation of injury by magnetic resonance imaging. *British Journal of Sports Medicine, 35*(6), 435-439; discussion 440.

Vieira, T. d. M. M., de Oliveira, L. F., and Nadal, J. (2009). An overview of age-related changes in postural control during quiet standing tasks using classical and modern stabilometric descriptors. *Journal of Electromyography And Kinesiology, 19*(6), e513-e519.

Voukelatos, A., Cumming, R. G., Lord, S. R., and Rissel, C. (2007). A randomized, controlled trial of tai chi for the prevention of falls: the Central Sydney tai chi trial. *Journal of The American Geriatrics Society, 55*(8), 1185-1191.

Widmaier, E. P., Raff, H., and Strang, K. T. (2004). *Human Physiology: the mechanisms of body function* (9th ed.). New York: McGraw-Hill.

Winter, D. (1995). Human balance and posture control during standing and walking. *Gait and Posture, 3*, 193-214.

Winter, J., Allen, T. J., and Proske, U. (2005). Muscle spindle signals combine with the sense of effort to indicate limb position. *The Journal of Physiology, 568(Pt 3)*, 1035-1046.

Wolf, S. L., Barnhart, H. X., Ellison, G. L., and Coogler, C. E. (1997). The effect of Tai Chi Quan and computerized balance training on postural stability in older subjects. Atlanta FICSIT Group. Frailty and Injuries: Cooperative Studies on Intervention Techniques. *Physical Therapy, 77*(4), 371.

Wolfson, L., Whipple, R., Derby, C. A., Amerman, P., and Nashner, L. (1994). Gender differences in the balance of healthy elderly as demonstrated by dynamic posturography. *Journal of Gerontology, 49*(4), M160-167.

Wong, A. M., and Lan, C. (2008). Tai chi and balance control. *Medicine And Sport Science, 52*, 115-123.

Woollacott, M. H. (1993). Age-related changes in posture and movement. *Journal of Gerontology, 48*, 56-60.

Wu, G. (2002). Evaluation of the effectiveness of Tai Chi for improving balance and preventing falls in the older population--a review. *Journal of The American Geriatrics Society, 50*(4), 746-754.

Wu, G., Zhao, F., Zhou, X., and Wei, L. (2002). Improvement of isokinetic knee extensor strength and reduction of postural sway in the elderly from long-term Tai Chi exercise. *Archives of Physical Medicine and Rehabilitation, 83*, 1364-1369.

Xu, D., Hong, Y., and Li, J. (2008). Tai Chi exercise and muscle strength and endurance in older people. *Medicine and Sport Science, 52*, 20-29.

Xu, D., Hong, Y., Li, J., and Chan, K. (2004). Effect of tai chi exercise on proprioception of ankle and knee joints in old people. *British Journal of Sports Medicine, 38*(1), 50-54.

Yamauchi, T., Islam, M. M., Koizumi, D., Rogers, M. E., Rogers, N. L., & Takeshima, N. (2005). Effects of Home-based well-rounded exercise in community-dwelling older adults. *Journal of Sports Science and Medicine, 4*(4), 563-571.

*Chapter 2*

# POSTURAL CONTROL: FROM PRESCRIPTION TO EMERGENCE

## R. Thouvarecq[*] and D. Leroy

CETAPS (EA3832) Faculty of Sports Sciences and Physical Education.
University of Rouen, Bd Siegfried, F76821 Mont Saint Aignan, France

## ABSTRACT

Studies of postural control using the theoretical framework of complex systems have multiplied over the past 20 years, challenging the traditional cognitive approach to this topic. According to Abernethy and Sparrow (1992), these opposing perspectives, generally concerning "motor control", reflect a paradigmatic crisis as defined by Kuhn (1964). This chapter develops this point of view on the basis of four points. (i) We briefly recall the theoretical origins and fundamental principles of these two approaches to motor function: both arose from the cybernetics research conducted in the 40s and 50s but can be distinguished by their respective control determinants. The cognitive framework assumes that motor function arises from the execution of prescribed programs that are controlled by feedback (Schmidt, 1975). The complex systems framework is based on the assumptions that coordination emerges from the interaction of constraints (Newell, 1986) and is self-organizing (Haken, Kelso, Bunz, 85). (ii) We then show the consequences of these two perspectives in posture research, with major but not exclusive reference to the proposals of Nashner and McCollum (1985) and Massion et al. (1992) for the cognitive perspective, and those of Bardy, Marin, Stoffregen, and Bootsma (1999) for the complex systems perspective. In both cases, recent developments are also considered. (iii) The limits of each perspective are then discussed. (iv) Last, we show the difficulty of reconciling these two approaches to postural control research and discuss the strong possibility that we are headed for a (probably) long period of so-called "normal science", particularly in that these two paradigms will have to coexist.Many studies on motor control, particularly regarding posture, have been published without a clear statement of the authors' ontological position. In most cases, the authors have based their work on cognitivist theory but this has been implicit. At times, internal contradictions are observed, suggesting that the lack of positioning may have been due to an inadequate

---
[*] Corresponding author: regis.thouvarecq@univ-rouen.fr.

understanding of the available theoretical perspectives. This issue is not without importance. In 1992, Abernethy and Sparrow published an article titled "The rise and fall of dominant paradigms in motor behavior research" and showed that the field of motor control research was in a period of paradigmatic crisis, as defined by Kuhn (1962). Essentially, since the early 1980s, the nearly exclusive domination of the cognitivist approach in motor behavior studies has been repeatedly contested by proposals based on complexity theory. In this chapter, we briefly review the ontological foundations of these two approaches and the insight into posture that each approach has contributed. We then examine the issue of whether these two approaches have points in common, at least in the field of posture research.

Both cognitivism and complexity theories were inspired by the Macy conference series held between 1946 and 1956 (see Dupuy, 1994, for a review), but they express radically different points of view regarding motor control1. Conversely, the study of motor behavior cannot proceed without a theoretical context]. In the cognitivist approach, the production and control of movement are assumed to be prescribed by a higher information-processing system. In turn, this system receives information from the environment and the musculoskeletal system through the sensory systems. Working from this perspective, Schmidt (1975) presented a model in the 1970s that was to become the reference. According to Schmidt (1975, 1988), the production and regulation of movement are not based on a single mental schema stored in memory, but on two schemas. Depending on the initial conditions and the goal, the recall schema containing the general rules for movement (the basis of the program) to be carried out permits movement initiation. This Generalized Motor Program (GMP) is applied to a set of similar movements that control certain segments. Once parameterized (segments, force, speed direction), the program issues a series of instructions (composed of invariants and parameters) that will be applied to the musculoskeletal system in the form of muscle contractions (and relaxation) that in turn will provoke feedback from the proprioceptive system (essentially via the neuromuscular spindles), the vestibular system, and so on. The muscle contractions have an effect on the environment, which is then captured by the external receptors (mainly vision). The recognition schema is evoked at the same time as the recall schema. This schema contains information on the expected proprioceptive and exteroceptive feedback. The comparison of these two types of information (proprioceptive and exteroceptive, the "subjective reinforcement")—that is, that which is perceived and that which is expected—then allows for movement correction, if there is sufficient time. Within this framework, representations have a major role and the main research focus is on the information processing that will result in prescriptions and the regulation of muscle activity.

In contrast, complex systems theories do not accord an important role to representations. Instead of a hypothesized higher information-processing system, complexity theories focus on notions of self-organization and emergence. In research on perception and action, three approaches can be distinguished, not contradictory but instead focused on slightly different topics. The first grew out of Gibson's work (1958, 1979) and is focused on the subject-environment relationship. This approach provides an alternative to the notion of action guided by the actor's internal representations and emphasizes perception-action coupling and the theory of affordances. Dynamical systems theory (Turvey, 1990), which built on the works of Bernstein (1967) and Von Holst (1969), has been more concerned with how motor coordination emerges from organismic, task and environmental constraints (Newell, 1986). Last, the synergetic approach (Haken, 1985) applies a model validated in other fields to the study of motor coordination (Kelso and Schoner, 1988). These three approaches share the same ontology and, although

---

[1] The research questions and fields of application of both cognitivist and complexity theories extend well beyond motor behavior research, a mere epiphenomenon in this debate (see, for example, Varela, 1993).

proposals for their integration have been made (Warren, 2006), this remains far from evident (Michaels, 1998). These two paradigms have provided the general theoretical framework for much of the research on postural control.

## COGNITIVISM THEORY AND POSTURE

Upright posture poses a mechanical problem because the center of gravity (CoG) projection has to remain within the base of support. In quiet stance, the CoG is the center of mass (CoM), the point where body mass is equally distributed (Robertson et al., 2004). However, upright immobility never really occurs because the individual is constantly swaying. Force platform time recordings of positions in the center of pressure (CoP), or the barycenter of ground reaction forces, show that the CoP oscillates within an ellipse oriented in the posterior-anterior axis, although it is never perfect. The most often used indices of CoP displacement, in addition to the 95% confidence ellipse (which usually contains 95% of the recorded points) are the displacement distance, its variations around a mean point on the anterior-posterior and mediolateral axes, and speed. Thus, a small ellipse and low variance are assumed to indicate efficient postural regulation and rapid CoP displacement is assumed to indicate high energy cost to maintain posture (Vuillerme and Nougier, 2003), which is thus inefficient. Regarding these measures, the norms obtained in standardized conditions are used for the clinical evaluation of postural disorders (Association Française de Posturologie, 1985). The causes for permanent sway are many. First, standing upright against downward gravitational pull requires constant muscle tone, particularly in the extensors. Yet muscle tone is not always equally distributed (Paillard, 1976). In addition, the smallest action added to posture, such as extending an arm to grab an object, will have the mechanical consequences of displacing mass and forward acceleration of the CoG. If these are not compensated in some way, the CoG will move outside of the base of support, resulting in a fall or a step forward (reactional adjustment as compensation) (Bouisset and Zattara, 1987). Conversely, dropping a heavy object will also modify the distribution of mass (Aruin, Forest and Latash, 1998) and cause imbalance. Last, the upright individual's environment can also cause an expected or unexpected disturbance in balance that will have to be compensated. All of these postural activities are directly determined by gravity, as is demonstrated by modifications in the distribution of postural muscle tone (Clement et al., 1984) and postural organization (Lestienne and Gurfinkel, 1988) in microgravity situations.

From the cognitivist perspective, postural regulation is a problem of information processing. Therefore, in order to understand it, it is essential to understand how information is perceived and used to maintain the CoG projection within the base of support and the processing mechanisms that allow this. According to Collins and De Luca (1993, 1995), postural regulation comprises two mechanisms, similar to those of movement control: an open loop for very short-term regulation and a closed loop for longer-term regulation relative to reference values, whether or not the posture is perturbed by external forces (Massion, 1992). But it is also essential to understand how posture itself is a source of information in the service of action. The head, truck, and legs form a succession of superposed modules, each mobile with regard to the others (Amblard, 1998; Mergner and Rosemeier, 1998) and at least three allocentric frames of reference are available. These are accessible through plantar cutaneous receptors, visual receptors and the vestibular system. Knowledge about these allocentric references and about modules relative positioning obtained principally from muscle and joint receptors and the proprioceptive system and are the basis for orienting and constructing movement (Massion, 1994; Paillard, 1971). Using the above-described cybernetic model, posture can thus be conceived as a source of information, probably the most important, to constitute the "initial conditions" for movement. This dual function (to maintain balance and provide the initial conditions for additional movement) and the notion that complementary modules of information processing may coexist led to the hypothesis that two systems are involved in postural control (Massion, 1994; Massion et al., 1998). In this conception, and in contradiction to the theory of the inverted pendulum articulated around the ankle (Nashner and McCollum, 1985), each body segment (head, trunk, legs) is controlled relative to its own position in space and relative to the adjacent segments. The head is the most important module since it contains visual and vestibular receptors and its stability in space serves as a reference for top-down control. The two systems make use of two types of representation: a postural body schema that includes a representation of the body configuration in relation to the external world and a second level that is responsible for organizing postural control on the basis of information available in representation form (Massion, 1992). Postural control, which is produced by information processing, is thus obtained on the basis of four elements: a regulated reference value, the body schema, error messages, and postural reactions.

The hypothesis of a regulated reference value was first presented in 1899 by Babinski (as reported by Massion, 1984), who suggested that the coordinated movements of the hips, neck and knees work to maintain the CoG projection on the ground at the same point. According to several authors (Gollhofer, Horstmann, Berger and Dietz, 1989; Horak and Nashner, 1986; Massion, 1997), maintaining the CoG projection within the base of support is the key central nervous system-controlled variable in maintaining upright posture. However, when a suprapostural task is performed—that is, a task added to posture—the question changes. For Massion (1997), the regulated reference value does not correspond only to the CoG projection, as this would exclude changes in body geometry. He used the example of a person holding a liquid-filled glass: if the only controlled variable is the CoG position and not the hand in relation to gravity, it is likely that the contents will spill. Lacquaniti (1992) suggested that the reference value concerned body geometry above all. In an animal study with cat (thus, not upright), this author hypothesized two types of regulated reference: first, segment geometry and body orientation in space and, second, stabilization through the exertion of contact forces, which contributes to regulating CoG position (Danis, Krebs, Gill-Body and Sahrman, 1998). To confirm this hypothesis, it was necessary to remove gravitational forces and work in microgravity. The experiments in these conditions clearly indicated the simultaneous existence of these two reference values, one geometric and the other kinetic (Massion et al., 1995). Another problem deals specifically with the perturbations to posture during movement. Moving the chest forward, raising the arm, and then grabbing an object provoke an acceleration of the CoG in the forward direction. If this is not compensated by an action in the opposite direction, the individual will fall. This compensation can be observed even before the movement is initiated via the activation or inhibition of specific muscle groups (Bouisset and Zattara, 1987). The parameters of these anticipated postural adjustments (APAs), which determine the spatial and time organization and the amplitude of the muscle action (Aruin and Latash, 1995; van der Fits, Klip, van Eykern and Hadders-Algra, 1998), depend on the voluntary action that will be performed, its anticipation, and thus its representation, as is indicated by the fact that there is little link between sensory deficit and APA functioning (Forget and Lamarre, 1990). The coordination between voluntary movement and APAs thus occurs through two hierarchical and parallel control processes (Massion, 1992). In the first, a copy of the central command that will provoke voluntary movement toward the system responsible for APA allows adjustment of this movement as well as the synchronization with action. It is used for example in the unloading type of task (Paulignan, Dufosse, Hugon and Massion, 1989). In the second process, postural control and movement control are controlled by a higher order. In this case, movement only begins when the postural dynamics have been established. In both cases, APAs occur during multi-joint movements (Minvielle and Audiffren, 2000).

Postural regulation is also based on a representation of the body in space, the second element in the model proposed by Massion et al. (1998). This internal representation of the body is not a new notion. Paillard (1986a) mentioned the thinking of Head and Holmes on this topic in a publication in 1911. It is easily validated by the capacity of individuals with closed eyes—and thus no external reference except gravity—to point to a part of their own body with very great precision. This representation is often confused with the generic term of body schema and Paillard (1986b) thus distinguished between the identified body and the situated body. The first concerns the knowledge we have of our own body shape independently of its position. The second, for which the term body schema is more appropriate, concerns the body position in space and serves as a self-centered reference point in motor control and maintenance of stable body position (Gurfinkel and Levik, 1991). Perception, particularly proprioception, seems to be dominant in the ongoing construction of this schema and its consequences on postural regulation, as shown in studies of stimulation by tendon vibration. These experiments have shown that when visual information is not available, ankle tendon vibrations in a free standing subject induce illusory forward body tilt and a compensatory postural action in the opposite direction (Roll, Vedel and Roll, 1989). Moreover, although the lack of gravity perturbs body orientation in space (Clement et al., 1984), it does not perturb the orientation of gestures relative to the reference point, which in this case is the longitudinal axis of the body (Gurfinkel et al., 1993).

The third element for postural regulation is error detection. Indeed, evaluating the difference between the prescribed and actual position is a way to maintain balance, according to the cybernetic model (Nashner and Berthoz, 1978). The cognitive framework assumes that information processing is linear, proceeding through a series of successive steps, and modular. Moreover, Broadman and especially Penfield (Penfield and Rasmussen, 1950) were among the first to report that nervous system anatomy suggests specialized areas, particularly regarding perception, and so-called associative areas. Information about errors is thus first processed in an intra-modality mode and then in an inter-modality mode. The respective influences of visual, proprioceptive, tactile and vestibular inputs and their integration have been the focus of many studies. The visual system locates and identifies light stimuli through central and peripheral vision, the retinotectal and geniculo-striate pathways, and the dorsal and ventral corticocortical pathways paillard langage). The influence of visual input on postural control is determined by the Romberg quotient (Njiokiktjien and Van Parys, 1976), which is calculated as the ratio between the CoP sway area when the subject's eyes are open and the area when they are closed (multiplied by 100). Closing the eyes greatly increases the sway area, reducing the coefficient. However, a perturbation of vision—for example, by modifying the nature of light (continuous versus stromboscopic) as demonstrated by Amblard and Cremieux (1976)—causes a greater deterioration in postural control than does it absence. Nevertheless, the condition that seems to most degrade postural control is when the subject is asked to keep his or her eyes open in the dark (Hafström et al., 2001). According to these authors, when the eyes are open, the system "expects" to receive information and thus does not immediately give compensatory weight to other sensory systems. But when individuals remain in darkness for prolonged periods (more than 20 minutes), postural control noticeably changes (Rougier, 2003), suggesting a shift from dominant visual control to vestibular-kinesthetic control. Moreover, posture is also disturbed by a moving visual scene in what is called the vection phenomenon, whose intensity depends on the manipulated variables: the area of the scene, the speed, and so on (Dietz, 1992). When an individual has to fix a visual target, the distance between the target and the individual also influences the postural parameters (Paulus, Straube and Brandt, 1984). The visual system alone, however, does not detect movement if the movement is due to the individual's displacement (passive, in particular) or a displacement of the environment, as seen in vection experiments (Lee and Lishman, 1975). This confirms the importance of the step of multisensory integration.

The role of the kinesthetic system in postural control has also been widely studied, in particular with tendon vibration experiments and, more indirectly, with fatigue studies (Vuillerme, Danion, Forestier and Nougier, 2002). Even defining this system is difficult. Etymologically, the name means sensation (esthesis) of movement (kine). From a functional approach, the definition of kinesthesia necessarily includes muscle, joint and tendon receptors, as well as vestibular, tactile and visual receptors. To study the relative influence of the visual and kinesthetic systems, and assuming that the first integrates the second, the rules for logical reasoning and the experimental methodology proposed by Claude Bernard cannot be applied. Roll (1994) suggested that kinesthesia be integrated into a more general system for knowledge of body properties, somesthesia, which would also include proprioception (linked to muscle and joint receptors). McCloskey (1978), on the other hand, defined kinesthesia more restrictively, limiting it to the receptors distributed in the muscle-joint system. Other authors integrated the kinesthetic system (in the sense of McCloskey, 1978) and the tactile system into the same functional perception which they termed haptic (Gentaz, Baud-Bovy and Luyat, 2008). Paillard (1976) distinguished the sense of movement (kinesthesia) from the sense of position (statesthesia). More recently, Gandevia, Refshauge and Collins (2002) proposed that in addition to movement, position and force detection, proprioception should include the conscious aspects of motor command timing. On the basis of receptors and nerve pathways, classic neuroanatomy suggests a distribution of the sensory systems that isolates—at least for the initial processing steps—the visual system from the proprioceptive and tactile systems. All this debate is important because the problem with definitions reveals a deeper problem, which is the great difficulty of determining the link between a functional multimodality kinesthesia and the study of how each one of the modalities affects postural control. In this context, considering kinesthesia and proprioception as synonyms is unhelpful and consensus is today far from evident. This confusion is particularly detrimental for cognitive theory per se as, within this theoretical framework, functioning can only be understood with the clear distinction of each of the steps. Moreover, the kinesthetic system is assumed to be both a sixth sense (of movement) (Berthoz, 1997), in addition to the five other "single-modality" senses, and the first sense, in that it is used to calibrate the other senses (Roll, 2003). Tendon vibration of the muscles (but not their antagonists) is again one of the best means to evaluate the influence of muscle receptors on posture in the absence of vision (Roll and Vedel, 1982). Mechanical tendon stimulation provokes muscle stretching, thus stretching the neuromuscular spindles, which creates the "illusion" of activity in the concerned segment. As early as 1972, Eklund showed that tendon vibration applied to the limbs or trunk induced postural tilting in the direction of the stimulated muscle. However, Hlavacka, Mergner and Krizkova (1996) observed that vibration can also induce tilting in the opposite direction of the stimulated muscle—in their case, the gastrocnemius—which permits knee flexion and is very involved in antigravity functions. Tendon vibration was also applied to the arms (Cordo, Gurfinkel, Bevan and Kerr, 1995), the oculomotor muscles (Roll, Roll and Velay, 1991), and the neck muscles, whose proprioceptive afferents provide information about head position in relation to the trunk (Mergner, Huber and Becker, 1997) and in all cases provoked postural reactions (Ivanenko, Grasso and Lacquaniti, 1999; Kavounoudias, Gilhodes, Roll and Roll, 1999). These studies clearly demonstrated that the proprioceptive system plays a major role in the feedback and error detection processes of postural regulation. However, Isableu and Vuillerme (2006) observed that those individuals with the smallest sway area in normal situations were the most destabilized by a soft support surface. This suggested that the influence of kinesthetic information in postural control varies between individuals. The influence of cutaneous mechanico-reception in postural control, particularly plantar, has also been explored by locally anesthetizing the receptors involved in this modality; this resulted in increased postural instability (Thoumie and Do, 1996), particularly in the mediolateral axis when vision was not available (Meyer, Oddson and De Luca, 2004). The other method has been to vary the support surface by using foam, such as used in rehabilitation (Chiang and Wu, 1997; Isableu and Vuillerme, 2006), to degrade the somatosensory plantar input or by stimulating the receptors by placing the subjects on planks covered with small balls (Okubo, Watanabe and Baron, 1980). The results indicated that in the first case postural control was disturbed and in the second the area of postural sway was diminished in comparison with the area observed on a smooth surface. Specific stimulation of a part of the sole of the foot systematically provoked tilting in the direction opposite (backward if the front of the foot is stimulated, and contralaterally if the side of the foot is stimulated). This seems to indicate correction mechanisms with plantar origins (Kavounoudias, Gilhodes, Roll and Roll, 1999). The other stimulation technique consisted of adding tactile input by asking the subject to touch a surface with a finger without exerting force (the force must be less than 1 Newton), while maintaining upright posture (Holden, Ventura and Lackner, 1994). In this situation, the CoP ellipse area and speed of displacement diminished. However, in this specific case, the stimulation was not naturally or directly involved in maintaining posture. Thus, in the strictest sense, information was added that is not there when one simply stands upright. This method thus provides more information on sensory integration and the addition of information than on the role of skin mechanical receptors in postural control.

The vestibular system is also involved in postural control. It is the first to become functional during embryogenesis and it is constantly being stimulated except in situations of microgravity. This system detects linear and angular accelerations of the head. Exploration of its involvement in postural maintenance is principally carried out through clinical case studies because of the difficulty of suppressing the stimulations detected by this system and its anatomical position. Although some studies have reported that postural regulation is deteriorated in patients with vestibular lesions (Allum et al., 1998), this does not suggest that vestibular input has a major influence on postural control in the healthy individual, especially when other sensory input (visual, kinesthetic) is available (Dietz, 1992). According to Fitzpatrick and McCloskey (1994), in natural posture, the amplitude of head oscillations does not reach the activation threshold for vestibular receptors. Although not simple, it is possible to experimentally stimulate the vestibular system. Galvanic vestibular stimulation, which consists of varying the intensity of electrodes (anode or cathode) applied to the mastoid process, induces a perception of deviation in the gravitational axis and a disturbance in postural balance (Hkavacka, Krizkova and Horak, 1995; Hlavacka, Mergner and Krizkova, 1996). This association between perception of the gravitational axis and postural disturbance has been observed by other means. At the end of the 1940s, Witkin (1950) seated subjects experimentally deprived of vision on a platform turning on its axis. In these conditions of no vision and centrifugal force, he observed postural deviation. Because of the addition of rotation, the vestibular system detected both gravitational and rotational accelerations. The subjects thus had the illusion of leaning outward and sought to reorient the trunk toward the interior, thereby indicating the influence of this sensory system. It should be noted, however, that in this case, the subjects were seated and not standing and that the experimental situation was far from ecological (in the sense of "natural") in that the gravitational-inertial forces were quite removed from those of everyday experience. These data clearly indicate that each of these sensory systems influences postural control in one way or another. However, although these inputs from different sources are first processed independently, they are used simultaneously in control processes. And although each system has an important role to play, it is only after all the input has been integrated that a single postural regulation system, itself integrated into a single and global system of information processing, will detect errors.

The surplus of information and its many sources lead to redundancies that can be seen as inter-modality conflicts, as in the case of motion sickness. Yet these redundancies are not without utility. First, they ensure posture in the absence of input from one of the sensory systems: for example, we are able to stand in total darkness, although perhaps with less stability, and astronauts are able to organize their posture in the absence of gravity. However, although the absence of input from a sensory system can be compensated for, the relative importance of the sensory systems seems hierarchical, with vision being the most important, according to the experiments of Nashner and Berthoz (1978). Their subjects stood on a moving platform but visual indicators did not signal this because a "box" had been placed over their heads and this "box" was moving in phase with the platform. The authors thus observed no postural reaction. But when the environment was fixed (the "box" did not move), a postural reaction was observed. However, the greatest sensory redundancy in postural regulation seems to be due to the fact that posture itself is a source of input. In 1995, Simoneau, Ulbrecht, Derr and Cavanagh tested the relative and combined influences of visual, vestibular, and somatosensory input. Although the methodology used to perturb the somatosensory (comparison between subjects with and without neuropathy) and vestibular (maintenance of head straight or inclined backward at 45°) input can be debated, the results yielded information on sensory integration in the service of postural regulation. According to the authors, a disturbance in vestibular input increased instability by 4%, in visual input by more than 40%, and in somatosensory input by more than 65%, which (in sum) equals 110%. When the three were simultaneously disturbed, the increase in instability was 250%. The 140% difference was thus due to the input from three sources simultaneously. In other words, the information received and processed by each sensory system is then combined (Oie, Kiemel and Jeka, 2001; Oie, Kiemel and Jeka, 2002) and, in nonpathological situations or situations of artificial disturbance, the result of this combination is used to detect errors in postural regulation. Adding supplementary information to what is normally available in upright posture also reduces postural sway. As noted earlier, finger contact (without mechanical pressure) with a solid surface reduced sway by 50% in positions with one foot in front of the other (Jeka and Lackner, 1995). This type of result was also observed during unipedal standing (Holden, Ventura and Lackner, 1994) or with feet together (Clapp and Wing, 1999). Haptic and proprioceptive data about arm position provide more information about sway, thereby reducing it and thus energy cost. The notion that "light touch" with a stable surface has an influence because it provides additional information about a new reference frame seems confirmed by the observation that an increase in the size of the contact surface had no effect on sway, whereas the surface needed to be rigid (Lackner, Rabin and DiZio, 2001). Patients with sensory deficits can partially compensate for them by adding "light touch." Thus, light touch improved postural regulation in patients with superficial leg neuropathies, particularly when the postural task was difficult, vision was not available, and the support surface was narrow (Dickstein, Shupert and Horak, 2001). Patients with vestibular lesions regulated posture better without vision than subjects without this pathology in the same situation but without finger contact (Lackner et al., 1999). These observations suggest that the error detection system, although it can do without light contact information to regulate balance, can also directly integrate it as a new reference frame, particularly when the postural task is difficult.

Beside, the regulated reference value, the body schema, the error detection messages system, postural reactions strategies is the fourth process involved in postural regulation. Postural strategy refers to the musculoskeletal mechanisms controlled by the information-processing system to maintain balance. Although posturographic data about CoP displacements provide kinetic information, they give no information about the kinematics. The human body has many joint modules that function synergistically, so there is more than one way to move the CoG forward. For this reason, balance (keeping the CoG projection within the support base) should be distinguished from posture (the way this is accomplished) (Massion, 1984). As early as 1899, Babinski observed that when patients were asked to perform a dorsiflexion of the trunk and neck, it was accompanied by knee flexion to maintain balance. These synergies also appear during breathing movements (Gurfinkel and Elner, 1973). This raises the question of how posture is organized in response to expected and unexpected disturbances, given the great number of possibilities that are mechanically available. In other words, the question is whether relatively stable patterns of muscle activation are implemented. The publications of Nashner and McCollum (1985) and Horak and Nashner (1986) are references on this topic, not least because of the sheer number of times they have been cited, whether as sources of inspiration or targets for criticism, as expressed by Bardy, Marin, Stoffregen and Bootsma (1999), for example.

Nashner and McCollum (1985) analyzed postural organization using a three-segment model (leg, thigh, trunk) plus one (the foot resting on the support surface), articulated in the sagittal plane around three points (ankle, knee and hip) by three pair of muscles (abdominal/paraspinal, quadriceps/hamstrings, tibial/gastrocnemius). After formally describing the types of coordination possible and their mechanical consequences, the authors suggested two hypotheses. According to the first, coordination requires a limited number of muscles that function synergistically, and thus the number of coordination strategies is limited. According to the second, the mode of nervous system control will involve a minimal number of calculations for precision. With these two hypotheses, the authors are firmly situated in the cognitivist camp and the first hypothesis expresses a "Bersteinian" perspective of simplified control. They demonstrated three (more one) strategies, using perturbation. In the ankle strategy, posture is organized as an inverted pendulum around the ankle axis, with the body behaving as a rigid block. Control of the CoG position in the anterior-posterior axis is thus quite simplified (Fujisawa et al., 2005). This strategy is used for slight body sway with a wide support surface but for mechanical reasons it cannot be used for great sway: the angular moment at the ankle is limited by the length of the foot relative to the height (and size) of the center of mass. In the hip strategy, postural stability is organized around the hip. This strategy is used for narrow support surfaces or perturbations with high frequency or amplitude. According to these authors, these two strategies are functionally distinct: either one or the other is used, and when both are used simultaneously, postural regulation fails. In fact, subjects capable of using a pure hip strategy generally succeed in maintaining balance on a narrow surface, whereas those who alternate between hip and ankle strategies often lose their balance (25 to 75% of the cases). The ankle strategy seems to be used for low frequencies, of less than 0.2 Hz (Nashner, Shupert, Horak and Black, 1989) or small amplitudes of less than 20° (McCollum and Leen, 1989) and the hip strategy is used when the perturbations are greater (means). A third strategy was also assumed, the "vertical strategy," in which the objective is to lower the center of gravity using the hips, knees, and ankles simultaneously. The last strategy to conserve balance is to take a step in the same direction as the CoG displacement. The determinants for changing from ankle to hip strategy or vice versa have nevertheless continued to be debated because of the theoretical problem they raise. From the cognitivist perspective, an important point to settle is whether these two strategies correspond to two radically different schemas or a single schema with variations. Schmidt provided an element of response when he suggested that a "behavioral unit"—that is, what determines behavior—is more abstract than muscle synergies and thus is situated at the level of programs. From this perspective, the choice of muscles used depends on the program and does not define it. According to Kuo (1995) and Kuo and Zajak (1993), the explanation may be related to energy cost: from a biomechanical point of view, the ankle strategy maintains posture despite perturbation with low energy cost, which is evidenced by ankle stiffening, according to the authors. However, they also point out that, more than a pure ankle strategy, a mixed strategy is used to minimize "nervous system" work; that is, the cost of control. Also, ankle stiffening, which should compensate for a lack of visual information, is not seen in the blind (Rougier and Farenc, 2000), simply because the cost of constant maintenance would be too high. Studies in no gravity (space flight) seem to indicate the primacy of strategies over synergies because strategies remain stable throughout flight, whereas synergies were modified (Lestienne and Gurfinkel, 1988). Although Nashner and McCollum (1985) have frequently been cited, other empirical works have partially contradicted their results. Runge, Shupert, Horak and Zajac (1999) questioned the hypothesis of two distinct strategies (hip and ankle). By varying the speed of displacement toward the back of the platform on which subjects were placed, they observed a continuum wherein the hip strategy was added to the ankle strategy, but they did not observe a "pure" hip strategy. Gatev, Thomas, Thomas and Hallett (1999) showed that ankle strategies dominated during "normal" posture maintenance. But with the reduction in the support surface the hip mechanisms became much more important, at least in the sagittal plane. According to the authors, the constant control of sway keeps a precise representation of posture up to date.

Although the debate is often sharp concerning the functioning of the four main elements of upright posture maintenance: regulated reference values, body schema, error detection, and postural reactions, the model used in the cognitive framework is widely accepted, with some studies of postural regulation providing support for the hypothesis of a single information-processing system. The attentional cost of postural control was first thought to be negligible but works from the mid 1980s onward have disproved this hypothesis using the dual-task paradigm as applied to posture (Kerr, Condon and McDonald, 1985). The difficulty of allocating attention to a task appears even more marked when posture is difficult to maintain, such as on a narrow surface (Lajoie, Teasdale, Bard and Fleury, 1993), and it varies as a function of the task (Kerr, Condon and McDonald, 1985). The attentional requirements for postural balance also seem greater in the elderly than in younger people when sensory input is disturbed (no vision or on a soft surface) (Teasdale, Bard, LaRue and Fleury, 1993). Although some results do not allow firm conclusions to be drawn (Stoffregen et al., 2007), the overall finding is that postural regulation implicates information-processing systems and thus requires attentional resources (Woollacott and Shumway-Cook, 2002). These resources are shared with other functions, which validates the hypothesis of a single processing channel. The inner coherence of cognitivist theory and its sheer weight in the field of posture research has not hindered the development of other theories, presented further on. But one of the great strengths of this theory is its relevance for nervous system physiology and pathology, although it must be said that sometimes this relationship has appeared to be a circular co-justification.

Nervous system anatomy indicates cybernetic functioning. In addition to the central control of local feedback loops that ensure muscle tone, posture is regulated by many subcortical structures (striatum, lateroventral thalamus, subthalamic nucleus, substancia nigra, pallidum, red nucleus) of the extra-pyramidal system in association with the cortex (Paillard, 1986b) regarding the efferent pathways, with the final common pathway being the alpha motor neuron (Schmidt, 1988). Gamma motor neurons ensure that neuromuscular spindles are adjusted to the current length of the muscle. Each sensory system involved in postural control has its own afferent pathway projecting to specific cortical areas with lateral subcortical projections. The pathways from the peripheral vestibular apparatus are an exception because they are not projected by a specifically differentiated pathway toward a "vestibular cortical area" (although the posterior insula is sometimes attributed this function, Brandt, Dieterich and Danek, 1994) but toward subcortical structures after a step to the vestibular nuclei. This pathways and these projections can no doubt be explained by the phylogenetic age of this sensory system. In contrast, the vestibular nuclei receive visual and proprioceptive information. The influence of each of the four elements involved in postural control and their interactions have been mapped to biological components of the nervous system, mainly through studies in pathology. However, the danger is that the cognitive approach becomes a caricature, with the study of human functioning a kind of "nephrenology" with each zone of the central nervous system corresponding to a function. Quite to the contrary, cognitive researchers assume that each zone contributes to a vast functional network (Mazoyer, 2002).

The specific effects of perceptual system deficits on posture have been thoroughly described. Although the data from subjects with visual deficits are not the same as the data from subjects without visual deficit and eyes closed, they are still very informative. The congenitally blind have an unusual posture with the head tilted forward, which in two thirds of the cases causes spinal cord deformity (Martinez, 1977). This is often associated with asymmetric gait and, in blind youth, frequent rocking. The head position observed in blind individuals can be explained by the 30° tilt of the horizontal canals when the seeing eye is on the horizontal axis, and the oscillations would stimulate the vestibular system (which detects accelerations and not positions) to compensate the lack of visual information (Berthoz, 1974. In patients with retinitis pigmentosa, a degenerative disorder that first affects peripheral vision and then causes blindness, postural sway is known to be great (Geruschat and Turano, 2002). Bullinger (2004) demonstrated that when sensory flow (visual, for example) was cut off in children, they increased the available flows to generate the covariations needed to construct body image and orientation in space. In Parkinson's disease, a central nervous system disorder, the nigro-strial dopaminergic pathways degenerate, provoking the well-described motor symptoms (rigidity, akinesia, rigidity). The vestibular-proprioceptive system is affected as well, causing postural disturbances that can be quite specific, as in the patient reported by Sachs (1985) who leaned forward without realizing it. Another interesting argument for the cognitivist hypothesis from postural studies in pathology concerns the case of "contraversive pushing."

"Pusher syndrome" is seen in patients with unilateral cortical lesions and is characterized by pushing in the direction opposite the unaffected hemisphere, which provokes an imbalance and a tendency to fall in the direction of the lesion. Paradoxically, although the subjective postural vertical may show great error in these patients, the subjective visual vertical remains intact (Karnath, Ferber and Dichgans, 2000). This suggests different systems of gravitational information processing at the central level. However, the severe hemispatial neglect—that is, ignoring half of one's body (contralateral to the lesion, in the right hemisphere in this study, Lafosse et al., 2005)— conversely suggests higher order processes for body image with the same subsystems as used in postural balance. These results may seem contradictory but are not if one looks at the evolving nature of the cognitivist theory over the years. Cognitivist researchers have consistently used data from nervous system physiology but they have never claimed to be able to make a direct link between functional psychological models and the structural models from neurosciences. Moreover, the components of the central nervous system, which is considered to be a single processing system, are involved in many functions to ensure overall coherence. Developments in brain imaging (PET, fMRI, MEG) clearly show that cognitive processes often make use of large networks involving a great number of cortical and subcortical structures. Therefore, it is unsurprising that deficits affecting the motor system also affect the higher processes. As Paillard observed (1986c), motor behavior involves a high number of structures that function in a circular manner (cybernetic) by definition, and some of them, like the associative cortex or the zones in front of the central sulcus, are also involved in a high number of executive functions.

Cognitivist theory is not able to answer all questions about postural regulation, it contains contradictions about the relationships between system elements, and it can be criticized on a number of other points. However, it is based on an extraordinary quantity of experimental findings accumulated over more than half a century of research. During this time, it has developed into a nearly exclusive ontological framework providing, overall, a coherent model for understanding postural regulation.

## COMPLEX SYSTEMS AND POSTURE

From the perspective of complexity theory, postural coordination does not result from prescriptions given by on the basis of information gathered from the perceptual modalities that is then integrated into internal representations and feedback loops. Posture is understood as a coupling between perception and action, and from this perspective studying each of the steps proposed by cognitivist theory has little relevance. A radical split thus occurred when Stoffregen and Riccio (1988) challenged the classical notion of orientation (Mittelstaedt, 1983) by positing that verticality results from the combined input from the perceptual systems, with each able to indicate the gravitational axis (Howard and Templeton, 1966), and that this combined input serves as the basis for postural control. Their arguments were based on several points, particularly concerning the vestibular system. The otoliths have traditionally been considered as graviceptors, in the service of postural regulation among other tasks. Stoffregen and Riccio (1988), however, observed that these receptors detect acceleration and thus concluded that, once the head is moving, vestibular information cannot be used to distinguish between forces due to motion and gravity. Moreover, they reviewed the studies of vertical perception in immersion, which, according to them, is the best way to isolate the somesthetic senses. They showed that the vestibular system alone cannot determine the gravitational axis. They therefore deduced that vertical perception (which in itself does not exist) cannot be used to understand the determinants of postural regulation and that instead posture regulation should be examined in relation to the qualities of the support surface: size, resistance to deformation, the amount of friction to prevent slipping, and its relation to gravitational forces, which may require the application of forces to maintain the posture. Some surfaces have affordances for standing and others do not, and from an ecological perspective, these authors noted that information emerges from the interaction between body and surface. These same authors (Riccio and Stoffregen, 1990) also proposed that kinematic aspects should be taken into account because a change in orientation may be linked to a variety of movements (for example, detected head movement can be due to movement in the neck joint or the chest). They further suggested that, more than the traditional quantitative analysis based on the CoP, geometric analyses of the configurations and transitions were called for to understand postural regulation.

Another original assumption of the ecological approach is that posture maintenance as an end in itself is very rare (Balasubramaniam, Riley and Turvey, 2000; Bardy, Marin, Stoffregen and Bootsma, 1999). For these theorists, upright posture is in the service of and is constrained by tasks (called suprapostural), such as grabbing an object or fixing and reading a text (Smart et al., 2004). It is also a means to facilitate visual search (Stoffregen, Pagulayan, Bardy and Hettinger, 2000). The efficiency of a postural strategy is thus defined in terms of the consequences for action, and stability is defined as a state in which uncontrolled movements in perception/action coupling (and the flow that they generate) are minimized (Sparrow and Newell, 1998). The action of orienting the body in relation to the ground thus emerges from the interaction between three constraints, the support surface, the organismic properties, and the task goal, with this last being most important (Riccio and Stoffregen, 1990).

Postural control thus is not understood as the permanent attempt to minimize sway but as a constant compromise between effort and stability. For example, to better detect a target, archers standing in profile sway more in the mediolateral direction and reduce movements in the anterior-posterior direction (Balasubramaniam, Riley and Turvey, 2000). This constant swaying generates multisensorial flow. The term multimodality suggests a certain independence between modalities and may seem contradictory to the arguments of Stoffregen and Bardy (2001) concerning "global array." However, this issue has not been dealt with in postural studies and the link between perceptual flow and postural action has usually been seen from the standpoint of a single optical flow based on the experimental procedure of the "moving room." Originally, subjects were placed placed in an environment whose walls or floor could be moved, generating optical flow. This was eventually replaced by virtual environments projected onto a screen or a mask. Many studies showed that generating optical flow with a moving room induced an "accompaniment" of the environment, without intentionality (Bardy, Warren and Kay, 1996; Baumberger, Isableu and FlUckinger, 2004; Stoffregen, 1985; Stoffregen, 1986). In addition, postural adaptations appeared whether the suprapostural task was to track the target (Stoffregen, Smart, Bardy and Pagulayan, 1999) or to simply gaze at it (Stoffregen, 1985). The movement, oriented in the same direction as the generated flow, tended to minimize the dilations and contractions in the optical flow, which demonstrated that optical expansion and parallax, specifying the speed, acceleration, and position of the body relative to the environment, are fundamental invariants of the visual control of posture (Bardy, Warren and Kay, 1996). Although these results demonstrate the perception/action coupling in postural regulation and the influence of invariants, important questions remain regarding multimodality from an ecological point of view. Since the manipulated flow was strictly visual (and thus without direct kinesthetic, vestibular or somatosensorial effect), it may seem surprising that action occurred in response to stimulation. In fact, the contradiction is merely superficial since, according to Stoffregen and Bardy (2001), the relative changes in the flows remain congruent during task performance and the generated movement also creates flow (Baumberger, Isableu and FlUckinger, 2004). This interpretation seems confirmed by the observation of the same result when the applied flow is acoustic (Stoffregen et al., 2009). Moreover, when subjects are asked whether a support surface will permit upright posture to be maintained based on its degree of inclination, the responses do not depend on the modality (visual or haptic) engaged (Regia-Corte, Luyat, Darcheville and Miossec, 2004), which suggests the intervention of amodal information.

A radically different methodology has also been used to explore the link between flow and postural movement. In this case, the focus is to determine the effect of multimodal perceptual disturbance on the time structure of postural regulation (Riley, Balasubramaniam and Turvey, 1999; Clark and Riley, 2006; Riley and Clark, 2003; Schmit, Regis and Riley, 2005). The dependent variable is the CoP and the perceptual manipulations consist of varying the availability of vision (eyes open vs. closed), the nature of the visual environment (fixed vs. one that follows postural sway), and the support surface (rigid vs. soft). Recurrence Quantification Analysis (RQA) is used to process the CoP movements. The principle is to create a coordinate system by taking the measured signal and a number of time-lagged copies of the signal. Then the proximity of the points in time and space are determined. For a given point, the number of points situated within a sphere of fixed radius is determined and so on for the next points, which can be represented by a recurrence graph. For example, white noise (without dynamic structure) would give a uniform distribution of these neighbors. Three indices are particularly interesting. First, the percent recurrence (%REC) is the number of recurrent points expressed as a percentage of the number of potentially recurrent points multiplied by 100. A %REC equal to 100 corresponds to the repetition of the same point or a flat signal. Second, percent determinism (%DET) is the percentage of recurrent points falling on upward diagonal line segments, which indicates the degree with which the recurrent points form repeated chains of data. These are represented by lines on the recurrence graphs. For example, a totally predictable signal would have a %DET of 100. Last, the third index is TREND, which indicates the signal deviation (or drift). A non-zero TREND (most often negative) indicates a nonstationary signal. In their study, Riley, Balasubramaniam and Turvey (1999) asked standing subjects to look at a 3D array of vertical bars (3 rows of 9) placed either in front of them or to the side (the eyes-closed condition was added). After RQA on the signals (anterior-posterior displacement of CoP), their results indicated that the signal was not stochastic and that determinism depended on the conditions. One of the most striking results was that in the eyes-closed condition, determinism increased, as did the variability and amplitude of CoP displacement, which according to the authors was counterintuitive. In other words, the greater the amplitude and variability of the signal, the more deterministic it was! According to these authors, in addition to the variability and amplitude of CoP motions, changes in time structure have an adaptive function. Riley and Turvey (2002) suggested that these time structure changes in CoP motions are linked to behavioral changes in the organization of degrees of freedom. However, the use of "perturbation" and what exactly constitutes it are still matters of debate. In a response to an article by Creath et al. (2005), Bardy, Lagarde, Oullier and Stoffregen (2007) even questioned the very idea of perturbation. They noted that no clear definition of what is and what is not a perturbation has yet been given. Thus, for example, tracking a target with the head while in upright position may or may not be a perturbation, depending on the research question, which in turn depends on the ontological and theoretical framework for the study.

These studies provide data on the relationships between information flows and the forces exerted, the constraints affecting quiet stance, and the way posture is established (for example, being on a boat changes the distance and angle between the feet) (Stoffregen, Chen, Yu and Villard, 2009). But they provide little insight into how a postural response is actually produced. The classic explanation is ankle strategies for small perturbations and hip strategies for bigger or more frequent perturbations (Nashner and McCollum, 1985). This explanation at least resolves in part the question of managing degrees of freedom (Bernstein, 1996; Turvey, 1990). However, these strategies are not compatible with complex systems theory. According to Bardy, Marin, Stoffregen and Bootsma (1999), ambiguity regarding the simultaneous use of ankle and hip strategies can be seen in the literature. Researchers interested in biomechanical (McCollum and Leen, 1989) or pathological (Horak, Nashner and Diener, 1990) aspects, or postural control (Horak and Nashner, 1986; Nashner, Shupert, Horak and Black, 1989), have emphasized the exclusivity of one or the other, whereas the works of Nashner and McCollum (1985) to which they refer were focused on dominance and not unicity. Moreover, some empirical data have shown concomitant activity of the ankles and hips (Bardy, Marin, Stoffregen and Bootsma, 1999; Horak, Nashner and Diener, 1990; Stoffregen et al., 1997). Classically, hip rotation during ankle strategy-type activity has been assumed to be uncontrolled nonfunctional noise (Horak and Nashner, 1986). As noted by Bardy, Marin, Stoffregen and Bootsma (1999), the ambiguousness of the data is undoubtedly because chosen analyzed variables at different levels, such as muscle (Nashner and McCollum, 1985), joint movements (Horak and Nashner, 1986), or the forces generated by postural activity on the support surface (Horak, Nashner and Diener, 1990), are related in equivocal ways (Bernstein, 1967). A series of studies was thus published, advancing the idea that postural coordination should be described from a macroscopic and dynamic point of view (Bardy, Marin, Stoffregen and Bootsma, 1999; Marin et al., 1999; Oullier, Bardy, Stoffregen and Bootsma, 2002). In these studies, postural coordination was summarized as simultaneous ankle and hip movements acting like asymmetric coupled oscillators. Subjects standing with the hands behind the back were asked to use the head to track a target oscillating at different amplitudes (the control parameter, which could also be the frequency) in the anterior-posterior axis. The relative phase (order parameter) was calculated from the angular movements of the hips and ankles collected with goniometers. Two spontaneous coordination modes emerged. For small oscillation amplitudes, an in-phase mode (closer to 20° of relative phase) was observed, with hips and ankles oscillating in the same direction. For the largest amplitudes, the anti-phase mode (180°) occurred.

These results constitute empirical evidence that the theory of the "inverted pendulum" for small perturbations is incorrect. They also concord with the results in bimanual coordination studies (Kelso, 1988) and can be interpreted as the emergence of patterns due to specific constraints. Two modes of postural coordination emerge in these conditions. However, in hip/ankle coupling, the in-phase relationship is not established at 0° but at around 20°, and in contrast to oscillators in bimanual coordination, the hip/ankle system is not symmetric: the differences in the mass and length of the body segments result in lower stability and precision in the coupling (Kelso and Jeka, 1992; Baldissera, Cavallari, Marini and Tassone, 1991). Fourcade, Bardy and Bonnet (2003) interpreted this finding by pointing out that, in contrast to what happens in bimanual coordination, leg and trunk movements have mechanically reciprocal influences in the service of balance maintenance.

In addition to the two types of relative phase, Bardy, Marin, Stoffregen and Bootsma (1999) and Marin et al. (1999) sought to show that hip/ankle coordination emerges not from stimulation but from an interaction between types of constraints, as suggested by Newell (1986) for motor behavior in general and Riccio and Stoffregen (1990) for posture in particular. In the same type of protocol with two factors—that is, mass added at either the neck or knees and four amplitudes of visual target movement—Bardy, Marin, Stoffregen and Bootsma (1999) showed that only two patterns (phase and anti-phase) emerged and that the mode depended on the interaction of the two imposed constraints. The same conclusions were drawn by these authors when they varied the length of the support surface and by Marin et al. (1999) when they varied the characteristics of the support surface (on rollers or a more or less soft surface). In all cases, when the conditions for maintaining posture became more precarious, coordination shifted from in-phase to anti-phase. The results were the same when the target movement frequency was manipulated. Moreover, with the same protocol, Oullier, Bardy, Stoffregen and Bootsma (2002) showed similar results when subjects used the head to track target movement and when they simply watched it oscillate, although hip/ankle coupling was weaker and the joint movement amplitude was smaller in the second condition. Postural regulation can be seen as a complex system with coordination modes emerging from interactions between organismic, environmental and task constraints, with the last raising the issue of intention. Intentionality is important to consider because it concerns a voluntary act (and learning), whereas the "(bio)mechanization" of the dynamical approach to both motor behavior and motor and postural control is a frequent criticism from of the perspective of complexity theory in psychology. Several studies (Faugloire, Bardy and Stoffregen, 2006;

Faugloire, Bardy, Merhi and Stoffregen, 2005; Faugloire, Bardy and Stoffregen, 2009) have shown that intention was an aid in producing different types of coordination, with the help of feedback or not. Learning new patterns (135°) was not greatly affected by the stability of the initial patterns observed in pretests but, on the other hand, these last were influenced over the long term by the learning of "non-spontaneous" coordination modes (Faugloire, Bardy and Stoffregen, 2006). Learning new patterns improved general performance, as reflected by greater homogeneity in the production of a range of patterns (Faugloire, Bardy and Stoffregen, 2009). However, it should be noted that when subjects were asked to adopt different types of hip/ankle coordination, anti-phase appeared spontaneously in contrast to in-phase (Faugloire, Bardy, Merhi and Stoffregen, 2005). In this study, the instructions concerned coordination and not a task (visually tracking a target in most of the above-cited studies), and the authors concluded that the instructions (and thus the intention) strongly influenced the postural behavior. In addition, the interaction between intention and the control parameter led to greater change in the stability of postural organization, which is known to be greater for high and low values of the control parameter and lower for mid-range values (Bardy, Marin, Stoffregen and Bootsma, 1999; Marin et al., 1999). An initial conclusion that can be drawn from these empirical studies is that postural coordination displays a certain number of elements that characterize dynamical systems: multi-stability (relative phase around 180° and 20°) and instability for midrange values of the control parameter (although at this stage nothing shows that this instability precedes a transition). However, to be a true dynamical system, postural coordination should also display three other signatures: transitions, hysteresis and modification of relaxation time.

Bardy, Oullier, Bootsma and Stoffregen (2002) thus increased and decreased the oscillation frequency of a visually tracked target. The analyses of hip/ankle relative phase and the estimated point method (Zanone and Kelso, 1992) revealed two stable states, two attractors, and sudden shifting from in-phase to anti-phase (or the converse when frequency was decreased). Moreover, a detailed study of transition frequencies and the behavior of the order parameter surrounding the frequencies showed hysteresis and critical fluctuations. In a second experiment, they perturbed the system by imposing a sudden 180° change in direction of the anterior-posterior target displacement. In line with their hypothesis, the relaxation time (time needed to return to stable state) increased with the approach of frequencies corresponding to phase transitions, and stability was greater in in-phase compared with the anti-phase pattern. Postural coordination thus displays the characteristics expected of a dynamical system and can be considered as such. However, the processes underlying the emergence of postural coordination remain largely unknown. In great part, this is because, as noted above, it is impossible to return from final global behavior to initial conditions in a complex system, but several possible explanations have been advanced (Oullier et al., 2006; Bardy, Oullier, Bootsma and Stoffregen, 2002). Transitions can be explained by mechanical limitations at different levels of the postural system. For example, limitations in the joints (Yang, Winter and Wells, 1990), maximal sway frequencies (Buchanan and Horak, 1999), or sway amplitudes (Riccio and Stoffregen, 1990) would provide ample explanation for the need to shift from one pattern to the other.

This explanation alone is nevertheless not sufficient. According to Bardy, Marin, Stoffregen and Bootsma (1999), a single coordination mode can be used in several biomechanical conditions and several different modes can be used for a single condition. Moreover, if we resituate the debate in terms of models, it seems difficult to explain transitions in a dynamical model on the basis of classical Newtonian mechanics (Beek, Peper and Stegeman, 1995). Another explanation of postural behavior is energy cost. Hoyt and Taylor (1981) studied gait patterns in horses and showed that the natural gait pattern always corresponded to the lowest energy cost, whatever the speed. This principle can thus reasonably be applied to postural transitions: when a pattern becomes inefficient, the system changes to another and, as suggested by Corna et al. (1999), this will be the least costly pattern to maintain balance in a given set of conditions. This explanation alone, however, is not sufficient either, for at least three reasons. First, if we assume that posture is usually not an end in itself but instead serves to facilitate a suprapostural task (Stoffregen, Smart, Bardy and Pagulayan, 1999), then the individual's problem is to find the best compromise between task success and energy cost (Sparrow and Newell, 1998) rather than to focus on efficiency only (Riccio and Stoffregen, 1990). Second, Diedrich and Warren (1995) showed a strong association between energy cost and transition from one coordination mode to another in walking, but they also showed that, as the transition approached, there was not necessarily a correspondence between the two. The third reason can be drawn from daily experience. Everyone has at some point "held back" the transition from walking to running or has observed this principle in athletic walkers. This example is certainly debatable, especially as this is a question of "spontaneous posture", but it at least shows that energy cost, although a factor in transition, is not alone to determine it. This type of explanation concerns changes in the available information. Indeed, postural organization can be modified by manipulating the available information (Allum et al., 1998; Horak, 2006) and optical stimulation induces oscillations in the direction of the stimulus (Megrot, Bardy and Dietrich, 2002). However, the inverse argument—that is, that transitions occur without modifications in information—also leads to the rejection of a determinant role of information in transitions. The observation that no single reason is sufficient to explain postural behavior and its determinants is in fact another indication that postural regulation should be understood as a complex system. From this perspective, Newell's suggestion (1986) that postural coordination emerges from the interactions between constraints (Riccio and Stoffregen, 1990) seems justified. According to complex systems theories in general, it is futile to attempt to understand a phenomenon from each of its parts or the relationships between the parts. Although not exempt from criticism and limitations, the theory of perception/action coupling and dynamical modeling as a means to understand postural control provides an alternative to the cognitive viewpoint that is convincing and empirically documented.

## TWO IRRECONCILABLE APPROACHES

Each of these two approaches seem convincing but each has limitations both as general theories and as applied to postural control. The limitations are not exactly the same, however, but depend on the paradigm. The limitations of cognitivist theory mainly concern the contradiction between what the theory assumes and the observed results, which of course calls the theory itself into question (Stoffregen and Riccio, 1988, Riccio and Stoffregen, 1990, Bardy et al., 2002). And if cognitive theory has to abandon its fundamental assumptions, like prescription or strategies (Nashner and Mc Collum, 1986), in order to fit empirical fact, then it will not only lose its meaning but it will be discarded. This has nevertheless not stopped the accumulation of data in a theoretical framework which, although called into question, has long been considered to be the most convincing. Conversely, criticisms of the complex approach concern particularly the absence of response to certain key questions or the conceptual and technical incapacity to even address them. Everyday discrete and meaningful movements, implicit learning, and some aspects of development are examples of issues on which complexity research is silent, but entire fields seem to be ignored, as well, like neuropsychology. In contrast to cognitive theory, complexity theory offers a high level and precision of explanation but with few concrete applications that go beyond generalities. One example is the link between cortical activity and movement. Although studies in this field have been published (e.g., Kelso, 1998), they remain quite exploratory and we are far from the day when brain surgery will be performed for patients with Parkinson's disease (Guridi et al., 2000). Certainly, this is a neurological issue but the underlying model is cognitivist (information computation), reflected by the executive function tests that evaluate the effects of these operations (Jahanshahi et al., 2000). Yet despite the gaps in complexity theory, there is no proof, to our knowledge, that these questions cannot be dealt with in the future and no indication in the data to date that the theoretical hypothesis is invalid.

Overall, the cognitivist framework is well-regarded in the research community (and not only among postural control researchers). Many remain attached to the paradigm in which they were trained, the number of disciplines that use its models is impressive (robotics, artificial intelligence, neurosciences, medicine, etc.), and it has yielded a certain number of undeniable technical results. But it has also benefited from a certain inertia in the growth of knowledge and, despite all its strengths, it continues to be challenged (Varela, 1993). The complexity alternative theory, which was originally developed and supported in disciplines like psychology and the neurosciences, has avoided the internal contradictions of cognitive theory. It is incomplete, of course, and requires much more experimental validation, but it offers perspectives that, in so far as they have not been disproved, are quite convincing.

Today we have two rich but contradictory paradigms for the study of motor behavior in general and posture in particular. The question now is how to articulate them. The first solution would be to disregard the boundaries of each framework and to use both freely to answer pragmatic questions about posture. In this case, the research question would dictate the choice of framework. This would work for technical activity but not for epistemic activity. Only two other possibilities can be suggested. The first would be to reconcile the two paradigms by creating a hybrid model and the second would be to continue to debate and point out contradictions in the other until one of them emerges as the dominant model or a completely new one emerges. The path of reconciliation is based on the attractive argument that the two paradigms deal with the same process but at different levels. In this case, the dynamical approach would explain automatic activities in which neither (or very little) planning nor cognitive control is necessary. The cognitivist approach thus would explain intentional action and cognitive processes could possibly be found to supervise underlying dynamical processes. Abernethy and Sparrow (1992) noted a certain number of experimental findings that seem to corroborate this, like the cortical supervision of subcortical control of automatic walking. They even suggested that in this type of hybrid model, the cerebellum would be of major importance because of its anatomic position and functional roles. They further pointed out that this idea of hybrid model is not new. Schmidt (2003) suggested revising the schema theory (yet without specifying that he was integrating dynamical concepts) to create a model that would include a maximum of empirical data and that would not be contradicted by any of them. Attempts at hybridization are also seen in the proposals to "mix" affordances and representations, as was done by Norman (1999), or to add calibration processes to the visual guidance of action, as proposed by Gibson and his successors (Fajen, 2005). However, Abernethy and Sparrow (1992) did not seem convinced by their own arguments and instead suggested that a paradigmatic crisis was underway. This seems almost unavoidable given that the two paradigms are in competition for the greatest recognition and that certain contradictions cannot be resolved. Take, for example, the role of representation, as just mentioned. As Newell noted, the arguments against the metaphor of symbolic computation are not necessarily directed against memory or representations of action, but instead question a particular form of representation, the symbolic motor representation (Newell, 2003). This representation, from which action will be prescribed, is the basis for the cognitive model of motor behavior or posture. It thus appears that we are in a period in which, to use Newell's expression (2003), "the two paradigms have agreed to disagree" (p. 385) and we will remain there at least for the time being. The end of the crisis will be followed by a period of normal science in which the two paradigms cohabit. Although this description from Newell may very well be accurate, it does not mean that the "two camps" will stop claiming to be right. But without doubt, greater depth in the research and the limitations that each school brings to light concerning the other will force the scientific community at a given moment to choose between them, although this is not exactly the description of "normal science" given by Kuhn.

To conclude, as long as these two paradigms remain side by side, with the scientific community unable to unify around a single one, researchers on the determinants of postural behavior will first need to specify the ontological framework for their studies. As contributors to a broader theoretical perspective, they will in this way bring elements of meaning, which is after all the main objective of scientific work. A formal statement of ontology might sometimes seem unnecessary, as in some publications this will be evident. Moreover, some might think that readers should be responsible for discerning the theoretical position. This crisis in paradigms forces researchers to make a choice because studying posture cannot be separated from a more global understanding of motor behavior as a single entity. Researchers thus cannot consider the issue of paradigms as secondary without running the risk of developing research programs compromised by internal contradictions. However, it is clear in postural research that the two approaches have striking limitations. And since the proponents of neither can claim to present the "truth", the choice of paradigm will be based on both scientific argument and subjective factors.

However, the attempt to reconcile these two theoretical perspectives is at an impasse today. Therefore, future research on motor behavior or posture, especially for those directing research, requires a choice between two solutions. The first is to choose one paradigm or the other based on the study objective, the situation, the collaborative set-up, or other considerations. In this case, it is sufficient to remain within the strict framework chosen, given the known limitations of each perspective. However, this solution raises at least two problems. The first is that it is difficult (though not impossible) to ensure the coherence of a corpus of research that shifts between two paradigms. But the second problem, which is more important if we consider that doing research is above all about contributing meaning, concerns the researcher's conviction as to the interest of the paradigm that has been chosen. It is possible to do research using a paradigm without particular conviction, simply by saying that this is a necessary step, that the studies will each in their measure contribute to pushing back the limitations to the theory or, conversely, to establish them just a little bit more. As already demonstrated, the research questions raised within the two paradigms are not the same, nor are the methods. It is thus likely that studies will be developed in fields for which the theoretical coherence of a paradigm is at odds with the facts. If this is done with full awareness, it can be a form of distancing from positivism, which tends to underlie the cognitive sciences. Another solution would be to take an ontological stand. As seen in the introduction, this is based on beliefs or a gamble about the "nature of things." In the narrow field of motor behavior study, this would mean clearly stating one's beliefs from the outset or betting on either the cognitivist or the complexity hypothesis being correct. A bet is by nature irrational and implies great subjectivity. However, scientific arguments contribute to the choice.

## ACKNOWLEDGMENTS

Preparation of this article was supported by the project "RISC" with High-Normandy Regional grant from GRR TLTI and with European (FEDER) grant.

## REFERENCES

Abernethy, B. and Sparrow, W.A. (1992). The rise and fall of dominant paradigms in motor behavior research. In J. J. Summers (Ed.), *Appraches to the study of motor control and learning*. : Elsevier. pp. 3-45.

Allum, J. H., Bloem, B. R., Carpenter, M. G., Hulliger, M. and Hadders-Algra, M. (1998). Proprioceptive control of posture: a review of new concepts. *Gait and Posture, 8 (3)*, pp. 214-242.

Amblard, B. (1998). Les descripteurs du contrôle postural. Annales de réadaptation et de médecine physique, 41, pp. 225-237.

Amblard, B. and Cremieux, J. (1976). Role of visual information concerning movement in the maintenance of postural equilibrium in man. *Agressologie: Revue Internationale de PhysioBiologie et de Pharmacologie Appliquees Aux Effets De L'agression, 17*, pp. 25-36.

Aruin, A. S. and Latash, M.L. (1995). Directional specificity of postural muscles in feed forward postural reactions during fast voluntary arm movments. *Experimental Brain Research, 106 (2)*, pp. 291-300.

Aruin, A. S., Forest, W. R. and Latash, L. (1998). Anticipatory postural adjustments in conditions of postural instability. *Electroencephalography and Clinical Neurophysiology, 109 (4)*, pp. 350-359.

Association Française de Posturologie, (1985). Normes 85 : Association Posture et Equilibre.

Balasubramaniam, R., Riley, M. A. and Turvey, M.T. (2000). Specificity of postural sway to the demands of a precision task. *Gait and Posture, 11 (1)*, pp. 12-24.

Baldissera, F., Cavallari, P., Marini, G. and Tassone, G. (1991). Differential control of in-phase and anti-phase coupling of rhythmic movements of ipsilateral hand and foot. *Experimental Brain Research, 83*, pp. 375-380.

Bardy, B. G., lagarde, J., Oullier, O. and Stoffregen, T.A. (2007). On perturbation and pattern coexistence in postural coordination dynamics. *Journal of Motor Behavior, 28 (1)*, pp. 326-334.

Bardy, B. G., Marin, L., Stoffregen, T. A. and Bootsma, R.J. (1999). Postural coordination modes considered as emergent phenomena.. *Journal of Experimental Psychology: Human Perception and Performance, 25*, pp. 1284-1301.

Bardy, B. G., Oullier, O., Bootsma, R. J. and Stoffregen, T.A. (2002). Dynamics of human postural transitions. *Journal of Experimental Psychology. Human Perception and Performance, 28 (3)*, pp. 499-514.

Bardy, B. G., Warren, W. H. and Kay, B.A. (1996). Motion parallax is used to control postural sway during walking. *Experimental Brain Research, 111*, pp. 271-282.

Baumberger, B., Isableu, B. and FlUckinger, M. (2004). The visual control of stability in children and adults: Postural readjustments in ground optical flow. *Experimental Brain Research, 159*, pp. 33-46.

Beek, P. J., Peper, C. E. and Stegeman, D.F. (1995). Dynamical models of movement coordination. *Human Movement Science, 14*, pp. 573-608.

Bernstein, N. A. (1967). The co-ordiantion and regulation of movements. : Pergamon Press.

Bernstein, N. A. (1996). On dexterity and its development. In M. Latash and M. Turvey (Eds.), *On dexterity and its development*.: Lawrence Elbraum Associates. pp. 9-236.

Berthoz, A. (1974). Occulomotricité et proprioception. *Revue d'Electroencéphalographie et de Neurophysiologie Clinique de Langue Française, 4*, pp. 569-586.

Berthoz, A. (1997). Le sens du mouvement. : Odile Jacob.

Bouisset, S. and Zattara, M. (1981). A sequence of postural movements precedes volontary movement. *Neuroscience Letters, 22*, pp. 263-270.

Bouisset, S. and Zattara, M. (1987). Biomechanical study of the programming of anticipatory postural adjustments associated with voluntary movement. *Journal of Biomechanics, 20*, pp. 735-742.

Brandt, T., Dieterich, M. and Danek, A. (1994). Vestibular cortex lesions affect the perception of verticality. *Annals of Neurology, 35 (4)*, pp. 383-384.

Buchanan, J. J. and Horak, F.B. (1999). Emergence of postural patterns as a function of vision and translation frequency. *Journal of Neurophysiology, 81*, pp. 2325-2339.

Bullinger, A. (2004). Le développement sensori-moteur de l'enfant et ses avatars. Eres.

Chiang, J. and Wu, G. (1997). The influence of foam surfaces on biomechanical variables contributing to postural control. Gait and Posture, *5 (3)*, pp. 239-245.

Clapp, S. and Wing, A.M. (1999). Light touch contribution to balance in normal bipedal stance. *Experimental Brain Research, 125 (4)*, pp. 521-524.

Clark, S. and Riley, M.A. (2006). Multisensory information for postural control: Sway-referencing gain shapes center of pressure variability and temporal dynamics. *Experimental Brain Research, 176 (2)*, pp. 299-310.

Clement, G., Gurfinkel, V. S., Lestienne, F., Lipshits, M. I. and Popov, K.E. (1984). Adaptation of postural control to weightlessness. *Experimental Brain Research, 57*, pp. 61-72.

Collins, J. J. and De Luca, C.J. (1993). Open-loop and closed-loop control of posture: a random-walk analysis of center of pressure trajectories. *Experimental Brain Research, 95 (2)*, pp. 308-318.

Collins, J. J. and De Luca, C.J. (1995). The effects of of visual input on open loop and closed loop postural control mechanisms. *Experimental Brain Research, 103 (1)*, pp. 151-163.

Cordo, P., Gurfinkel, V. S., Bevan, L. and Kerr, G.K. (1995). Prprioceptive consequences of tendon vibration during movement. *Journal of Neurophysiology, 74 (4)*, pp. 1675-1688.

Corna, S., Tarantola, J., Nardone, A., Giordano, A. and Schieppati, M. (1999). Standing on a continuously moving platform: is body inertia counteracted or exploited? Experimental Brain *Research, 124*, p. 331–341.

Creath, R., Kiemel, T., Horak, F., Peterka, R. and Jeka, J. (2005). A unified view of quiet and perturbed stance: simultaneous co-existing excitable modes. *Neuroscience Letters, 377*, pp. 75-80.

Danis, C. G., Krebs, D. E., Gill-Body, K. M. and Sahrman, S. (1998). Relationship between standing posture and stability. *Physical Therapy, 78 (5)*, pp. 502-517.

Dickstein, R., Shupert, C. and Horak, F.B. (2001). Fingertip touch improves postural stabilityn in patients with peripheral neuropathy. *Gait and Posture, 14 (3)*, pp. 238-247.

Diedrich, F. J. and Warren, W.H. (1995). Why Change Gaits? Dynamics of the Walk-Run Transition. *Journal of Experimental Psychology: Human Perception and Performance, 21 (1)*, pp. 183-202.

Dietz, V. (1992). Human neuronal control of automatic functional movements: interaction between central programs and afferent input. *Physiological review, 72 (1)*, pp. 33-69.

Dupuy, J. P. (1994). Aux origines des sciences cognitives. La Découverte.

Eklund, G. (1972). General features of of vibration induced effects on balance. *Upsala Journal of Medical Sciences, 77 (2)*, pp. 112-124.

Fajen, B. R. (2005). Perceiving possibilities for action: On the necessity of calibration and perceptual learning for the visual guidance of action. *Perception, 34*, pp. 717-740.

Faugloire, E., Bardy, B. G. and Stoffregen, T.A. (2006). Dynamics of learning new postural patterns: influence on preexisting spontaneous behaviors. *Journal of Motor Behavior, 38 (4)*, pp. 299-312.

Faugloire, E., Bardy, B. G., Merhi, O. and Stoffregen, T.A. (2005). Exploring coordination dynamics of the postural system with real-time visual feedback. *Neuroscience Letters, 374*, pp. 136-141.

Faugloire, E., Bardy, E. and Stoffregen, T.A. (2009). (De)Stabilization of required and spontaneous postural dynamics with learning. *Journal of Experimental Psychology: Human Perception and Performance, 35 (1)*, pp. 170-187.

Fitzpatrick, R. and McCloskey, D.I. (1994). Proprioceptive, visual and vestibular thresholds for perception of sway during standing in humans. *Journal of Physiology, 478*, pp. 173-186.

Forget, R. and Lamarre, Y. (1990). Anticipatory postural adjustments in the absence of normal peripheral feedback. *Brain Research, 508 (1)*, pp. 176-179.

Fourcade, P., Bardy, B. G. and Bonnet, C. (2003). Modeling postural transitions in human posture. In S. Rogers and J. Effken (Eds.), *Studies in perception and action Studies in perception and action VII.* : Lawrence Erlbaum. pp. 99-103.

Fujisawa, N., Masuda, T., Inakoa, Y., Fukuoka, H., Ishida, A. and Minamitani, H. (2005). Human standing control depending on adopted startegies. *Medical and Biological engineering and computing, 43 (1)*, pp. 107-114.

Gandevia, S. C., Refshauge, K. M. and Collins, D.F. (2002). Proprioception: peripheral inputs and perceptual interactions. *Advances in Experimental Medicine and Biology, 508*, pp. 61-68.

Gatev, P., Thomas, S., Thomas, K. and Hallett, M. (1999). Feedforward ankle strategy of balance during quiet stance in adults. *Journal of Physiology, 514 (3)*, pp. 915-928.

Gentaz, E., Baud-Bovy, G. and Luyat, M. (2008). The haptic perception of spatial orientations. *Experimental Brain Research, 187 (3)*, pp. 331-348.

Geruschat, D. and Turano, K.A. (2002). Connecting research on retinis pigmentosa to the paractice of orientation and mobility. *Journal of visual impairment and Blindness*, 96, pp. 69-85.

Gibson, J. J. (1958). Visually Controlled Locomotion and visual orientation in animals. *British Journal of Psychology*, 49, pp. 182-194.

Gibson, J. J. (1979). The ecological approach to visual perception. Lawrence Erlbaum Publisher.

Gollhofer, A., Horstmann, G. A., Berger, W. and Dietz, V. (1989). Compensation of translational and rotational perturbations in human posture: stabilization of the center of gravity. *Neuroscience Letters*, 105, pp. 73-78.

Gurfinkel, V. S. and Elner, A.M. (1973). On two types of static disturbances in patients with local lesions of the brain. *Agressologie: Revue Internationale de Physio-Biologie et de Pharmacologie Appliquees Aux Effets De L'agression*, 14D, pp. 65-72.

Gurfinkel, V. S. and Levik, Y. (1991). Perceptual and automatic aspects of the postural body Scheme. In J. Paillard (Ed.), *Brain and Space*. : Oxford University Press. pp. 145-182.

Gurfinkel, V. S., Lestienne, F., Levik, Y. S., Popov, K. E. and Lefort, L. (1993). Egocentric references and human spatial orientation in microgravity, II. Body centred coordiantes in the task of drawing ellipses with prescribed orientation. *Experimental Brain Research , 95 (2)*, pp. 343-348.

Guridi, J., Rodriguez-Oroz, M. C., Lozano, A. M., Moro, E., Albanese, A., Nuttin, B., Gybels, J.et al. (2000). Targeting the basal ganglia for deep brain stimulation in Parkinson's disease. *Neurology*, 55, p. S21-8.

Hafström, A., Fransson, P. A., Karlberg, M., Ledin, M. and Magnusson, M. (2001). Readiness to receive visual information affects postural control and adaptation. In J. Duysens, C. M. Bouwien, B. Smit-Engelsman and H. Kingma (Eds.), *Control of posture and gait*. : International Society of Posture and Gait Research. pp. 285-289.

Haken, H. (1985). Synergetics : an interdisciplinary approach to phenomena of self organization. *Geoforum; Journal of Physical, Human, and Regional Geosciences, 16 (2)*, pp. 205-211.

Haken, H., Kelso, J. S. and Bunz, H. (1985). A Theoretical Model of Phase Transitions in Human Hand Movements. *Biological Cybernetics*, 51, pp. 347-356.

Hkavacka, F., Krizkova, M. and Horak, F.B. (1995). Modification of human postural response to leg muscle vibration by electrical vestibular stimulation. *Neuroscience Letters, 189 (1)*, pp. 9-12.

Hlavacka, F., Mergner, T. and Krizkova, M. (1996). Control of body vertical by vestibular and propiroceptive inputs. *Brain Research Bulletin, 40 (5-6)*, pp. 431-434.

Holden, M., Ventura, J. and Lackner, J. (1994). Stabilization of posture by precision contact of the index finger . *Journal of vestibular research, 4 (4)*, pp. 285-301.

Horak, F. B. (2006). Postural orientation and equilibrium: what do we need to know about neural control of balance to prevent falls? *Age and Ageing, 35-S2*, p. iI7-ii11.

Horak, F. B. and Nashner, L.M. (1986). Central programming of postural movements: adaptation to altered support-surface configurations. *Journal of Neurophysiology, 55 (6)*, pp. 1369-1381.

Horak, F. B., Nashner, L. M. and Diener, H.C. (1990). Postural strategies associated with somatosensory and vestibular loss. *Experimental Brain Research, 82*, pp. 167-177.

Howard, I. P. and Templeton, W.B. (1966). Human spatial orientation. John Wiley.

Hoyt, D. F. and Taylor, C.R. (1981). Gait and energetics of locomotion in horses. *Nature, 292*, pp. 239-240.

Isableu, B. and Vuillerme, N. (2006). Differential integration of kinaesthetic signals to postural control. *Experimental Brain Research, 174*, pp. 763-768.

Ivanenko, Y. P., Grasso, R. and Lacquaniti, F. (1999). Effect of gaze on postural responses to neck proprioceptive and vestibular stimulation in humans. *Journal of Physiology, 519*, pp. 301-314.

Jeka, J. J. and Lackner, J.R. (1995). The role of haptic cues from rough and slippery surfaces in human postural control. *Experimental Brain Research, 103 (2)*, pp. 267-276.

Karnath, H. O., Ferber, S. and Dichgans, J. (2000). The neural representation of postural control in humans. *The Proceedings of the National Academy of Sciences (US), 97 (25)*, pp. 13931-13936.

Kavounoudias, A., Gilhodes, J. C., Roll, R. and Roll, J. (1999). From balance regulation to body orientation: two goals for muscle proprioceptive information processing? . Experimental Brain *Research, 124 (1)*, pp. 80-88.

Kelso, J. S. and Jeka, J.J. (1992). Symmetry breaking dynamics of human multilimb coordination. *Journal of Experimental Psychology: Human Perception and Performance, 18*, pp. 645-668.

Kelso, J. S. and Schoner, G. (1988). Self-organiszation of coordinative movement patterns. *Human Movement Science, 7*, pp. 27-46.

Kelso, J. S., Fuchs, A., Lancaster, R., Holroyd, T., Cheyne, D. and Weinberg, H. (1998). Dynamical cortical activity in the humain reveals motor equivalence. *Nature, 392*, pp. 814-818.

Kerr, B., Condon, S. and McDonald, L.A. (1985). Cognitive spatial processing and the regulation of posture. *Journal of Experimental Psychology, 11*, pp. 617-622.

Kuhn, T. (1962). The Structure of Scientific Revolutions. University of Chicago Press.

Kuo, A. D. (1995). An optimal control model for analyzing human postural balance. *IEEE Transactions on Bio-Medical Engineering, 42 (1)*, pp. 87-101.

Kuo, A. D. and Zajak, E. (1993). Human standing posture: multi-joint movement strategies based on biomechanical constrainsts. In J. H. J. Allum, D. J. Allum-Mecklenburg, F. P. Harris and R. Probst (Eds.), *Progress in Brain Research 97*. Elsevier. pp. 349-358.

Lackner, J. R., DiZio, P., Jeka, J., Horak, F., Krebs, D. and Rabin, E. (1999). Precision contact of the fingertip reduces postural sway of individuals with bilateral vestibular loss. *Experimental Brain Research, 126 (4)*, pp. 459-466.

Lackner, J. R., Rabin, E. and DiZio, P. (2001). Stabilization of posture by precision touch of the index finger xith rigid and flexible filaments. *Experimental Brain Research, 139 (4)*, pp. 454-464.

Lacquaniti, F. (1992). Automatic control of limb movement and posture. Current Opinion in *Neurobiology, 2 (6)*, pp. 807-814.

Lafosse, C., Kerckhofs, E., Troch, M., Vereeck, L., Van Hoydonck, G., Moeremans, M., Broeckx, J.et al. (2005). Contraversive pushing and inattention of the contralesional hemispace. *Journal of Clinical and Experimental Neuropsychology: Official Journal of the International Neuropsychological Society, 27*, pp. 460-484.

Lajoie, Y., Teasdale, N., Bard, C. and Fleury, M. (1993). Attentional demands for static and dynamic equilibrium. *Experimental Brain Research*, *97*, pp. 139-144.

Lee, D. N. and Lishman, J.R. (1975). Visual proprioceptive control of stance. *Journal of Human Movement Studies*, 1, pp. 87-95.

Lestienne, F. G. and Gurfinkel, V.S. (1988). Postural control in weightlessness: a dual process underlying adaptation to an unusual environment. *Trends in Neurosciences*, *11*, pp. 359-363.

Marin, L., Bardy, B. G., Baumberger, B., Fluckiger, M. and Stoffregen, T.A. (1999). Interaction between task demands and surface properties in the control of goal-oriented stance. *Human Movement Science*, *18*, pp. 31-47.

Martinez, F. (1977). Les informations auditives permettent-elles d'établir des rapports spatiaux ? Données expérimentales et cliniques chez l'aveugle congénital. *l'Année Psychologique*, *77*, pp. 179- 204.

Massion, J. (1984). Postural changes accompanying voluntary movements. Normal and pathological aspects. *Human Neurobiology*, *2*, pp. 261-267.

Massion, J. (1992). Movment, Posture, and equilibrium: interaction and coordination. *Progress in Neurobiology*, *38 (1)*, pp. 35-56.

Massion, J. (1994). Postural control system. *Current Opinion in Neurobiology*, *4 (6)*, pp. 877-887. Massion, J. (1997). Cerveau et motricité. Presses Universitaires de France.

Massion, J., Amblard, B., Assaiente, C., Mouchnino, L. and Vernazza, S. (1998). Body orientation and control of coordinated movements in microgravity. *Brain Research Review*, *28 (1-2)*, pp. 83-91.

Massion, J., Gurfinkel, V., Lipshits, M., Obadia, A. and Popov, K. (1992). Strategy and synergy: two levels of equilibrium control during movement. Effects of the microgravity. Comptes Rendus de *L'academie des Sciences. Serie III, Sciences de la Vie*, *314*, pp. 87-92.

Massion, J., Popov, K., Fabre, J. C., Rage, P. and Gurfinkel, V. (1995). Body orientation and center of mass control in microgravity. *Acta Astraunotica*, *36 (8-12)*, pp. 763-769.

Mazoyer, B. (2002). L'imagerie cérébrale foctionnelle : apports, limites et perspectives. In O. Houdé, B. Mazoyer and N. Tzourio-Mazoyer (Eds.), *Cerveau et psychologie.* : Presses Universitaires de France. pp. 605-609.

McCloskey, D. I. (1978). Kinesthetic sensibility. *Physiological Review*, *58 (4)*, pp. 763-820.

McCollum, G. and Leen, T.K. (1989). Form and exploration of mechanical stability limits in erect stance. *Journal of Motor Behavior*, *21*, pp. 225-244.

Megrot, F., Bardy, B. G. and Dietrich, G. (2002). Dimensionality and the dynamics of human unstable equilibrium. *Journal of Motor Behavior*, *34*, pp. 323-328.

Mergner, T. and Rosemeier, T. (1998). Interaction of vestibular, somatosensory and visual signals for postural control and motion perception under terrestrial and microgravity conditions: a conceptual model. *Brain Research Review*, *28 (1-2)*, pp. 118-135.

Mergner, T., Huber, W. and Becker, W. (1997). Vestibular-neck interaction and transformation of sensory coordinates. *Journal of vestibular research*, 7 (4), pp. 347-367.

Meyer, P. F., Oddson, L. I. and De Luca, C.J. (2004). The role of plantar cutaneous sensation in unperturbed stance. *Experimental Brain research,* 156 (4), pp. 505-512.

Michaels, C. (1998). The ecological/dynamical approach, manifest destiny and a single movement science. In A. A. Post, J. R. Pijpers, P. Bosh and M. S. J. Boschker (Eds.). Print Parners Ipskamp. pp. 65-68.

Minvielle, G. and Audiffren, M. (2000). Study of anticipatory postural adjustments in an air pistol-shooting task. *Perceptual and Motor Skills*, *91*, pp. 1151-1168.
Mittelstaedt, H. (1983). A new solution to the problem of the subjective vertical. D*ie Naturwissenschaften*, *70*, pp. 272-281.
Nashner, L. and Berthoz, A. (1978). Visual contribution to rapid motor responses during postural control. *Brain Research*, *150 (2)*, pp. 403-407.
Nashner, L. and McCollum, G. (1985). The organization of human postural movements: a formal basis and experimental synthesis. *Behavioral and Brain Sciences*, *8*, pp. 135-172.
Nashner, L. M., Shupert, C. L., Horak, F. B. and Black, F.O. (1989). Organization of posture controls: An analysis of sensory and mechanical constraints. *Progress in Brain Research*, 80, pp. 395-418.
Newell, K. M. (1986). Constrainst on the development of coordination. In M. G. Wade and Whiting H T (Eds.), *Motor development in children: aspects of coordination and control*. Martinus Nijhoff. pp. 341-371.
Newell, K., Liu, Y. T. and Mayer-Kress, G. (2003). A dynamical systems interpretation of epigenetic landscapes for infant motor development. *Infant Behavior and Development*, *26 (4)*, pp. 449-472.
Njiokiktjien, C. J. and Van Parys, J.A. (1976). Romberg's sign expressed in a quotient II. Pathology. Agressologie: *Revue Internationale de Physio-Biologie et de Pharmacologie Appliquees Aux Effets De L'agression*, *17*, pp. 19-23.
Norman, D. A. (1999). Affordances, Conventions and Design. *Interactions*, *I.3*, pp. 38-42.
Oie, K. S., Kiemel, T. and Jeka, J.J. (2001). Human multisensory fusion of vision and touch: detecting non linearity with small changes in the sensory environment. *Neurosciences Letters*, *315 (3)*, pp. 113-116.
Oie, K. S., Kiemel, T. and Jeka, J.J. (2002). Multisensory fusion: simultaneous re-weighting of vision and touch for the control of human posture. *Cognitive Brain Research*, *14 (1)*, pp. 164-176.
Okubo, J., Watanabe, I. and Baron, J.B. (1980). Study on influences of the plantar mechanoreceptor on body sway. *Agressologie: Revue Internationale de Physio-Biologie et de Pharmacologie Appliquees Aux Effets De L'agression*, *21*, pp. 61-69.
Oullier, O., Bardy, B. G., Stoffregen, T. A. and Bootsma, R. (2002). Postural coordination in looking and tracking tasks. *Human Movement Science*, *21*, pp. 147-167.
Oullier, O., Marin, L., Stoffregen, T., Bootsma, R. J. and Bardy, B.G. (2006). Variability in coordination postural dynamics. In K. Davids, S. J. Bennett and K. M. Newell (Eds.), *Movement system variability*. : Champaign: Human kinetics publishers. pp. 25-47.
Paillard, J. (1971). Les déterminants moteurs de l'organisation de l'espace. *Cahiers de psychologie*, *14 (4)*, pp. 261-316.
Paillard, J. (1976). Tonus, posture et mouvement. In C. Kayser (Ed.), *Physiologie,* 3ème édition. : Flammarion. .
Paillard, J. (1986a). Le corps et ses langages d'espace. In J. Paillard (Ed.), *Pour une psychophysiologie de l'action*. Actio. pp. 153-168.
Paillard, J. (1986b). Les attitudes dans la motricité. In J. Paillard (Ed.), *Pour une psychophysiologie de l'action*. Actio. pp. 11-29.
Paillard, J. (1986c). L'acte moteur. In J. Paillard (Ed.), *Pour une psychophysiologie de l'action*. Actio. pp. 81-98.

Paulignan, Y., Dufosse, M., Hugon, M. and MAssion, J. (1989). Acquisition of co-ordiantion between posture and movement in a bimanual task. *Experimental Brain Research, 77 (2)*, pp. 337- 348.

Paulus, W. M., Straube, A. and Brandt, T. (1984). Visual stabilization of posture. Physiological stimulus characteristics and clinical aspects. *Brain : a Journal of Neurology, 107*, pp. 1143-1163.

Penfield, W. and Rasmussen, T. (1950). The cerebral cortex of man. Macmillan, New-York.

Regia Corte, T., Luyat, M. and Darcheville, J. (2004). La perception d'une affordance pour la posture verrticale par les systèmes perceptivo-moteurs visuel et haptique. *L'année psychologique,* 104, pp. 169-202.

Riccio, G. E. and Stoffregen, T.A. (1990). Gravitoinertial force versus the direction of balance in the perception and control of orientation. *Psychological Review, 97*, pp. 135-137.

Riley, M. and Turvey, M.T. (2002). Variability and determinism in motor behavior. *Journal of Motor Behavior, 34 (2)*, pp. 99-125.

Riley, M. A. and Clark, S. (2003). Recurrence analysis of human postural sway during the sensory organization test. *Neuroscience Letters, 342 (1-2)*, pp. 45-48.

Riley, M. A., Balasubramaniam, R. and Turvey, M.T. (1999). Recurrence quantification analysis of postural fluctuations. *Gait and Posture, 9 (1)*, pp. 65-78.

Robertson, Caldwell, Hamill, Karen and Whittlesley (2004). Research methods in biomechanics. *Human kinetics publishers.*

Roll, J. (1994). Sensibilités cutanées et musculaires. In M. Richelle, J. Requin and M. Roberts (Eds.), *Traité de psychologie expérimentale.* : Presses Universitaires de France. pp. 483-542.

Roll, J. P. (2003). Physiologie de la kinestèse. La propriocepton : sixième sens ou sens pemier ? *Intellectica, 36/37*, pp. 49-66.

Roll, J. P. and Vedel, J.P. (1982). Kinaesthetic role of muscle afferent in man, studied by tendon vibration and microneurography. *Experimental Brain Research, 47(2)*, pp. 177-190.

Roll, J. P., Vedel, J. P. and Roll, R. (1989). Eye, head and skeletal muscle spindle feedback in the elaboration of body references. *Progress in Brain Research, 80*, p. 113-23; discussion 57-60.

Roll, J., Roll, R. and Velay, J. (1991). Proprioception as a link between body space and extra-personal space. In J. Paillard (Ed.), *Brain and space.* : Oxford University Press. pp. 113-132.

Rougier, P. (2003). Adaptation of control mechanisms involved in upright undisturbed stance maintenance during prolonged darkness. *Neurophysiologie Clinique, 33 (2)*, pp. 86-93.

Rougier, P. and Farenc, I. (2000). Adaptative effects of loss of vision on upright undisturbed stance. *Brain Research, 871 (2)*, pp. 165-174.

Runge, C. F., Shupert, C. L., Horak, F. B. and Zajac, F.E. (1999). Ankle and hip postural strategies defined by joint torque. *Gait and Posture, 10 (2)*, pp. 161-170.

Sacks, O. (1985). The Man Who Mistook His Wife for a Hat, and Other Clinical Tales. Summit books.

Schmidt, R. A. (1975). A schema theory of discrete motor skill learning. *Psychological Review, 82*, pp. 225-260.

Schmidt, R. A. (1988). Motor control and learning: a behavioral emphasis (2nd ed.). Champaign, Human kinetics.

Schmidt, R. A. (2003). Motor schema theory after 27 years: reflections and implications for a new theory. *Research Quarterly for Exercise and Sport, 74 (4)*, pp. 366-375.

Schmit, J. M., Regis, D. I. and Riley, M.A. (2005). Dynamic patterns of postural sway in ballet dancers and track athletes. *Experimental Brain Research, 163 (3)*, pp. 370-378.

Simoneau, G. G., Ulbrecht, J. S., Derr, J. A. and Cavanagh, P.R. (1995). Role of somatosensory input in the control of human posture. *Gait and Posture, 3*, pp. 115-122.

Smart, J. L. J., Mobley, B. S., Otten, E. W., Smith, D. L. and Amin, M.R. (2004). Not just standing there: The use of postural coordination to aid visual tasks. *Human Movement Science, 22 (6)*, pp. 769-780.

Sparrow, W. H. and Newell, K.M. (1998). Metabolic energy expenditure and the regulation of movement economy. *Psychonomic Bulletin and Review, 5*, pp. 173-196.

Stoffregen, T. and Riccio, G.E. (1988). An Ecological Theory of Orientation and the Vestibular System. *Psychological Review, 95 (1)*, pp. 3-14.

Stoffregen, T. A. (1985). Flow structure versus retinal location in the optical control of stance. *Journal of Experimental Psychology: Human Perception and Performance, 11 (5)*, pp. 554-565.

Stoffregen, T. A. (1986). The role of optical velocity in the control of stance. *Perception and Psychophysics, 39 (5)*, pp. 355-360.

Stoffregen, T. A. and Bardy, B.G. (2001). On specification and the senses. *Behavioral and Brain Sciences, 24 (2)*, pp. 213-261.

Stoffregen, T. A., Adolph, K., Thelen, E., Gorday, K. M. and Sheng, Y.Y. (1997). Toddlers' postural adaptations to different support surfaces. *Motor Control, 1*, pp. 119-137.

Stoffregen, T. A., Chen, F., Yu, Y. and Villard, S. (2009). Stance width and angle at sea: effects of sea state and body orientation. *Aviation, Space, and Environmental Medicine, 80*, pp. 845-849.

Stoffregen, T. A., Pagulayan, R. J., Bardy, B. G. and Hettinger, L.J. (2000). Modulating postural control to facilitate visual performance. *Human Movement Science, 19*, pp. 203-220.

Stoffregen, T. A., Smart, L. J., Bardy, B. G. and Pagulayan, R.J. (1999). Postural stabilisation of looking. *Journal of Experimental Psychology: Human Perception and Performance, 25*, pp. 1641- 1658.

Stoffregen, T. A., Villard, S., Kim, C., Ito, K. and Bardy, B.G. (2009). Coupling of head and body movement with motion of the audible environment. *Journal of Experimental Psychology. Human Perception and Performance, 35*, pp. 1221-1231.

Stoffregen, T., Hove, P., Bardy, B., Riley, M. and Bonnet, C. (2007). Postural stabilization of perceptual but not cognitive performance. *Journal of Motor Behavior, 39 (2)*, pp. 126-138.

Teasdale, N., Bard, C., LaRue, J. and Fleury, M. (1993). On the cognitive penetrability of postural control. *Experimental Aging Research, 19*, pp. 1-13.

Thoumie, P. and Do, M.C. (1996). Changes in motor activity and biomechanics during balance recovery following cutaneous and muscular deafferentation. *Experimental Brain Research, 110 (2)*, pp. 289-297.

Turvey, M. T. (1990). Coordination. American Psychologist, 45 (8), pp. 938-953. van der Fits, I., Klip, A. W., van Eykern, L. and Hadders-Algra, M. (1998). Postural adjustments accompanying fast pointingmovements in standing, sitting and lying adults. *Experimental Brain Research,* 120 (2), pp. 202-216.

Varela, F., Thompson, E. and Rosch, E. (1993). The embodied mind. MIT Press.

von Holst, E. (1969). Relative coordiantion as a phnomenon and as a method of analysis of central nervous system (1939). In , *Selected Papers of Erich von Holst: The Behavioural Physiology of Animals and Man, London.* Methuen.. pp. 33-135.

Vuillerme, N. and Nougier, V. (2003). Effect of light finger touch on postural sway after lower limb muscular fatigue. *Brain Research Bulletin, 84 (10)*, pp. 1560-1563.

Vuillerme, N., Danion, F., Forestier, N. and Nougier, V. (2002). Postural sway under muscle vibration and muscle fatigue in human: effetcts of changes in sensory inputs. *Neuroscience Letters, 333 (2)*, pp. 131-135.

Warren, W. H. (2006). The dynamics of perception and action. *Psychological Review, 113 (2)*, pp. 358-389.

Witkin, H. A. (1950). Individual differences in ease of perception of embedded figures. *Journal of Personality, 19*, pp. 1-15.

Woollacott, M. and Shumway-Cook, A. (2002). Attention and the control of posture and gait: a review of an emerging area of research. *Gait and Posture, 16*, pp. 1-14.

Yang, J. F., Winter, D. A. and Wells, R.P. (1990). Postural dynamics in the standing human. *Biological Cybernetics, 62*, pp. 309-320.

Zanone, P. G. and Kelso, J.S. (1992). Learning and transfer as dynamical paradigms for behavioural change. In G. E. Stelmach and J. Requin (Eds.), *Tutorial in motor Behavior*. pp. 517-532.

In: Posture: Types, Assessment and Control
Editors: A. Wright and S. Rothenberg, pp. 63-97
ISBN 978-1-61324-107-3
© 2011 Nova Science Publishers, Inc.

*Chapter 3*

# INFLUENCE OF SPORT TRAINING ON SAGITTAL SPINAL CURVATURES

## P. A. López-Miñarro,[1] J. M. Muyor,[2] F. Alacid,[3] and P. L. Rodríguez[1]

[1]Department of Physical Education. University of Murcia, Spain
[2]Department of Physical Education. University of Almería, Spain
[3]Department of Sports Sciences. University of Murcia, Spain

## ABSTRACT

Sagittal spinal curvatures are geometric parameters which influence mechanical properties of spinal tissues. Sagittal alignment influences postural loading and load balance of the intervertebral disc.

Sagittal spinal curvatures may adapt gradually when training intensively for long periods. Theoretically, intensive training could lead to adaptations in the spine and might be an important factor associated with changes in the degree of spinal curvatures.

The spinal curvatures of an intensively trained athlete may differ in sagittal configuration from one sport to another. There have been studies on the sagittal spinal curvatures in female rhythmic gymnasts, young ballet dancers, soccer players, runners, Greco-Roman and free style wrestlers, cyclists, rowers, paddlers, skiers... Other studies have analyzed heterogeneous samples of athletes of differing in sports participation. All these studies revealed that specific and repetitive movements and postures of each sport influence spinal curvatures. These differences have been associated to specific spine positions during the training and competition activities. Furthermore, several studies have found some differences between athletes participating in different sports and with respect to control groups of age-matched sedentary subjects.

Sagittal alignment influences postural loading and load balance of the intervertebral disc in healthy subjects. Alterations in spinal curvatures may influence the development of low-back pain, which is a common injury among athletes. Greater spinal angles produce larger shear forces, larger contributions from passive components and greater intradiscal pressures on the thoracic and lumbar tissues. This is of special concern in young athletes, because an increased thoracic angle and/or kyphotic lumbar postures impose great demands on the immature spine, altering the spine's exposure to mechanical loadings during growth. Moreover, prolonged static and cyclic loading has been related to creep deformation in the lumbar viscoelastic tissues. These changes seem to be associated with microdamage to the collagen structure since it was shown to elicit spasms in spinal muscles.

Because the specific positions and movements of the sport training may influence the spine posture, the aim of this chapter is to analyze the influence of sport training in the thoracic and lumbar spinal curvatures of young and adult athletes.

## INTRODUCTION

In a normal spine there are four types of spinal curvatures that are important to balance, flexibility, and stress absorption and distribution. The spine performs a number of critical functions in the human body. As a structure, the spine is frequently defined by the vertebrae, discs, and surrounding soft tissues. When seen in sagittal profile the spine presents antero-posterior curves. The normal spine has lordotic curves in the cephalad and caudal regions with a kyphotic curve in-between. Curvature in the sagittal plane is termed as a kyphosis when its concavity is directed ventrally and as a lordosis when the concavity is directed dorsally. From a mechanical standpoint, physiological sagittal spinal curvature acts as a shock absorber. The resistance of a column to axial stress is directly proportional to the square of the number of curvatures plus one (resistance = $n^2+1$). If we take a straight column (number of curvatures = 0) as reference, structural resistance would be calculated as 1, while a column with 3 curvatures has a resistance equal to 10 [39].

Optimal alignment of the spine and its position in relation to the pelvis and lower extremities has marked clinical implications. Sagittal curvatures are geometric parameters that are known to have a significant influence on mechanical properties during compressive loading [4, 41]. The normal development of spine sagittal curvatures depends on the interaction between growth factors and the mechanical environment in which the spine grows [117].

Spinal curvatures are capable of considerable variation in the movements of the body and static postures. There are variations in the degree of normal curvature but this shape nevertheless allows equal distribution of forces across the spinal column. There is a positive correlation between thoracic kyphosis and lumbar lordosis [89]. Furthermore, changes in pelvic posture also affect spinal alignment [47]. Several studies have confirmed that some structural features of the pelvis modulate and determine the standing lumbar lordosis, as well as the sagittal pelvic alignment and spinopelvic balance [18, 46].

The shape of the human vertebrae is gender affected due to genetic, hormonal and environmental factors responsible for growth-spurt timing [97]. Differences in the anatomic development of the spine and the pelvis might cause individual variation in vertebropelvic alignment. Masharawi et al. [64] found that females have less kyphotic lower thoracic and lumbar vertebrae. This difference is a key element in female spine adaptations to lumbar hyperlordosis.

Spinal deformity involves a curvature or altered alignment that exceeds normal limits for a particular spinal region (figure 1). The causes of sagittal spine imbalance are multi-factorial. Theses changes in sagittal shapes of the trunk could be responsible for a global sagittal trunk imbalance.

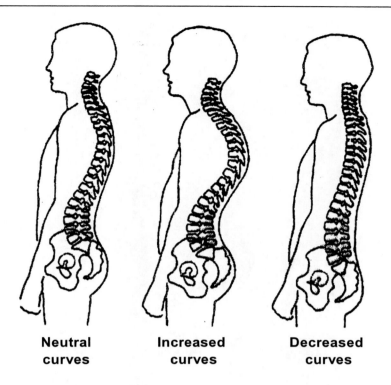

**Neutral curves**  **Increased curves**  **Decreased curves**

Figure 1. Different types of sagittal spinal curvatures.

The pelvis is considered to be the base for the spine, and its anteroposterior orientation affects the sagittal curves of the spine. The neutral position of the pelvis in standing has been defined as the posterior superior iliac spine and anterior superior iliac spine, and is approximately in the horizontal plane, a posture that produces the optimal degree of lumbar lordosis. Increased anterior pelvic tilt is associated to larger lumbar lordosis and compensatory increases in the thoracic and cervical curves above so maintaining the head above the feet.

There is minimal spinal muscle involvement required for maintaining static equilibrium in erect standing. A balanced sagittal alignment of the spine has been shown to strongly correlate with less pain, less disability, and greater health status scores [100]. Changes in spinal shape, however, are likely to disrupt this balance. An increase in sagittal curvatures may alter physiologic loading through the spine as a consequence of a shift in trunk mass, leading to increased flexion moments and compression and shear forces imposed on spine segments [4].

Several spinal deformities have been described. Thoracic hyperkyphosis is a sagittal deviation of the spine that presents itself as an anterior spinal curvature (figure 2). While the term "kyphotic" is occasionally used to describe someone with accentuated thoracic curvature, hyperkyphosis is preferred since kyphosis itself refers to the normal sagittal angle of thoracic curvature [76]. Thoracic kyphosis is defined as the primary sagittal spinal curve between T1 and T12. Thoracic kyphosis exceeding the normal range can be present at all ages, although its incidence increases with age.

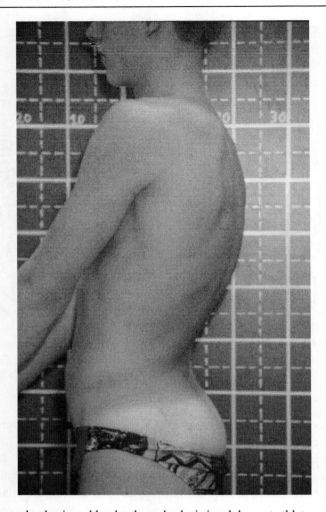

Figure 2. Thoracic hyperkyphosis and lumbar hyperlordosis in adolescent athlete.

There are varying reports in the literature on normal values for acceptable kyphosis or lordosis in the spine. Thoracic kyphosis is between 20° and 50°, and normal lumbar ranges from 31° to 79° from L1 to S1. Several reference values have been proposed for defining neutral and altered angles. Mejia et al. [68] proposed values between 20° and 45° as neutral thoracic kyphosis, values below 20° as thoracic hypokyphosis and values above 45° as thoracic hyperkyphosis.

On the other hand, lumbar hyperlordosis is an increased lumbar curve that exceeds the normal angle (figure 2). In lumbar curve, values between 20° and 40° were considered to be neutral, while values below 20° were considered to be hypolordotic and values above 40° were considered to be hyperlordotic [107].

Of the different thoracic elements, the vertebral bodies in particular accounted for most of the variability in kyphosis [27]. However intervertebral discs and posterior spinal musculature (muscles and ligaments) are other elements that may also be important in determining the whole kyphotic curvature of the thoracic region. It is important to differentiate between a simple postural thoracic hyperkyphosis or lumbar hyperlordosis that is flexible and reducible, from a true and structural deformity. Flexible deformities are primarily disc-based. In the majority of cases, these deformities are painless and flexible [89].

Alterations in spinal balance and curvature are deemed by many investigators to be involved in the development of a variety of spinal disorders, including acute and chronic low back pain [32, 104], and disc degeneration [96]. In a group of 124 normal and low back pain subjects, Harrison et al. [32] found that several lumbar morphological measurements, including segmental and total lumbar lordosis, were able to discriminate normal subjects from acute low back pain sufferers (hyperlordotic) and chronic low back pain sufferers (hypolordotic).

Sagittal spinal alignment is found to change as a child grows [10]. Widhe [113] found that kyphosis in relation to lordosis decreased with age in girls, but did not change in boys. Mellin and Poussa [69] also reported that thoracic kyphosis was less in girls compared to boys. The difference was most pronounced at the age of 13-14 years. One reason for this difference between the genders could be that the adolescent growth spurt and completion of growth is 2 years ahead in girls [113].

## THE SPINE AND SPORTS

The sagittal spinal curvatures are determined by individual features: genetic, psychomotor, functional, habits, etc. Sport exercises, often performed under high loads and aimed at shaping specific skills, may lead to postural changes especially when applied to very young subjects.

The spine plays an essential role in the contribution toward athletic performance. As the central pillar of the body, the structures of the spine are susceptible to adaptation and injury related with sports participation. The spine in athletes is subjected to compressive, shear, and lateral bending loads of large magnitude during training.

Excessive compressive loading of the spine is known to affect normal spinal development at the apophyses. Most athletic training and competition exposes the spine to large loads. This is because, according to Newton's laws, large muscle forces are required to rapidly accelerate or decelerate body segments. Intense training increases that exposure because it involves multiple, repeated loading cycles. In highly competitive sports, the spine of the growing athlete may be vulnerable because it is the conduit for transferring mechanical power between the upper and lower extremities during rapid and forceful movements. Consequently, it is subjected to large three-dimensional bending moments in flexion, extension, and axial rotation, with concomitantly large compression and shear forces.

Intense athletic training may alter the sagittal curvatures by increasing spine exposure to increased mechanical loading generated mainly by the trunk muscles. The capacity of the spine to withstand those forces, and the subsequent response of the spine to those forces and bending moments, will probably determine its sagittal shape [117].

With training, the spine adopts a sport-dependent posture. Each sport places the spine of athletes in specific postures. The exposure to years of systematic training may influence the sagittal curvatures [117]. Theoretically, intensive training could lead to adaptations in the spine and might be an important factor associated with changes in the degree of spinal curvatures (figure 3).

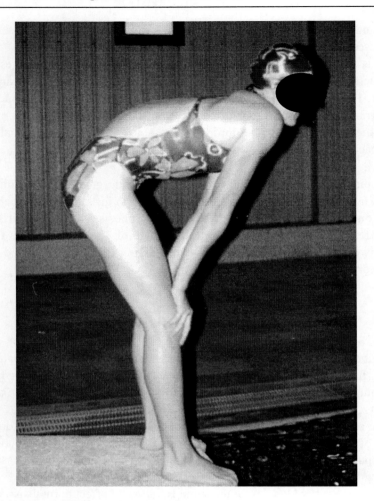

Figure 3. Lumbar kyphosis in a female swimmer.

A higher frequency of hyperkyphotic postures in the standing position has been found in sports where maintained trunk flexion postures are predominant, such as skiing, rowing, wrestling, volleyball, and canoeing, and in athletes who perform repetitive intervertebral flexions for muscle strengthening (table 1); however, in sports where specific exercises are performed for the improvement of body image and posture with frequent spinal extension positions (such as rhythmic gymnastics and dance), significant decreases in thoracic kyphosis have been observed [44, 74].

The increase in spinal curvatures might also be due to loss of disk height, which would tend to reduce the length of the anterior column of the spine, thereby increasing thoracic kyphosis and lumbar lordosis. A possible reason for this could be a long training with the spine in a static or cyclic flexed position. Several studies have justified an increased thoracic kyphosis in relation to specific training postures [1, 80, 117], although these studies did not measure the specific posture during sport training. Most studies have focused on the evaluation of spinal curvature in the standing, sitting, and flexion positions of the trunk, but not on the sports' specific exercise positions (table 1).

**Table 1. Studies on sagittal spinal curvatures in athletes**

| Study | Sport | Population | Variables | Position | Measurement System | Findings |
|---|---|---|---|---|---|---|
| Ohlén et al. [74] | Gymnasts | 64 female gymnasts (11.9 ± 2.7 years old). Mean training volume: 12.3 ± 2.6 hours per week. Mean experience: 4.3 ± 2.0 years | Thoracic and lumbar curves | Standing and total trunk forward bending | Debrunner kyphometer and Myrin´s inclinometer | Low back pain was reported by 20% of the females, and these females had a significantly greater lordosis. |
| Uetake et al. [109] | Heterogeneous sample: rugby, soccer, kendo, swimming, sailing, sprinting, distance running, jumping, throwing, and bodybuilding | 380 males (21.8 ± 4.0 years). Participation ranged from 4 to 17 years, and were ranked high in national competitions or in students' national competitions | Thoracic kyphosis and lumbar lordosis | Standing | Moire photograph | Sprinters, middle- and long-distance runners, jumpers, kendo participants and throwers had increased curves, whereas swimmers, bodybuilders, sailors, soccer players, rugby players and non-athletes had reduced curvatures. |

## Table 1. (Continued)

| Study | Sport | Population | Variables | Position | Measurement System | Findings |
|---|---|---|---|---|---|---|
| Boldori et al. [2] | Heterogeneous sample: swimming, tennis, soccer, artistic gym, classical dance, basket, and volleyball. | 3.765 students of the 4th and 6th class of primary schools | Thoracic kyphosis and lumbar lordosis | Standing | Orthopaedic screening | The incidence of hyperlordosis was significantly lower in boys playing soccer. Swimming males showed a higher incidence of thoracic hyperkyphosis compared to the control group. In females the incidence of hyperlordosis did not correlate with any of the sports considered, whereas the incidence in boys playing soccer and swimming showed a decrease. |
| Rajabi et al. [81] | Cyclists | - 120 male cyclists (Professional national team members, amateur club cyclists, and recreational cyclists). Minimum criterion of 5 years cycling. - 120 male non-cyclists | Thoracic kyphosis | Standing | Modified Electrogoniometer | The thoracic kyphosis angle measured in the cyclists group was greater than for the non-cyclists. |

| Study | Sport | Population | Variables | Position | Measurement System | Findings |
|---|---|---|---|---|---|---|
| Wojtys et al. [117] | Heterogeneous sample: American football, gymnastics, hockey, track, swimming, volleyball, weight lifting, and wrestling | 2.270 children (407 girls and 1.863 boys) between 8 and 18 years of age. Regular extracurricular athletic training and competition for at least 1 year (4 or more days per week, and at least 3 months per year). | Thoracic kyphosis and lumbar lordosis | Standing | Optical raster-stereographic method | Larger angles of thoracic kyphosis and lumbar lordosis were associated with greater cumulative training time. Gymnasts showed the largest curves. Lack of sports participation, in contrast, was associated with smaller curves. |
| Wodecki et al. [116] | Soccer players | 31 soccer players and 47 non-athletes. Soccer players were licensed members of a soccer club and participated in regular sports activities (at least 4 hours per week for at least 2 years). | Thoracic kyphosis, lumbar lordosis, and sacral tilt | Standing | Radiography | Spinal alignment was characterized by a less pronounced thoracic kyphosis and a more pronounced sacral tilt and lumbar lordosis in soccer players. |

**Table 1. (Continued)**

| Study | Sport | Population | Variables | Position | Measurement System | Findings |
|---|---|---|---|---|---|---|
| Nilsson et al. [72] | Dancers | 23 students of first-year at Ballet School (age: 10 years). Training volume: 10 hours/week | Thoracic and lumbar curves | Standing and sagittal range of motion | Debrunner Kyphometer and Myrin´s inclinometer | Dancers showed high mobility of the thoracic spine, and reduced lumbar and thoracic curves in standing. |
| Alricsson and Werner [1] | Skiers | 15 young cross-country elite skiers at 13.6±0.9 year (pre-test) and after 5 year (post-test). | Thoracic kyphosis | Standing | Debrunner's kyphometer | The skiers increased their thoracic kyphosis in the post-test (+9.4°) but no change was shown for lumbar lordosis. |
| Stutchfield and Coleman [105] | Rowers | Twenty-six male rowers' 20.6±1.5 years. Universitary population with more than 2 years' rowing experience and rowing training at least six times per week | Lumbar curve | Trunk flexion in sitting | Schober method | Participants with low back pain showed significantly reduced lumbar flexion |
| Kums et al. [44] | Rhythmic Gymnasts | - Elite female rhythmic gymnasts aged 13-17 years (n= 32) competing at national level. Volume training: 6-7 | Thoracic kyphosis and lumbar lordosis | Standing | Spinal pantography | Thoracic kyphosis and lumbar lordosis were lower in gymnasts in comparison with the control group. |

| Study | Sport | Population | Variables | Position | Measurement System | Findings |
|---|---|---|---|---|---|---|
| | | hours/day during 8-12 years.<br><br>- Untrained age-matched controls. | | | | |
| Rajabi et al. [79] | Hockey players | - Elite female players (n=50; 22.7 ± 3.5 years) from national league for at least during 3 years.<br><br>- Control group (n=50; 23.1 ± 3.0 years). | Thoracic kyphosis | Standing | Modified Electrogoniometer | An increased thoracic kyphosis in hockey players in comparison with non-athletes group was found. |
| Rajabi et al. [80] | Wrestlers | - 30 free style wrestlers, 30 Greco-Roman wrestlers and 30 non-athletes between 18-29 years.<br><br>Competed at national or international level. Minimum criterion of 5 years wrestling. | Thoracic kyphosis | Standing | Modified Electrogoniometer | The thoracic kyphosis was highest in free-style wrestling, followed by non-athletes and then free-style wrestlers. The extent of kyphosis was not influenced by years of training. |

**Table 1. (Continued)**

| Study | Sport | Population | Variables | Position | Measurement System | Findings |
|---|---|---|---|---|---|---|
| López-Miñarro et al. [61] | Recreational weight lifters | 40 young males (mean age: 24.6 ± 5.6 years) | Thoracic kyphosis and lumbar lordosis | Standing and during bilateral curl bar exercise | Unilevel Inclinometer | Greater lumbar lordosis angle was found at the end of the concentric phase than in standing. |
| López-Miñarro et al. [55] | Recreational weight lifters | 193 young male adults (mean age: 25.3 ± 6.3 years) | Thoracic kyphosis | Standing and during triceps-pushdown exercise | Unilevel inclinometer | Thoracic kyphosis during triceps-pushdown exercise was significantly higher (+4°) than in standing. |
| López-Miñarro [62] | Recreational weight lifters | 150 young males (mean age: 22.3 ± 6.1 years) | Thoracic kyphosis | Standing and during several strength exercises for upper limbs | Unilevel Inclinometer | Thoracic kyphosis was significantly higher when performing strength exercises for upper limbs than in standing. |
| López-Miñarro et al. [50] | Paddlers and runners | 30 kayakers and 30 long distance runners highly-trained (13-14 years). | Thoracic and lumbar curves | Relaxed standing and maximal trunk flexion (sit-and-reach test) | Unilevel Inclinometer | The kayakers reached greater angles in maximal trunk flexion for both lumbar and thoracic curves. |
| Grabara and Hadzik [28] | Voleyball | 42 volleyball players and 43 untrained girls (aged 13-16 years) | Thoracic kyphosis, lumbar | Standing | Computer posturography | Volleyball players were predominantly kyphotic and their lumbar lordosis was |

| Study | Sport | Population | Variables | Position | Measurement System | Findings |
|---|---|---|---|---|---|---|
| | | | lordosis, and pelvic alignment | | | flattened, especially in those having longer training experience. |
| López-Miñarro et al. [56] | Recreational weight lifters | 66 young male adults (mean age: 24.7 ± 4.9 years) | Lumbar lordosis | Standing and during lat pulldown exercise | Unilevel inclinometer | The lat pulldown exercise showed a lower lumbar lordosis than standing, and a greater frequency of lumbar kyphotic and hypolordotic postures was found. |
| Föster et al. [23] | Rock Climbers | 46 performance-oriented sport climbers, climbing at a minimum UIAA grade 9 (redpoint) for at least 3 years and no intensive participation in any other sporting discipline.<br><br>34 recreational climbers (control group), climbing up to UIAA grade 7 and less than three times climbing training per week. | Thoracic kyphosis and lumbar lordosis | Standing erect, maximal extension and flexion. | Spinal Mouse | Spinal curvatures were characterized by an increased thoracic kyphosis and lumbar lordosis. The climbing ability level was strongly correlated to the postural adaptations. |

Table 1. (Continued)

| Study | Sport | Population | Variables | Position | Measurement System | Findings |
|---|---|---|---|---|---|---|
| López-Miñarro et al. [58] | Recreational weight lifters | 50 young male adults (mean age: 24.3 ± 5.4 years) | Lumbar lordosis | Relaxed standing and during standing triceps overhead extension exercise | Unilevel inclinometer | A greater percentage of hyperlordotic postures when performing the exercise was found than in the standing position. |
| López-Miñarro et al. [51] | Paddling | 45 elite kayakers (males and females), 20 elite canoeists (males) and 44 non-athletes (males and females) (13-14 years old). | Thoracic and lumbar curves | Relaxed standing and maximal trunk flexion (sit-and-reach test) | Unilevel Inclinometer | Paddling training did not influence thoracic standing posture, although it produced a reduced lumbar lordosis in standing and greater thoracic and lumbar angles in maximal trunk flexion. |
| López-Miñarro et al. [53] | Kayakers | 40 highly-trained young males (15.25 ± 0.72 years-old). | Thoracic and lumbar curves and pelvic tilt | Standing and sitting in the kayak. | Spinal Mouse | The kayakers adopted a lumbar flexed posture and posterior pelvic tilt in their kayak, although this position may not affect the sagittal configuration of lumbar and thoracic spine in standing. |

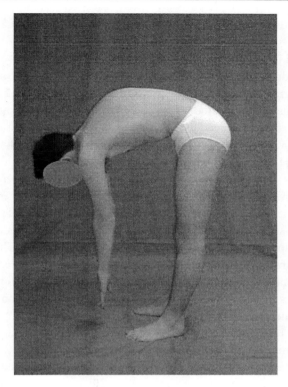

Figure 4. Increased thoracic kyphosis in the toe-touch test. Previous study in standing position showed neutral values.

Most studies concerning athlete population have analyzed the standing posture. However, other common positions in daily activities and sport training such as relaxed sitting and trunk flexion should also be analyzed. Usually a good posture is found while standing but an increased curvature is detected when trunk flexion with knees extended (sit-and-reach and toe-touch tests) are performed (figure 4).

It can be postulated that there might be an association between the normal development of the sagittal curvatures of the spine and the mechanical environment (excessive compressive loading of the anterior and tensile loading of the posterior portion of the vertebraes). The influence of mechanical loading (stress) on the thoracic vertebrae in the flexed position and its association with morphological adaptation of the thoracic elements and an accompanying increase in kyphosis is well established.

Concerning the mechanics of the spine, Harrington referred to the Hueter-Volkmann principle, which claims that abnormal pressures placed on the facets and the vertebral bodies over a period of time affect the vertebral bodies, the facets, and the growth endochondral plates. Actually, Volkmann developed the theory of bone and joint deformities caused by overloading of the growing skeleton, postulating that abnormal pressure ampres the growth of the epiphyseal plates in adolescents, whereas stretching stimulates it.

An increased thoracic kyphosis could be explained by a theory that the pressure on the anterior portion of vertebrae as a result of flexed kyphotic posture produces a "remodeling" or "reforming" of the bone, leading to the appearance of anterior compression. Volkmann's law indicates that pressure on an epiphysis delays the speed of growth in the affected area whilst tension in the posterior portion of the vertebral column increases the amount of the growth [80].

Wojtys et al. [117] reported that a high exposure of intensive athletic training might increase the risk of developing adolescent hyperkyphosis in certain sports. In elite cross-country skiers, Alricsson and Werner [1] found that the sagittal configuration of the spine changed in adolescents after a period of 5 years of intensive cross-country skiing (table 1). The skiers increased their thoracic kyphosis but no change was shown for their lumbar lordosis. In a clinical screening of the Norwegian national team cross-country skiers, increased thoracic kyphosis was found in 66% of the skiers [90].

Some differences in spinal curvatures between sports have been associated to spine positions during training activities. Rajabi et al. [80] studied the influence of different disciplines in a single sport. They found significant differences of thoracic kyphosis in standing among free-style wrestling, Greco-Roman style wrestling and non-athletes. These differences were related to the specific positions of each discipline. The free style routinely puts the spine in more flexed position while the Greco-Roman style uses the spine in an almost in erect position. López-Miñarro et al. [51] found no differences between male canoeists and kayakers in standing and sit-and-reach test, although important differences exist between both disciplines in both posture and technique.

Wojtys et al. [117] examined the association between cumulative hours of athletic training and the magnitude of the sagittal curvature in a sample of 2.270 children (407 girls and 1863 boys) between 8 and 18 years. They found an association between increased spinal curvatures with cumulative training exposure. A 300% increase in training hours was associated with a 5° increase in spinal curvatures. While the curvatures of the athletes were generally in the normal range, gymnasts were most affected, followed by those participating in American football, hockey, swimming, and wrestling. Both the thoracic and lumbar angles were significantly lower in the sedentary control group when compared with each of the athletic groups. The sports of football, gymnastics, hockey, swimming, and wrestling had significantly greater angles of thoracic and lumbar curvature when compared with track sports and volleyball. The gymnastics presented the largest spine curvature in both the thoracic (42°) and lumbar (52°) curves.

Among different sports, the position of the spine during training differs greatly from its anatomical standing position, and this is why some sports have received more attention in the research literature.

## Cycling

Cycling is currently a popular sport despite its diverse performance requirements, such as high physical demands, suitable climate, interaction with motor vehicles, bicycle design [13], and comfort [3]. In cycling, the primary posture is sitting on the bicycle with three support points: the seat, handlebars, and pedals [13]. This posture has been classified as anti-natural with respect to standing.

Usabiaga et al. [110] found that a cyclist's position involves a change from lumbar lordosis in standing to lumbar kyphosis while sitting on a bicycle. Slumped sitting has been associated with greater intradiscal pressure on the lumbar and thoracic spine [77, 94, 114, 115]. Moreover, prolonged sitting has been associated with creep deformation in the lumbar viscoelastic tissues [66]. Cyclists spend a large amount of time training on their bicycles to elicit a physiological training effect, and this training may influence their spinal curvature. Rajabi et al. [81] found a significantly greater standing thoracic kyphosis in cyclists than in sedentary individuals. The high physical demands, duration of training, and races that characterise cycling could accentuate the spinal curvature values in these athletes, given that high-intensity exercise can lead to modifications in the sagittal configuration of the spine.

The reported incidence of low back pain in cyclists is high (rates of up to 50%) and may be related to cyclists' positions on their bicycles [92]. However, the overall mechanical load on the spine would be reduced in cycling because weight is shifted onto the upper limbs [110].

Rajabi [81] stated that kyphotic posture in cycling is due to marked pressure on the anterior edge of the vertebra producing a "remodeling" or "reforming" of the bone, resulting in the appearance of anterior compression. However, when comparing the thoracic kyphosis between standing and sitting on a bicycle, a significant decrease was observed at the three different handlebar positions for elite cyclists [71]. It is likely that this difference is due to hand support on the handlebar, which leads to a scapular retropulsion and thoracic intervertebral extension (figure 5).

To obtain a more aerodynamic position, the cyclists flexed their hip and positioned the pelvis more horizontally. McEvoy et al. [65] reported that elite cyclists had a significantly greater anterior pelvic tilt angle than non-athletes due to a specific sport adaptation when tested during static long-term sitting.

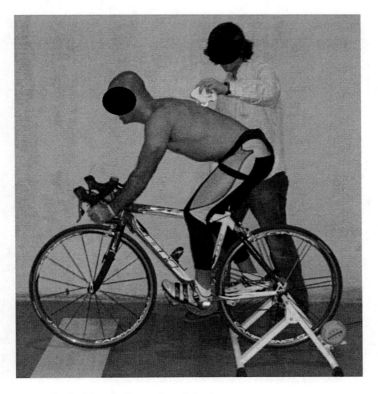

Figure 5. Spinal curvatures in the bicycle (lower handlebar).

Cycling produces specific adaptations in lumbar curvature when trunk flexion postures are assumed. Cyclists reach greater lumbar flexion than non-athletes during maximal trunk flexion and while sitting on the bicycle. However, cycling training does not appear to influence lumbar curvature during standing because neutral values were found. The frequency of hypolordotic postures in cyclists of different cathegories was reduced [71].

## Paddling

The two disciplines of flat-water paddling (kayaking and canoeing) are basically repetitive movements of the upper body. Paddlers maintain the same position and use the same muscles repetitively for long periods.

Both canoeing and kayaking differ in spinal postures and movements. The kayaker is sitting in the boat, with the knees slightly flexed, around 20 degrees, and performs symmetrical strokes (figure 6). The trunk is slightly flexed, to approximately, 10-15 degrees, and the stroke is characterized by significant trunk rotation. The fact that the kayakers are seated increases the tendency towards a kyphotic lumbar posture, unless there is well-developed hamstring muscle extensibility. Canoeing is characterized by kneeling in a canoe and performing dynamic strokes on one side only (figure 7). The stroke requires significant flexion and rotation of the trunk and a slight lateral inclination.

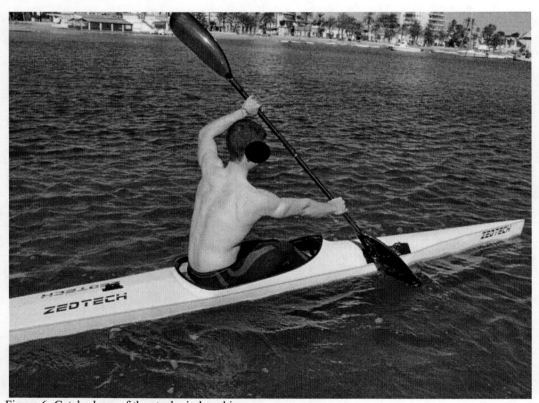

Figure 6. Catch phase of the stroke in kayaking.

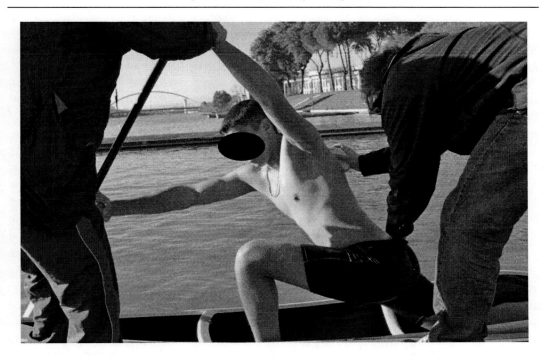

Figure 7. Catch phase position in the canoe.

As paddlers spend a large amount of time training in their boats to elicit a physiological training effect, this may influence their thoracic and lumbar spinal curvatures. The different position and stroke technique between kayakers and canoeists could be associated to specific adaptations in sagittal spinal curvatures.

López-Miñarro et al. [51] compared paddlers and non-athlete population (analyzed by gender) and found no significant differences in thoracic angle in standing. The mean values of thoracic and lumbar angles in standing were considered normal in terms of angle references for kayakers and canoeists. However, a previous study had found a high frequency of thoracic hyperkyphosis in canoeists and kayakers and explained this as an adaptation to the trunk position during stroke [49]. With regards to lumbar curve, lower lumbar angles in paddlers than in control age-matched subjects were found. When paddlers were classified into lumbar categories, only one case of hyperlordosis was detected. However, a higher frequency of lumbar hyperlordosis was found in the control groups, especially in the female control group (22.7%). The reduced lumbar lordosis in standing in paddlers could be related to the sitting posture in kayakers during the stroke because sitting on a horizontal surface involves posterior pelvic tilt and reduced lumbar lordosis [63]. In the case of canoeists, their dynamic trunk flexion and their gender (males) could explain why no cases of lumbar hyperlordosis were found.

Sagittal spinal curvatures in the sit-and-reach test have been analyzed in several studies (50-52, 59, 60, 87]. The paddlers reached larger thoracic and lumbar angles than non-athlete population and runners. These differences may be due to the increased physical demands placed on the spines of paddlers in the course of training and competition. The prolonged sitting and repeated flexion of the lumbar spine which characterizes kayaking and canoeing, respectively, might lead to the development of an increased spinal flexion in growing individuals due to creep deformation of the spinal tissues [75, 101].

On comparing the spinal curvatures between genders, the females showed lower thoracic kyphosis and greater lumbar lordosis in standing than males in both paddlers and control groups [51]. These differences are in concordance with previous studies in adolescents [69, 78, 113] and adult athletes [87]. When analyzing the spinal curvatures in the sit-and-reach, the females showed higher angles in lumbar curve and lower values in thoracic curve than males. The greater hamstring muscle extensibility of females and its influence on hip range of motion could explain these differences [87].

The analysis of posture in the specific position of training is very important. When sitting in the kayak, the posture was characterized by a reduced thoracic curve and a lumbar kyphotic curve [53]. They found a significant decrease of thoracic kyphosis (between 12-14°) when the kayakers were sitting in their kayak. At the catch phase of the stroke, smaller lumbar and thoracic curves than in the relaxed sitting in a stool were found. The reduction in thoracic kyphosis may have been mediated by active support from muscle activation of spinal extensors and may have beneficial effects for spinal loading. The lower thoracic kyphosis in the catch phase is also related to ventilatory capacity and scapula kinematics. Slump sitting reduces tidal volume, decreases forced vital capacity, and forced expiratory volume in 1 s and peak expiratory flow when compared to upright postures [45]. An increased thoracic kyphosis may bring the scapula in an anterior tilt and protracted position, so restricting subacromial space and shoulder range of motion [22, 40]. The increased thoracic kyphosis in standing in the current study is probably related more to growth variables and spinal posture in the daily activities than to the specific position in the kayak.

The flexed position of the lumbar spine which characterizes the position in the kayak might lead to the development of a decreased lumbar curvature over time in growing individuals. However, most paddlers had neutral angles. A few paddlers only showed hypolordotic posture in standing [51].

## Rowing

Rowing is a strenuous sport with a significant lumbar spinal injury rate amongst competitive participants of all standards. It has been speculated that the majority of spinal injuries are mechanical in origin and related to the training regime and rowing technique [102]. Low back injuries are a significant problem in rowers [34,36,85]. The amount of lumbar flexion that occurs during the rowing stroke has been suggested [83] as a factor that might influence the possibility of a lower back injury.

Hosea et al. [35] reported that the trunk moved from approximately 30° of flexion at the start of the drive phase (when the oar is placed in the water) to 28° of trunk extension at the finish of the drive phase.

Bending moments increase considerably as an athlete approaches the limit of their range of lumbar flexion, and stress on spinal structures is increased [15]. If a rower has relatively less total range of motion, then they may be operating closer to the elastic limits of their soft tissue structures (disc and ligaments), thus increasing the chance of injury.

Rowers attained relatively high levels of lumbar flexion during the drive phase of the rowing stroke, and these levels were increased during the duration of the trial [6].

Two studies have analyzed rower population. Howell [36] analyzed lumbar curvature in seventeen lightweight female rowers using the sit-and-reach test and found that 76% of the subjects exhibited hyperflexion of the lumbar spine. Greater lumbar flexion may be beneficial for rowers in increasing the available range of motion while generating power during the drive.

Excessive lumbar flexion may influence the potential for injury to spinal structures. An awareness of increased lumbar flexion and muscle fatigue in the erector spinae muscles may be important for injury prevention programs for rowers [6].

Stutchfield and Coleman [105] examined the relationships between low back pain, hamstring flexibility, and lumbar flexion in rowers. Their results showed that low back pain was highly prevalent in rowers. However, no association was observed between low back pain and hamstring flexibility, or between hamstring flexibility and lumbar flexion.

## Rhytmic Gymnastics

Dancers are normally involved in daily classes followed by several hours of training. In dance, fitness incorporates elements of body composition, joint mobility, cardiorespiratory fitness, coordination, and muscular strength. Rhythmic gymnastics is a very popular sport among girls and young women that includes many of the demands of both gymnastics and dance and requires significant flexibility, particularly extension, of the lower spine. The most talented girls are trained in professional clubs according to special training programs.

Gymnasts often adopted exaggerated postures such as sway-back or hyperlordosis. The sport demands both the coordination of handling various apparatus and the flexibility to attain positions not seen in any other sport. To attain perfection and reproducibility of their routines, the athletes must practise and repeat the basic elements of their routines thousands of times. In so doing, the athlete places herself at risk to a myriad of overuse injuries, of which the most common is low back pain [37].

The risk of low back injury in rhythmic gymnasts may be related to conditioning and proper technique. When rhythmic athletes perform a back scale (a position in which the back is fully extended and one leg points straight up and the second remains in contact with the floor), beginners or lesser performers tend to rise from this position by dropping their leg first in contrast to elite or high level performers who rise from their torso using their abdominal muscles. By dropping their leg to lift their torso, poor performers are using their lumbar spine as a fulcrum placing significant compressive forces on the vertebrae (especially the pars interarticularis). To reduce low back injuries, care must be taken to optimize abdominal strength and perform techniques properly [37].

Three studies have analyzed the spinal curvatures of female gymnasts. Óhlen et al. [74] found neutral thoracic kyphosis and lumbar lordosis in standing. These postures have been associated with specific exercises performed for the improvement of body image and posture with frequent spinal extension positions. Kums et al. [44] compared the spinal posture between elite gymnasts and untrained subjects. The thoracic kyphosis, lumbar lordosis and sacral inclination in standing were significantly lower in gymnasts in comparison with the control subjects. The authors hypothesized that spinal curvatures are largely determined by the specifics of training. Tsai and Wredmark [106] analyzed posture and spinal sagittal mobility in former female elite gymnasts in comparison with matched control subjects. The gymnasts had less thoracic kyphosis than the control subjects. No difference in thoracic range of motion was found. In the lumbar spine there was no difference as to either posture or sagittal motion.

## Weight Lifters

People of almost all ages participate in weight lifting for training and recreation. Weight training has many benefits, but if not properly executed can lead to chronic pain and serious injuries [16]. Adequate spine posture in weight-lifting activities is important for prevent chronic vertebral injuries. In order to buttress anterior shear forces on the spine and to reduce the risk of injury, a neutral posture must be preserved throughout the movement (figure 8) [7,29,67].

In a study on the sagittal thoracic and lumbar curvatures during relaxed standing in the context of health-related fitness, López-Miñarro et al. [54] found a high frequency of thoracic hyperkyphosis in recreational weight lifters while lumbar lordosis showed normal values. They found an average thoracic kyphosis of 46.34 ± 8.42° (lowest value: 22°; higher value: 72°). Briggs et al. [4] found that increases in thoracic kyphosis were associated with significantly higher spinal loads and trunk muscle forces in standing.

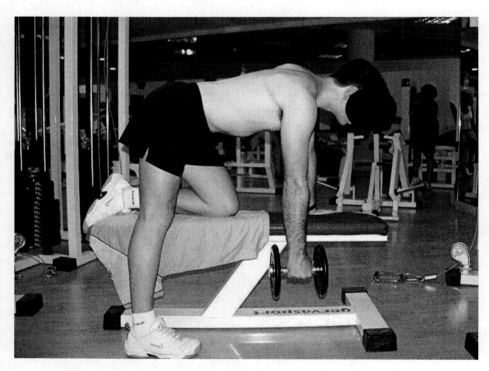

Figure 8. Active correction of spinal curvatures.

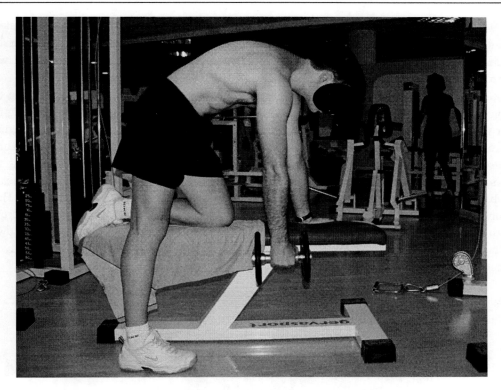

Figure 9. Increased thoracic kyphosis and lumbar kyphosis in a row exercise.

When weight training is performed bending forward or backward works the wrong muscles and can cause injury [103]. Studies have also shown a tendency to place the thoracic spine in kyphotic postures during the weight exercises [55, 56]. When kyphotic posture is adopted (figure 9) there is a greater intervertebral flexion. Flexing the spine substantially reduces the intrinsic strength and reduces the ability to sustain loads [67]. Indeed, a greater intervertebral flexion increases the intradiscal pressure and anterior shear [94, 114, 115].

Some studies have analyzed the spinal curvatures during strength exercises (table 1). López-Miñarro et al. [61] found that recreational weight lifters showed a greater lumbar lordosis angle and a high frequency of hyperlordotic postures when performing the standing bilateral curl bar exercise. López-Miñarro et al. [55] compared the thoracic posture between relaxed standing and triceps-pushdown exercise, and found that thoracic kyphosis during triceps-pushdown was significant higher than in standing. López-Miñarro [62] measured sagittal thoracic curvature when performing various strength exercises for upper limbs (standing biceps curl, seated row with anterior trunk restrained, triceps pushdown, and latissimus dorsi pulldown behind the neck position) with respect to the standing thoracic kyphosis. For standing thoracic kyphosis, the subjects were assigned to one of three groups (Group 1, < 40°; Group 2, 40°-50°; and Group 3, > 50°). The mean values of thoracic kyphosis in the exercises were higher than the thoracic kyphosis in standing, except for the seated row with trunk restrained, which showed the lowest values. The subjects of group 1 achieved greater increases of thoracic kyphosis when performing the exercises.

In another study, López-Miñarro et al. [56] evaluated the posture of thoracic spine during latissimus dorsi pulldown behind the neck position exercise. Thoracic kyphosis were 45.22 ±

8.29° in relaxed standing and 49.95 ± 9.51° in latissimus dorsi pulldown behind the neck position (p < 0.001). They found the highest percentage of subjects with thoracic hyperkyphosis when the latissimus dorsi pulldown behind the neck position exercise was performed.

The greater thoracic kyphosis angle during latissimus dorsi pulldown occurs during the concentric phase (figure 10). The concentric phase of the exercise is initiated by pulling the bar from overhead to the base of the neck at the first thoracic vertebrae. When the exercise becomes difficult towards the mid or end of a set, there is a temptation to "cheat", which causes subjects to flex their thoracic and cervical spine. Fees et al. [20] believe that the latissimus dorsi behind the neck pulldown, while popular in most fitness centres and health clubs is an unnecessary component of a strength program and should be avoided. They proposed the modified, seated with backrest support, front latissimus dorsi pulldown exercise with the torso leaning backwards about 30 degrees. In this position, there is a lower intradiscal pressure on the lumbar spine [115] and the thoracic kyphosis could probably be positioned in a more neutral position.

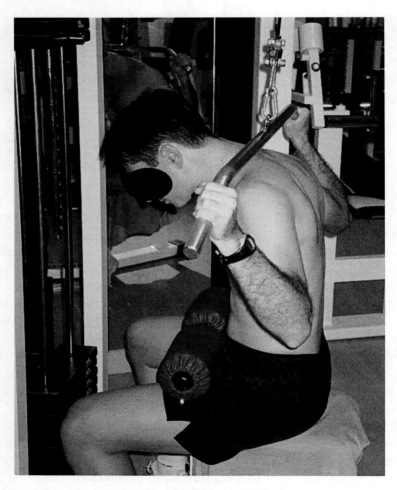

Figure 10. Increased thoracic kyphosis at the end of the concentric phase.

Other studies have evaluated the sagittal lumbar curvature. Scannell and McGill [95] demonstrated that the lumbar curvature assumed by subjects could be altered or adjusted through training. Such training may be a method to reduce low back injury risk.

López-Miñarro et al. [58] compared the lumbar lordosis while relaxed standing and during the standing triceps overhead extension exercise. Mean lumbar lordosis during the exercise (concentric and eccentric phases) and while standing were 37.36 ± 12.23°, 36.18 ± 12.25° and 30.81 ± 6.80°, respectively ($p < 0.05$). The post-hoc analysis showed significant differences ($p < 0.016$) between standing and both phases of the exercise. With regard to normality values, there was a greater percentage of hyperlordotic postures when performing the exercise (between 39.4% and 45.5%) than in the standing position (9,1%).

López-Miñarro et al. [54] analyzed the sagittal spinal curvatures of thoracic and lumbar spine in recreational weight lifters of private gyms (mean age: 24.6 ± 5.6 years) during relaxed standing and during the standing bilateral curl bar exercise. Mean thoracic kyphosis values while standing and during exercise were 46.00 ± 9.50° and 48.25 ± 9.80°, respectively ($p > 0.05$). With regard to lumbar lordosis, mean values were 30.52 ± 7.93° and 37.52 ± 9.32°, respectively ($p < 0.001$).

These studies show that better education of weight lifters and behaviour modification techniques are required. One of the biggest problems facing weightlifters today is that they do not know the proper techniques for performing simple weightlifting exercises [16]. Physicians who know the basic principles can prescribe exercise to effectively build muscle strength [43]. It is important for physicians to understand the proper technique so that they can instruct [82], because weight training is safe when done correctly. The spinal curvatures in the start position and during the exercise should be observed and controlled by the strength instructor. Weight training should be supervised closely at all times by knowledgeable specialists [30].

## HAMSTRING MUSCLES AND POSTURE

The hamstring muscle group comprises semitendinosus and semimembranosus medially, and biceps femoris, short and long heads, laterally. All muscles attach proximally to the ischial tuberosity, except for the short head of biceps femoris. Because the hamstring muscles originate in the ischial tuberosity of the pelvis, it is logical that tension in the hamstring muscles will have an influence on movement and posture of the pelvis [11, 14].

Clinical observations have suggested that the extensibility of the hamstring muscles may be also associated with specific sagittal spinal curvatures in trunk flexion. White and Sahrmann [112] stated that to compensate reduced hamstring extensibility if a maximal trunk flexion is performed, the adjacent segment (spine) presents a relatively higher range of motion. Reduced hamstring muscle extensibility is frequently reported and has been proposed as a predisposing factor for injuries [33], low back disorders [38] and changes in lumbopelvic rhythm [19, 25].

The reported incidence of reduced hamstring muscle length is high in children and adolescents. In a study on 459 children and adolescents, 75% of the boys and 35% of the girls over 10 years old had limited hamstring extensibility [5]. In another study on adolescents between 13 and 16 years old, using the passive knee extension test, Harreby et al. [31] found that tightness of the hamstring muscles is common in growing adolescents. Milne and Mierau

[70] observed a reduction in flexibility coinciding with the pubertal stage of rapid growth. However, Feldman et al. [21] registered no relation between growth and changes in hamstring muscle flexibility during the peri-pubertal period. The loss of hamstring muscle flexibility begins to manifest itself during the pre-pubertal period and reaches major significance in later growth stages.

The specific postures and movements of the sport could also influence hamstring muscle extensibility of athletes. Engaging in sports training and competitions commonly includes regular stretching, which has been assumed to result in better than average mobility. A few studies have evaluated hamstring muscle extensibility in athletes [9, 88, 111, 118], because it is an important factor in sports training. Decreased hamstring extensibility has also been reported in these studies. Earlier studies revealed significant differences between the playing positions in elite Australian Rules football [118], and junior elite volleyball players [17].

Some studies have compared the spinal and pelvic postures between subjects with reduced hamstring extensibility versus subjects with normal or improved extensibility. Congdon et al. [11] found significant differences in pelvic rotation between short and long hamstring subjects when maximal active straight leg raise was performed. Carregaro and Coury [8] found that the subjects with reduced hamstring flexibility presented higher trunk movement amplitudes and a restriction on pelvis movements during handling tasks. Gajdosik et al. [26] found differences in the mean flexion range of motion of the pelvis between men with or without decreased hamstring extensibility. Tully and Stillman [108] in a study on hip and spinal range of motion during toe-touch test in healthy subjects found that two distinct movement patterns emerged between successful and unsuccessful toe-touchers. Dewberry et al. [14] demonstrated that hamstring extensibility influences the motion of the pelvis. However, no association was found by Norris and Matthews [73] between hamstring muscle extensibility and pelvic tilt in people with extensibility of the hamstrings within normal limits, although they analyzed a submaximal flexion movement.

Decreased hamstring extensibility restricts pelvic tilting during maximal trunk flexion due to the attachment to the ischial tuberosity on the pelvis [25]. As the participant bends forward, the pelvis freely rotate forward until the passive tension in the hamstrings begins to influence pelvic rotation [98]. The subjects with lower hamstring extensibility showed an important posterior pelvic tilt in seated position with knees extended.

Hamstring extensibility did not influence the spinal curvatures while standing and slumped sitting [52]. The flexed position of both knees while sitting reduces the tension on hamstring muscles and limits its influence on pelvis and sagittal spinal curvatures.

Hamstring muscle extensibility influences the thoracic angle and pelvic position in maximal trunk flexion with knees extended. Flexion of the trunk requires coordinated lumbar and thoracic flexion together with an anterior pelvic tilt, described as lumbar-pelvic rhythm. Kendall et al. [42] and Sahrmann [91] reported an association between greater lumbar spinal flexion and reduced hamstring extensibility. The subjects with reduced hamstring extensibility showed greater thoracic angles and more posterior pelvic tilting in maximal trunk flexion [52]. Several studies have found that females reach lower thoracic angles when sit-and-reach tests are performed (51, 57, 59, 60). Given that females tend to have greater hamstring extensibility than males, it is possible that gender-specific postures are related to those differences inherent in extensibility.

A number of hamstring muscle length tests have been used previously but questions of validity and reliability have been raised for some procedures. The sit-and-reach test is a common hamstring muscle length test, although many authors contend that anthropometric factors such as limb length and/or scapular abduction, may influence the results [99]. López-Miñarro and Rodríguez [57] found that hamstring criterion-related validity of the sit-and-reach and toe-touch tests is related to hamstring muscle extensibility. These tests were not valid as measures of hamstring extensibility for subjects with reduced hamstring muscle extensibility. The straight leg raise test [42] is also used to assess hamstring muscle length. However, there is a lack of clarity about which structures limit the SLR test range. Davis et al. [12] and Fredriksen et al. [24] recommend using the passive knee extension angle as a measure of hamstring extensibility, because this test minimizes pelvis motion. However, the passive straight leg raise has been the most used test to determine the hamstring muscle extensibility.

Systematic hamstring stretching should be included in the training program to reduce the thoracic intervertebral flexion and improve anterior pelvic rotation when a maximal trunk flexion is performed. The stretching exercises for hamstring muscles should be performed maintaining an appropriate spinal alignment (Figure 11). However, stretching may be beneficial only if the technique employed and the stretch holding times are adequate. Some studies have found improvements in hamstring extensibility after a stretching program [84, 86, 93]. Li et al. [48] stated that hamstring stretching program may affect lumbar and hip motion during forward bending. Future studies should examine the effect of hamstring and postural program to avoid excessively kyphotic postures while trunk flexion in the athlete population.

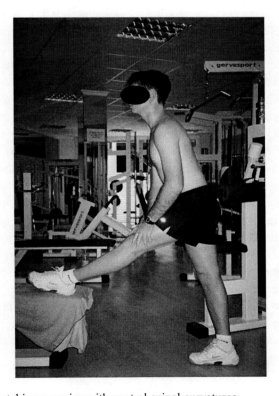

Figure 11. Hamstring stretching exercise with neutral spinal curvatures.

## LIMITATIONS OF STUDIES

Several methods that quantify spinal postures have been used to determine the spinal curvatures and pelvis position in athletes (table 1). External methods for measuring spinal ROM are commonly used because they are easy to apply, non-invasive and take little clinical time. The radiographic methods are considered the "gold standard" for measurement of spinal curvatures. However, the risk of radiation exposure limits its use for postural assessment. Moreover, these methods cannot be used to measure angular change during dynamic activities. The differences in measurements system make the comparison between studies more difficult.

Measurement error could be another explanation for the differences between studies. Test administrator training deficiencies were an important source of error. Measurement error is caused by differences between the information sought by the researcher and the information provided by the measurement process. Several sources of error measurement have been described. The lack of examiner's experience in using the device, causing a slippage or misplacement of the device, and the poor ability to identify bony landmarks were found to be the main source of error.

An interesting analysis when spinal curves are measured is to determine the internal consistency reliability. Reliability refers to the reproducibility of values of a test, assay or other measurement in repeated trials on the same individuals. Better reliability implies better precision of single measurements and better tracking of changes in measurements in research or practical settings. Intraclass correlation coefficients (ICC), and the associated 95% confidence intervals, according to the formula described by Shrout and Fleiss are usually used. However, few studies on spinal curvatures in athletes include ICC values.

The minimal detectable change (MDC) (SEM * 1.96 * $\sqrt{2}$) at the 95% confidence level should also be calculated to determine the real change when repeated measurement are performed. The MDC is the amount of change that is likely to be greater than the measurement error, which has been defined as "true change". López-Miñarro et al. [60] determined the MDC95% values in sagittal spinal measurement with a Unilevel inclinometer when different trunk flexion movements were performed. They found that changes of greater than 6° between tests would be required to reflect a real change in thoracic angle. A change angle less than this may occur as a result of measurement error associated with measurement of the spinal posture on separate occasions.

The differences in both age and competitive level between studies may distort the comparison of the results. Furthermore, some variability existed in the years of training between samples. The differences in training exposure might change the evolution of spinal curvatures. When compared between genders of same age, the different phase of growth between males and females is very important, because girls generally reach their skeletal maturity at an earlier chronological age than boys. For this reason, differences in spinal curvatures between males and females could be related to growth differences. Long-term studies are necessary, because sagittal spinal curvatures are known to change as a child grows [113].

## CONCLUSION

Several studies revealed that the specific, repetitive movements and postures of each sport influence spinal curvatures. Sports with a predominance of forward-bending postures have been associated with greater thoracic kyphosis in standing. However, ballet dancers and rhythmic gymnasts have shown reduced thoracic kyphosis and lumbar lordosis. These changes have been related to specific and repetitive postures during training. Yet, longitudinal studies including control group of age-matched non-athletes are necessary. Postural screening programs and postural retraining in paddlers with poor posture may be relevant. Postural activities should be incorporated into the training activities of athletes to improve the spinal posture.

## REFERENCES

[1] Alricsson M, Werner S. Young elite cross-country skiers and low back pain- A 5-year study. *Phys. Ther. Sport* 2006; 7, 181-184.
[2] Boldori L, Da Soldá M, Marelli, A. Anomalies of the trunk. An analysis of their prevalence in young athletes. *Minerva Pediatr.* 1999; 51, 259-264.
[3] Bressel E, Larson B. Bicycle seat designs and their effect on pelvic angle, trunk angle, and comfort. *Med. Sci. Sports Exerc.* 2003; 35, 327-332.
[4] Briggs AM, van Dieën J, Wrigley TV, Creig AM, Phillips B, Lo SK, Bennell K. Thoracic kyphosis affects spinal loads and trunk muscle force. *Phys. Ther.* 2007; 87, 595-607.
[5] Brodersen A, Pedersen B, Reimers J. Incidence of complaints about heel-, knee- and back-related discomfort among Danish children, possible relation to short muscles. *Ugeskr. Laeger.* 1994; 156, 2243-2245.
[6] Caldwell JS, McNair PJ, Williams M. The effects of repetitive motion on lumbar flexion and erector spinae muscle activity in rowers. *Clin. Biomech.* 2003; 18, 704-711.
[7] Callaghan JP, McGill SM. Intervertebral disk herniation: Studies on a porcine model exposed to highly repetitive flexion/extension motion with compressive force. *Clin. Biomech.* 2001; 16, 28-37.
[8] Carregaro RL, Coury HJC. Does reduced hamstring flexibility affect trunk and pelvic movement strategies during manual handling? *Int. J. Ind. Ergon.* 2009; 39, 115-120.
[9] Chandler TJ, Kibler WB, Uhl TL, Wooten B, Kiser A, Stone E. Flexibility comparisons of junior elite tennis players to other athletes. *Am. J. Sports Med.* 1990; 18, 134-136.
[10] Cil A, Yazici M, Uzumcugil A, Kandemir U, Alanay A, Alanay Y, Acaroglu RE, Surat A. The evolution of sagittal segmental alignment of the spine during childhood. *Spine* 2005; 30, 93-100.
[11] Congdon R, Bohannon R, Tiberio D. Intrinsic and imposed hamstring length influence posterior pelvic rotation during hip flexion. *Clin. Biomech.* 2005; 20, 947-951.
[12] Davis DS, Quinn RO, Whiteman CT, Williams JD, Young CR. Concurrent validity of four clinical tests to measure hamstring flexibility. *J. Strength Cond. Res.* 2008; 22, 583-588.

[13] De Vey Mestdagh K. Personal perspective: in search of an optimum cycling posture. *Appl. Ergon.* 1998; 29, 325-334.
[14] Dewberry MJ, Bohannon RW, Tiberio D, Murray R, Zannotti CM. Pelvic and femoral contributions to bilateral hip flexion by subjects suspended from a bar. *Clin. Biom.* 2003; 18, 1067-1076.
[15] Dolan P, Adams M. Influence of lumbar and hip mobility on the bending stresses acting on the lumbar spine. *Clin. Biomech.* 1993; 8, 185-192.
[16] Downing JH, Lander JE. Performance error in weight training and their correction. *JOPERD* 2004; 73, 44-52.
[17] Duncan MJ, Woodfield L, al-Nakeeb Y. Anthropometric and physiological characteristics of junior elite volleyball players. *Br. J. Sports Med.* 2006; 40, 649-651.
[18] During J, Goudfrooij H, Keessen W, Beeker TW, Crowe A. Toward standards for posture. Postural characteristics of the lower back system in normal and pathologic conditions. *Spine* 1985; 10, 83-87.
[19] Esola MA, McClure PW, Fitzgerald GK, Siegler S. Analysis of lumbar spine and hip motion during forward bending in subjects with and without a history of low back pain. *Spine* 1996; 21, 71-78.
[20] Fees M, Decker T, Snyder-Mackler, MJ. Upper extremity weight-training modifications for the injured athlete. A clinical perspective. *Am. J. Sports Med.* 1998; 26, 732-742.
[21] Feldman D, Shrier I, Rossignol M, Abenhaim L. Adolescent growth is not associated with changes in flexibility. *Clin. J. Sport Med.* 1999; 9, 24-29.
[22] Finley MA, Lee MY. Effect of sitting posture on 3-dimensional scapular kinematics measured by skin-mounted electromagnetic tracking sensors. *Arch. Phys. Med. Rehabil.* 2003; 84, 563-568.
[23] Föster R, Penka G, Bösl T, Schöffl V. Climber's back-form and mobility of the thoracolumbar spine leading to postural adaptations in male high ability rock climbers. *Int. J. Sports Med.* 2009; 30, 53-59.
[24] Fredriksen H, Dagfunrud H, Jacobsen V, Maehlum S. Passive knee extension test to measure hamstring muscle tightness. *Scand. J. Med. Sci. Sports* 1997; 7, 279-282.
[25] Gajdosik RL, Albert CR, Mitman JJ. Influence of hamstring length on the standing position and flexion range of motion of the pelvic angle, lumbar angle, and thoracic angle. *J. Orthop. Sports Phys. Ther.* 1994; 20, 213-219.
[26] Gajdosik RL, Hatcher CK, Whitsell S. Influence of short hamstring muscles on the pelvis and lumbar spine in standing and during the toe-touch test. *Clin. Biomech.* 1992; 1, 38-42.
[27] Goh S, Price RI, Leedman PJ, Singer KP. The relative influence of vertebral body and intervertebral disc shape on thoracic kyphosis. *Clin. Biomech.* 1999; 14, 439-448.
[28] Grabara M, Hadzik A. Postural variables in girls practicing volleyball. *Biom. Hum. Kin.* 2009; 1, 67-71.
[29] Gunning JL, Callaghan JP, McGill SM. Spinal posture and prior loading history modulate compressive strength and type of failure in the spine: a biomechanical study using a porcine cervical spine model. *Clin. Biomech.* 2001; 16, 471-480.
[30] Hamill BP. Relative safety of weightlifting and weight training. *J. Strength Cond. Res.* 1994; 8, 53-57.

[31] Harreby M, Nygaard B, Jessen T, Larsen E, Storr-Paulsen A, Lindahl A, Fisker I, Laegaard E. Risk factors for low back pain in a cohort of 1389 Danish school children: an epidemiologic study. *Eur. Spine J* 1999; 8, 444-450.
[32] Harrison DD, Cailliet R, Janik TJ, Troyanovich SJ, Harrison DE, Holland B. Elliptical modeling of the sagittal lumbar lordosis and segmental rotation angles as a method to discriminate between normal and low back pain subjects. *J. Spinal Disord.* 1998; 11, 430-439.
[33] Hartig D, Henderson J. Increasing hamstring flexibility decreases lower extremity overuse injuries in military basic trainees. *Am. J. Sports Med.* 1999; 27, 173-176.
[34] Hickey G, Fricker P, McDonald W. Injuries to elite rowers over a 10-yr period. *Med. Sci. Sports Exerc.* 1997; 29, 1567-1572.
[35] Hosea T, Boland A, McCarthy K, Kennedy T. *Rowing Injuries.* Forum Medicum, Inc., Pennsylvania, 1989.
[36] Howell DW. Musculoskeletal profile and incidence of musculoskeletal injuries in lightweight women rowers. *Am. J. Sports Med.* 1984; 12, 278-281.
[37] Hutchinson MR. Low back pain in elite rhythmic gymnasts. *Med. Sci. Sports. Exerc.* 1999; 31, 1686-1688.
[38] Jones MA, Stratton G, Reilly T, Unnithan VB. Biological risk indicators for recurrent non-specific low back pain in adolescents. *Br. J. Sports Med.* 2005; 39, 137-140.
[39] Kapandji IA. *Physiologie articulaire. 1. Membre supérieur.* Paris: Maloine, 5è édition, 1980.
[40] Kebaetse M, McClure P, Pratt NA. Thoracic position effect on shoulder range of motion, strength, and three-dimensional scapular kinematics. *Arch. Phys. Med. Rehabil.* 1999; 80, 945-950.
[41] Keller TS, Colloca CJ, Harrison DE, Harrison DD, Janik TJ. Influence of spine morphology on intervertebral disc loads and stresses in asymptomatic adults: implications for the ideal spine. *Spine J.* 2005; 5, 297-300.
[42] Kendall FP, McCreary EK, Provance PG, Rodgers MM, Romani WA. *Muscles: testing and function with posture and pain (5th ed.).* Baltimore: Lippincott Williams and Wilkins; 2005.
[43] Kraemer WJ. Strength training basics. Designing workouts to meet patients' goals. *PhysSportsmed* 2003; 31, 39-45.
[44] Kums T, Ereline J, Gapeyeva H, Pääsuke M, Vain A. Spinal curvature and trunk muscle tone in rhythmic gymnasts and untrained girls. *J. Back Musculoskeletal Rehabil.* 2007; 20, 87-95.
[45] Landers M, Barker G, Wallentine S, McWhorter JW, Peel C. A comparison of tidal volume, breathing frequency, and minute ventilation between two sitting postures in healthy adults. *Physiother. Theory Pract.* 2003; 19, 109-119.
[46] Legaye J, Duval-Beaupere G, Hecquet J, Marty C. Pelvis incidence: a fundamental pelvic parameter for three-dimensional regulation of spinal sagittal curves. *Eur. Spine J.* 1998; 7, 99-103.
[47] Levine D, Whittle MW. The effects of pelvic movement on lumbar lordosis in the standing position. *J. Orthop. Sports Phys. Ther.* 1996; 24, 130-135.
[48] Li Y, McClure PW, Pratt N. The effect of hamstring muscle stretching on standing posture and on lumbar and hip motions during forward bending. *Phys. Ther.* 1996; 76, 836-849.

[49] López-Miñarro PA, Alacid F, Ferragut C, García A. Valoración y comparación de la disposición sagital del raquis entre canoistas y kayakistas de categoría infantil. *Cult. Cien. Dep.* 2008; 9, 171-176.
[50] López-Miñarro PA, Alacid F, Muyor JM. Comparación del morfotipo raquídeo y extensibilidad isquiosural entre piragüistas y corredores. *Rev. Int. Med. Cienc. Act. Fís. Dep.* 2009; 36, 379-392.
[51] López-Miñarro PA, Alacid F, Rodríguez PL. Comparison of sagittal spinal curvatures and hamstring muscle extensibility among young elite paddlers and non-athletes. *Int. SportMed. J.* 2010; 11, 301-312.
[52] López-Miñarro PA, Alacid F. Influence of hamstring muscle extensibility on spinal curvatures in young athletes. *Sci. Sports* 2010; 25, 188-193.
[53] López-Miñarro PA, Muyor JM, Alacid F. Sagittal spinal curvatures and pelvic tilt in elite young kayakers. *Med. Sport* 2010; 63, 509-519.
[54] López-Miñarro PA, Rodríguez PL, Santonja F, Yuste JL, García A. Sagittal spinal curvatures in recreational weight lifters. *Arch. Med. Deporte* 2007; 122, 435-441.
[55] López-Miñarro PA, Rodríguez PL, Santonja FM, Yuste JL. Posture of thoracic spine during triceps-pushdown exercise. *Sci. Sports* 2008; 23, 183-185.
[56] López-Miñarro PA, Rodríguez PL, Santonja FM. Posture of the thoracic spine during latissimus dorsi pulldown behind the neck position exercise in recreational weight lifters. *Gazz. Med. Ital.* 2008; 168, 347-52.
[57] López-Miñarro PA, Rodríguez PL. Hamstring muscle extensibility influences the criterion-related validity of sit-and-reach and toe-touch tests. *J. Strength Cond. Res.* 2010; 24, 1013-1018.
[58] López-Miñarro PA, Rodríguez-García PL, Santonja F. Postura del raquis lumbar en el ejercicio de extensión de codo con mancuerna. *Rev. Int. Med. Cien. Act. Fís. Dep.* 2010; 37, 138-149.
[59] López-Miñarro PA, Sáinz de Baranda P, Rodríguez-García PL, Yuste JL. Comparison between sit-and-reach test and V sit-and-reach test in young adults. *Gazz. Med. Ital.* 2008; 167, 135-142.
[60] López-Miñarro PA, Sáinz de Baranda P, Rodríguez-García PL. A comparison of the sit-and-reach test and the back-saver sit-and-reach test in university students. *J. Sports Sci. Med.* 2009; 8, 116-122.
[61] López-Miñarro PA, Yuste JL, Rodríguez PL, Santonja F, Sáinz de Baranda P, García A. Disposición sagital del raquis lumbar y torácico en el ejercicio de curl de bíceps con barra en bipedestación. *Cult, Cien. Dep.* 2007; 7, 19-24.
[62] López-Miñarro PA. Comparación de la cifosis torácica entre varios ejercicios de acondicionamiento muscular para los miembros superiores. *Rev. And. Med. Dep.* 2009; 4, 110-115.
[63] Lord MJ, Small JM, Dinsay JM, Watkins RG. Lumbar lordosis: effects of sitting and standing. *Spine* 1997; 22, 2571-2574.
[64] Masharawi Y, Dar G, Peleg S, Steinberg N, Medlej B, May H, Abbas J, Hershkovitz I. A morphological adaptation of the thoracic and lumbar vertebrae to lumbar hyperlordosis in young and adult females. *Eur. Spine J.* 2010; 19, 768-773.
[65] McEvoy MP, Wilkie K, Williams MT. Anterior pelvic tilt in elite cyclists -A comparative matched pairs study. *Phys. Ther.* 2007; 8, 22-29.

[66] McGill SM, Brown S. Creep response of the lumbar spine to prolonged full flexion. *Clin. Biomech.* 1992; 7, 43-46.
[67] McGill SM. *Low back disorders. Evidence-Based prevention and rehabilitation.* Champaign, IL: Human Kinetics; 2002.
[68] Mejia EA, Hennrikus WL, Schwend RM, Emans JB. A prospective evaluation of idiopathic left thoracic scoliosis with MRI. *J. Pediatr. Orthop.* 1996; 16, 354-358.
[69] Mellin G, Poussa M. Spinal mobility and posture in 8- to 16-year-old children. *J. Orthop. Res.* 1992; 10, 211-216.
[70] Milne RA, Mierau DR. Hamstring distensibility in the general population: relationship to pelvic and back stresses. *J. Manipulative Physiol. Ther.* 1979; 2, 146-150.
[71] Muyor JM. Evaluación del morfotipo raquídeo en el plano sagital y extensibilidad isquiosural del ciclista. *Thesis disertation.* Almería, Spain, 2010.
[72] Nilsson C, Wykman A, Leanderson J. Spinal Sagittal mobility and joint laxity in young ballet dancers. *Knee Surg. Sports Traumatol. Arthroscopy* 1993; 1, 206-208.
[73] Norris CM, Matthews A. Correlation between hamstring muscle length and pelvic tilt during forward bending in healthy individuals: An initial evaluation. *J. Body. Mov. Ther.* 2006; 10, 122-126.
[74] Ohlén G, Wredmark T, Spandfort E. Spinal sagittal configuration and mobility related to low-back pain in the female gymnast. *Spine* 1989; 14, 847-850.
[75] Olson MW, Li L, Solomonow M. Flexion-relaxation response to cyclic lumbar flexion. *Clin. Biomech.* 2004; 19, 769-776.
[76] Perriman DM, Scarvell JM, Hughes AR, Ashman B, Lueck CJ, Smith PN. Validation of the flexible electrogoniometer for measuring thoracic kyphosis. *Spine* 2010; 35, E633-E640.
[77] Polga DJ, Beaubien BP, Kallemeier PM, Schellhas KP, Lee WD, Buttermann GR, Wood K. Measurement of in vivo intradiscal pressure in healthy thoracic intervertebral discs. *Spine* 2004; 29, 1320-1324.
[78] Poussa MS, Heliövaara MM, Seitsamo JT, Könönen MH, Hurmerinta KA, Nissinen MJ. Development of spinal posture in a cohort of children from the age of 11 to 22 years. *Eur. Spine J.* 2005; 14, 738-742.
[79] Rajabi R, Alizadeh M, Mobarakabadi L. Comparison of thoracic kyphosis in group of elite female hockey player and a group on on-athletic female subjects. *24th Universiade Banhkok. FISU Conference* 9-12, August, pp. 366-370, 2007.
[80] Rajabi R, Doherty P, Goodarzi M, Hemayattalab R. Comparison of thoracic kyphosis in two groups of elite Greco-Roman and free style wrestlers and a group of non-athletic subjects. *Br. J. Sports Med.* 2007; 42, 229-232.
[81] Rajabi R, Freemont A, Doherty P. The investigation of cycling position on thoracic spine. A novel method of measuring thoracic kyphosis in the standing position. *Arch. Phys. Bioch.* 2000; 1, 142.
[82] Reeves RK, Laskowski ER, Smith J. Weight training injuries. Part 2: Diagnosing and managing chronic conditions. *PhysSportsmed.* 1998; 26, 54-63.
[83] Reid D, McNair P. Factors contributing to low back pain in rowers. *Br. J. Sports Med.* 2000; 34, 321-325.
[84] Reid DA, McNair PJ. Passive force, angle, and stiffness changes after stretching of hamstring muscles. *Med. Sci. Sports Exerc.* 2004; 36, 1944-1948.

[85] Reid R, Fricker P, Kestermann O, Shakespear P. A profile of female rowers injuries and illnesses at the Australian Institute of Sport. *Excel* 1989; 5, 17-20.

[86] Rodríguez-García PL, Santonja F, López-Miñarro PA, Sáinz de Baranda P, Yuste JL. Effect of physical education programme on sit-and-reach score in schoolchildren. *Sci. Sports* 2008; 23, 170-175.

[87] Rodríguez-García PL, López-Miñarro PA, Yuste JL, and Sáinz de Baranda P. Comparison of hamstring criterion-related validity, sagittal spinal curvatures, pelvic tilt, and score between sit-and-reach and toe-touch tests in athletes. *Med. Sport* 2008; 61, 11-20.

[88] Rolls A, George K. The relationship between hamstring muscle injuries and hamstring muscle length in young elite footballers. *Phys. Ther. Sport* 2004; 5, 179-187.

[89] Roussouly P, Nnadi C. Sagittal plane deformity: an overview of interpretation and management. *Eur. Spine J.* 2010; 19, 1824-1836.

[90] Rusko H, Howard GK, Kuipers H, Renström P. Cross country skiing. In H. Rusko (Ed.), *Handbook of Sport Medicine and Science*. Oxford: Blackwell Science, 2003.

[91] Sahrmann SA. *Diagnosis and treatment of movement impairment syndromes*. St. Louis: Mosby, 2002.

[92] Salai M, Brosh T, Blankstein A, Oran A, Chechik A. Effect of changing the saddle angle on the incidence of low back pain in recreational bicyclists. *Br. J. Sports Med.* 1999; 33, 398-400.

[93] Santonja Medina FM, Sainz de Baranda Andújar P, Rodríguez García PL, López Miñarro PA, Canteras Jornada M. Effects of frequency of static stretching on straight-leg raise in elementary school children. *J. Sports Med. Phys. Fitness* 2007; 47, 304-308.

[94] Sato K, Kikuchi S, Yonezawa T. In vivo intradiscal pressure measurement in healthy individuals and in patients with ongoing back problems. *Spine* 1999; 24, 2468-2474.

[95] Scannell JP, McGill SM. Lumbar posture – should it, and can it, be modified? A study of passive tissue stiffness and lumbar position during activities of daily living. *Phys. Ther.* 2003; 83, 907-917.

[96] Schlegel JD, Smith JA, Schleusener RL. Lumbar motion segment pathology adjacent to thoracolumbar, lumbar, and lumbosacral fusions. *Spine* 1996; 21, 970-981.

[97] Scoles PV, Latimer BM, DigIovanni BF, Vargo E, Bauza S, Jellema LM. Vertebral alterations in Scheuermann's kyphosis. *Spine* 1991; 16, 509-515.

[98] Shin G, Shu Y, Li Z, Jiang Z, Mirka G. Influence of knee angle and individual flexibility on the flexion-relaxation response of the low back musculature. *J. Electrom. Kinesiol.* 2004; 14, 485-494.

[99] Simoneau GG. The impact of various anthropometric and flexibility measurements on the sit-and-reach test. *J. Strength Cond. Res.* 1998; 12, 232-237.

[100] Smith A, O'Sullivan P, Straker L. Classification of sagittal thoraco-lumbo-pelvic alignment of the adolescent spine in standing and its relationship to low back pain. *Spine* 2008; 33, 2101-2107.

[101] Solomonow M. Ligaments: a source of work-related musculoskeletal disorders. *J. Electromyogr. Kinesiol.* 2004; 14, 49-60.

[102] Stallard MC. Backache in oarsmen. *Br. J. Sports Med.* 1980; 14, 105-108.

[103] Stamford B. Weight training basics Part 2: A sample program. *PhysSportsmed* 1998; 26, 91-92.

[104] Steinberg EL, Luger E, Arbel R, Menachem A, Dekel S. A comparative roentgenographic analysis of the lumbar spine in male army recruits with and without lower back pain. *Clin. Radiol.* 2003; 58, 985-989.
[105] Stutchfield BM, Coleman S. The relationships between hamstring flexibility, lumbar flexion, and low back pain in rowers. *Eur. J. Sport Sci.* 2006; 6, 255-260.
[106] Tsai L, Wredmark T. Spinal posture, sagittal mobility, and subjective rating of back problems in former female elite gymnasts. *Spine* 1993; 18, 872-875.
[107] Tüzün C, Yorulmaz I, Cindaş A, Vatan S. Low back pain and posture. *Clin. Rheumatol.* 1999; 18, 308-312.
[108] Tully EA, Stillman BC. Computer-aided video analysis of vertebrofemoral motion during toe touching in healthy subjects. *Arch. Phys. Med. Rehab.* 1997; 78, 759-766.
[109] Uetake T, Ohsuki F, Tanaka H, Shindo M. The vertebral curvature of sportsmen. *J. Sports Sci.* 1998; 16, 621-628.
[110] Usabiaga J, Crespo R, Iza I, Aramendi J, Terrados N, Poza J. Adaptation of the lumbar spine to different positions in bicycle racing. *Spine* 1997; 22, 1965-1969.
[111] Wang SS, Whitney SL, Burdett RG, Janosky J. Lower extremity muscular flexibility in long distance runners. *J. Orthop. Sports Phys. Ther.* 1993; 17, 102-107.
[112] White SG, Sahrmann SA. A movement system balance approach to management of musculoskeletal pain. In: Grant R, editor. *Physical Therapy of the Cervical and Thoracic Spine*. Churchill: Livingstone; 1994. pp. 339-357.
[113] Widhe T. Spine: posture, mobility and pain. A longitudinal study from childhood to adolescence. *Eur. Spine J.* 2001; 10, 118-123.
[114] Wilke HJ, Neef P, Caimi M, Hoogland T, Claes LE. New in vivo measurements of pressures in the intervertebral disc in daily life. *Spine* 1999; 24, 755-762.
[115] Wilke HJ, Neef P, Hinz B, Seidel H, Claes LE. Intradiscal pressure together with anthropometric data - a data set for the validation of models. *Clin. Biomech.* 2001; 1, S111-S126.
[116] Wodecki P, Guigui P, Hanotel MC, Cardinne L, Deburge A. Sagittal alignment of the spine: comparison between soccer players and subjects without sports activities. *Rev. Chir. Orthop. Reparatrice Appar. Mot.* 2002; 88, 328-336.
[117] Wojtys E, Ashton-Miller J, Huston L, Moga PJ. The association between athletic training time and the sagittal curvature of the immature spine. *Am. J. Sports Med.* 2000; 28, 490-498.
[118] Young WB, Newton RU, Doyle T, Chapman D, Cormack S, Stewart G, Dawson B. Physiological and anthropometric characteristics of starters and non-starters and playing positions in elite Australian Rules football: a case study. *J. Sci. Med. Sport* 2005; 8, 333-345.

Chapter 4

# HUMAN STANDING POSTURE: MATHEMATICAL MODELS, THEIR BIOFIDELITY AND APPLICATIONS

### *P. B. Pascolo, G. Pagnacco and R. Rossi**

*Industrial Bioengineering Lab, DICA Department, University of Udine, Italy*

### ABSTRACT

In the last decades, several mathematical models of increased complexity have been developed with the goal of better understanding human standing posture and the mechanisms that control it. The sophistication and biofidelity of the models has increased from simple one-link inverted pendulum to full three-dimensional multi-link models. Although models have and continue to provide invaluable insights, they are still at this time too simple to allow the modeling of many pathological conditions and therefore much more work is needed in this field.

**Keywords**: Postural sway, equilibrium stability model, biofidelity, mathematical models

### INTRODUCTION

Standing is the static posture most commonly evaluated in balance assessments. This is because of its ubiquitous nature and because the act of precariously balancing two thirds of our body mass some distance from the ground "over two spindly structures" imposes critical

---

[*] Manuscript received on January 26, 2011
  PBP is with the Industrial Bioengineering Lab., DICA Department, University of Udine, 33100 Udine, Italy. (e-mail: paolo.pascolo@uniud.it).
  GP is with the Electrical and Computer Engineering Department, University of Wyoming, Laramie, WY, 82071, U.S.A.
  RR is with the Industrial Bioengineering Lab., DICA Department, University of Udine, 33100 Udine, Italy.

demands on the postural control system [Winter, 1987; Winter et al., 1990a]. The maintenance of a static posture, such as standing or sitting, produces spontaneous involuntary body movements termed postural sway that result from the neuromuscular corrective mechanisms acting to preserve that posture. To maintain standing balance, the postural control system integrates information from the visual, vestibular, and proprioceptive systems. Johassons [Johassons, 1991] reviewed a variety of topics related to human postural control, including biomechanics, neurophysiology, evaluation methods, and postural control models.

Postural stability is affected by the size and position of the body base of support, the height of the Center of Gravity (COG) above that base, the multi-segmented structure of the body, and the characteristic mobility of the supporting joints. Stability is maintained through the effort of many body structures, including the skin, joint capsules, ligaments, tendons and muscles. Stability control is provided by the central nervous system, which receives input from vestibular, visual, and proprioceptive sensors such the muscle spindles, and integrates these inputs to generate the overall tonic muscular activity.

Engineering analysis of posture have included measurements of elapsed standing times, ground reaction forces, center of pressure paths, joint angle trajectories, and muscle activation patterns during repeated stereotypical disturbances [Cordo and Nashner, 1982; Friendliet al., 1984; Woollacottet al.,1984; Chandler et al.,1990]. Similar biomechanical techniques have also been applied to the study of standing as restored to people with spinal cord injuries by external bracing or FNS (Functional Neuromuscular Stimulation) [Cybulski and Jaeger, 1986].

Over the years, various methods have been devised to quantify postural stability [Fregly, 1974; Jarret, 1976; Andres, 1979]. The most common measures of postural sway are based on the measurement of the ground reaction forces and the displacement of the Center of Pressure (COP) as the subject stands on one or more platforms equipped with force transducers (force platforms). The COP is defined as the centroid of the vertical force distribution [Elftman, 1934; Cavanagh, 1980], or as the intercept of the resolved wrench axis with the force plate surface [Shimba, 1984; Soutas-Little, 1990]. These two definitions are equivalent if horizontal forces between the feet and the ground are negligible. Using force platforms, the entire activity of the postural control system is studied by observing how well the subject maintain the COP within the foot support base.

Under static conditions, the COP coincides with the vertical projection of the COG. Generally, the displacement of the COP is greater in magnitude and frequency than the displacement of the COG [Winter, 1990b]. The COG is a function of body segment position [Riley et al., 1990], whereas the COP is the centroid of the applied body forces acting on the support surface. The COP movements are driven by the neuromuscular control signal (vector of joint torques) acting to position the COG [Murray et al., 1967; Riley et al., 1990; Ruder et al.,1989] and preserve a stable posture, whereas the COG position is the variable being controlled [Patlaet al.,1989]. Only for a statically stable body is the projection of the COG coincident with the COP [Schenkman, 1989]; otherwise there is a difference due to dynamic effects [Murray et al., 1967; Gurfinkel, 1973; Spaepenet al., 1977; Koozekananiet al., 1980; Shimba, 1984].

Evaluation of a patient's ability to maintain postural stability has been a routine part of the neurological examination since the Romberg's test was introduced over a century and a half ago [Romberg, 1853]. Earlier studies of postural stability were primarily based on the measurement of static equilibrium during quiet standing [Harris, 1986]. In static posturography, the sensory inputs from visual, proprioceptive, and vestibular system are overlapping and partially redundant. As a result, some investigators have suggested that dynamic equilibrium testing may provide a more sensitive method for detecting various balance disorders [Nashner and Wollacott, 1979; Andres and Anderson, 1980]. The premise is that translational and/or rotational perturbations of the patient's support base and visual surrounding activate all of the sensorimotor control mechanisms and are more likely to unmask subtle abnormalities of the system.

Clinical and experimental protocols for COP measurement are highly variable. For instance, different stances are evaluated in different studies, depending on the sensory and motor performance as well as the physical ability of the patient or study population. Most evaluations are variations of the Romberg's test and involve having the subject stand on the platform on both feet with eyes open or with eyes closed. The forces and moments applied by the subject are acquired over a fixed time interval [Kapteynet al., 1983]. Most studies include several repetitions of each stance, such as tandem stance [Patlaet al., 1989; Goldie et al., 1989], standing on a compliant surface [Bhattacharya et al., 1987], and standing on one leg [Lichtenstein et al., 1988; Frank et al., 1989; Hasanet al., 1990a; Hasanet al., 990b; Robin et al., 1991]. A few investigators use the force signals [Goldie et al., 1989] or the vertical torques [Soutas-Little et al., 1991] for balance assessment. More commonly, the acquired force and moment data are used to compute the COP coordinates.

One population group that has been a focus of balance studies is the elderly [Sheldon, 1963; Murray et al., 1975; Hasselkus and Shambes, 1975; Overstallet al., 1977; Imms and Edholm, 1981; Brocklehurstet al., 1982; Era and Heikkinen, 1985; Ring et al., 1988], for whom falls result in high morbidity and mortality rates [Miller, 1978; Weiss et al., 1983; Baker and Harvey, 1985]. Some of the studies [Overstallet al.,1977; Ring et al., 1988] have shown the reliability of sway measurement in detecting subjects likely to be at risk of falling, while others [Brocklehurstet al.,1982; Lichtenstein et al.,1988] have examined clinical correlates.

Although measures of postural sway can describe how a person stands, they provide little insight into the mechanisms used to maintain the desired posture. In other words, they are a measure of the outcome, not a description of how such a result is obtained. For that it is necessary to model the standing human in terms of its biomechanics as well as its neuromuscular control system. Creating models offers a way to better understanding the system being modeled, as for a model to be able to represent and functionally replicate a real system it has to contain most or all the elements that make the real system work as it does. It also allows to investigate how changes can produce results sometimes observed in reality, for instance how a specific pathology might affect human postural stability.

Hence, over the years, several mathematical models of human postural stability have been created. Sometimes these were created to investigate specific aspects or theories of the overall topic of human postural control. Other times, more general models capable of providing insight into more complicate issues of the interaction of different aspects have been developed.

## MATHEMATICAL MODELS

To better understand how a person can maintain an erect posture and especially to investigate the control strategies involved, mathematical models have been developed over the years [Smith, 1957;Hemamiand Jaswa, 1978;Stockwell, 1981; Winter, 2003]. These have increased their level of complexity and sophistication starting from very simple, one-degree of freedom inverted pendulum models without an active control system [Smith, 1957], all the way to 3-D, multi-link models with active musculature [Loram, 2005; Winter, 2003]. This increase in the complexity and sophistication of the models has been necessary to improve their biofidelity and has been possible thanks to the better understanding of human physiology as well as the advances in the computational tools available to researchers.

Although the models are several, they can be grouped in "families" based on their main characteristics: following is an overview of these "families" of models, their characteristics, and their limitations, in order of their increased complexity and biofidelity.

### One-Link Inverted Pendulum Model

The simpler way to model a standing human being is to use a planar (2-D), one-degree of freedom inverted pendulum [Smith, 1957; Winter et al., 1998; Morasso and Sanguineti, 2002; Loram and Lakie, 2002; Peterka et al., 2002; Bottaro et al., 2005]. In this model, the only joint considered is the ankle joint, and the entire body is modeled as a single mass m connected to the ankle joint by a mass-less rigid link. The ankle joint constrains the movement of the system so that only rotation of the joint is allowed. Therefore, the only movement the model can have is a planar oscillation θ around the ankle in the sagittal plane.

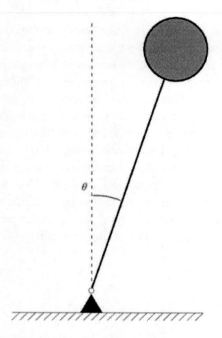

Figure 1. One-link inverted pendulum model [Pascolo 2009].

The hypothesis behind this model is that the simplest postural control strategy employed by humans is the so called "ankle strategy", consisting in maintaining the desired posture only by controlling the torque in the ankle joint. Under this assumption, a standing person can be assimilated to a rigid body with an equivalent mass, lumped in the location of the subject's center of mass, and rotating around the ankle joint. The effects of the mass and inertia distribution as well as the possible rotation around the other joints (knee, hip, and spine) are neglected.

When looking at the mathematical formulation of this model, the equation describing the equilibrium around the ankle joint is:

$$J \cdot \ddot{\theta} = m \cdot g \cdot h \cdot sin\theta - C_a + Z_{eq} \qquad (1)$$

where $\theta$ (Figure 1) is the clockwise rotation angle, $h$ is the link length (the distance between the COM and the ankle joint), $m$ and $J = J_g + m \cdot h^2$ are respectively the mass of the body as a lumped mass (without considering the feet) and its moment of inertia with respect to the ankle joint, $C_a$ is the torque due to the muscle activation and internal stiffness, torque that can be considered as a pure moment applied to the ankle joint, and $Z_{eq}$ represents the effects of internal as well as external perturbations. Often times, the internal perturbations, such as the effect of the breathing cycle [Hunter, 1981], cardiac activity [Buizza, 2003], visceral contractions, etc., are neglected, whereas some models include external perturbations such as the movements of the support surface [Welch, 2008].

It is possible to obtain the equations relating the movement of the center of pressure with the angle $\theta$ by considering the reaction forces on the ankle joint:

$$\begin{cases} F_v = m \cdot g - F_{i,v} - R_{eq,v} = m \cdot g - m \cdot a_v - R_{eq,v} \\ F_h = F_{i,h} - R_{eq,h} = m \cdot a_h - R_{eq,h} \end{cases} \qquad (2)$$

where $F_v$ and $F_h$ are respectively the vertical and horizontal ground reaction forces, $F_{i,v} = m$ and $F_{i,h} = m$ are the vertical and horizontal components of the inertia of the mass, $R_{eq,v}$ and $R_{eq,h}$ and are the vertical and horizontal components of the resultant internal and external perturbations.

Considering the kinematics of the model:

$$\begin{cases} a_v = h \cdot (-\ddot{\theta} \cdot sin\theta - \dot{\theta}^2 \cdot cos\theta) \\ a_h = h \cdot (-\ddot{\theta} \cdot cos\theta - \dot{\theta}^2 \cdot sin\theta) \end{cases} \qquad (3)$$

Furthermore, assuming small oscillations $sin\ \theta \approx 0$. In conditions of upright static posture

$m \cdot g \gg -m \cdot a_v - F_i$, so Eq. (2) becomes:

$$\begin{cases} F_v \approx m \cdot g \\ F_h \approx m \cdot h \cdot \ddot{\theta} \cdot \cos\theta - R_{eq,h} \end{cases} \quad (4)$$

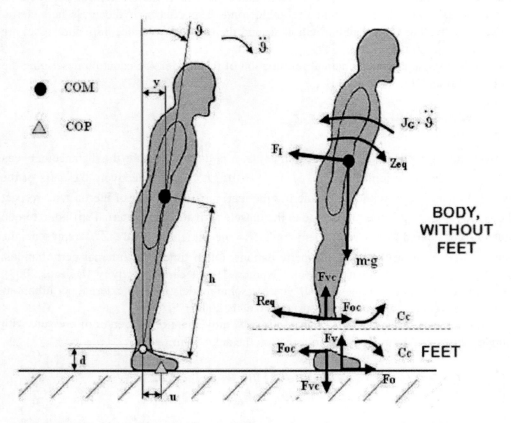

Figure 2. Forces and moments applied to the one-link inverted pendulum model[Pascolo, 2009]

Considering the equation representing the equilibrium of moments around the ankle joint relative to the foot (see Figure 2):

$$C_a = F_v \cdot u + F_h \cdot d \quad (5)$$

where $d$ represents the constant vertical distance of the ankle joint from the support surface and $u$ is the variable horizontal distance between the location of the COP and the ankle joint.

Substituting Eq. (5) into Eq. (4) and then into Eq. (1):

$$J_G \cdot \ddot{\theta} + m \cdot h^2 \cdot \ddot{\theta} - m \cdot h \cdot d \cdot \cos\theta \cdot$$
$$= m \cdot g \cdot h \cdot \sin\theta - m \cdot g \cdot u + R_{eq,h} \cdot d + \quad (6)$$

Considering that $h \gg d$, then $m \cdot h^2 \cdot \ddot{\theta} \gg m \cdot h \cdot d \cdot \cos\theta \cdot \ddot{\theta}$. Furthermore, because of small oscillations, $\sin\theta \approx 0$. Also, shear forces are commonly very small, therefore $R_{eq,h} \cdot d \ll$. Under these assumption Eq. (6) can be simplified as:

$$J_G \cdot \ddot{\theta} = m \cdot g \cdot (y - u) + Z_{eq} \qquad (7)$$

where y represents the horizontal displacement of the COM.

But under the hypothesis of small oscillations, $\ddot{y} = h \cdot \ddot{\theta}$, therefore:

$$\ddot{y} = \alpha(y - u) + \tilde{Z}_{eq} \qquad (8)$$

This equation shows how the horizontal acceleration $\ddot{y}$ of the COM is closely proportional to the horizontal distance COM-COP (Figure 3).

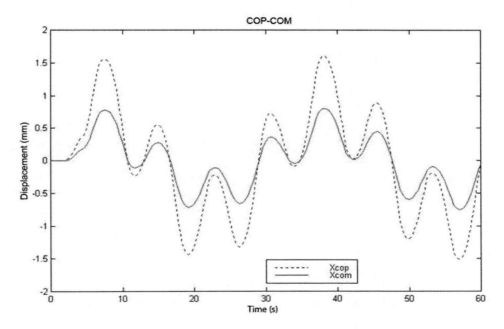

Figure 3. Anterior-posterior COP-COM plot for the one-link inverted pendulum model[Roiatti, 2003].

The major limitations of the one-degree of freedom inverted pendulum model arise from the underlying hypothesis that the principal strategy used in maintaining the erect standing posture in humans is the so called ankle strategy. This is a rough and crude simplification as it fails to consider motor strategies based on rotations of other joints and body segments, including but not limited to knee, hip, trunk, shoulder, elbow and neck joints. Although it can be experimentally observed that the angle of rotation of the ankle is often larger than that around the aforementioned joints, they are nevertheless important [Pinter, 2008]. Furthermore, the oscillation frequency around these joints is often higher than that around the ankle joint [Valk Fai, 1973]. As the angular velocity is proportional to the oscillation frequency and the angular acceleration is proportional to the square of the frequency, the magnitude of these kinematic variables can become large even in other joints besides the ankle which have smaller angles of rotation. Considering the kinetics of the system, the kinetic energy depends on the square of the angular velocity and the inertial torques are proportional to the segment's angular acceleration, so that both are proportional to the square of the frequency of oscillation and therefore can be significant if the frequency is high even if the amplitudes are small.

It is also clear how this model does not consider stability outside the sagittal plane, as the movements are constrained to occur in this plane only, whereas in reality a person's sway occurs both in the sagittal and the coronal plane.

Another limitation, although this is not proper of the type of model but rather is caused by some further common simplifications, is that often when using this model the terms $m \cdot h \cdot d \cdot \cos\theta \cdot \ddot{\theta}$ and $R_{eq,h} \cdot d$ in (6) are neglected. This is equivalent to neglecting the term $F_h \cdot d$ in (5), but although $F_h \ll F_d$ it must be considered that $d$ is in the range of $70 \div 80$ mm and $u$ is $30 \div 50$ mm, so in (5) $F_h \cdot d$ is comparable $F_h \cdot u$, thus neglecting those two terms in (6) can be an over-simplification resulting in less then realistic results.

As the only degree of freedom of this model is the rotation around the ankle joint, control mechanisms providing the necessary joint stabilization torque can be modeled in several relatively simple ways. These can range from a very simple linear torsional spring, to a non-linear torsional spring, to a spring and damper system, all the way to an active feedback-based actuator system, either linear or non-linear. It is also possible to provide the stabilization torque using geometrically linear passive or active elements to represent the relevant tendon and muscles [Gurfinkel, 1972].

Regarding the comparison of simulations conducted using this type of model and experimental observations, some studies [Winter, 1998] have shown how, considering Eq. (8) with a negligible $Z_{eq}$, the horizontal acceleration $\ddot{y}$ of the COM is closely proportional to the horizontal distance COM-COP i.e.$(y - u)$. Other studies [Roiatti, 2001] on the other hand suggest that such a proportional relationship does not exist in reality further suggesting the over-simplification of this type of model.

As with other models of postural dynamics, one way of estimating its biofidelity is to compare the results of the simulations using the model and experimental COP recordings. Figure 3 shows the results for a feedback control system and Figure 4 some experimental results.

Qualitatively it is rather clear how the experimental COP movement appears to be much more complex and perturbed than the model's.

Concluding, it is clear how, although this model has the advantage of being simple and easily understandable and implementable, it is only a first approximation of the real system and as such it can only provide some basic qualitative insights into the inner workings of the postural mechanisms in humans.

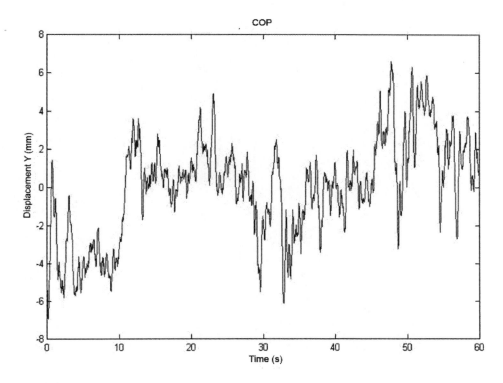

Figure 4. Anterior-posterior COP plot obtained using experimental data[Roiatti, 2003].

## Multi-Link Inverted Pendulum Model

For a more in depth investigation of the mechanics and the control strategies of the standing human posture it is necessary to overcome some of the limitations of the single inverted pendulum model. This has brought the development of models consisting of two or more segments, allowing the studying of how the increased number of degrees of freedom affect the postural control strategies.

In several studies [Aramakiet al., 2001; Creathet al., 2005; Alexandrovet al., 2005] the analysis of the experimental kinematic data of several body joints collected during static erect standing from healthy middle aged subjects in the absence of external perturbations has shown how important it is to consider not only the ankle strategy, i.e. the rotation of the ankle joint, but also the hip strategy, i.e. the rotation of the hip joint. If a model is to be used in investigating such strategy it is necessary for it to incorporate at least two degrees of freedom, i.e. to incorporate both the ankle and the hip joint.

The first model to incorporate both the hip and the ankle joint is the double inverted pendulum [Hemami, 1978]. Similarly to the single inverted pendulum previously examined, this model is usually two-dimensional and its movements are constrained to the sagittal plane. It consists of three bodies (feet, lower extremities, and the rest of the body above the hip) represented by two rigid segments (the feet are constrained to the support surface and therefore not considered) connected by two rotational joints (the ankle and the hip) as illustrated in Figure 5.

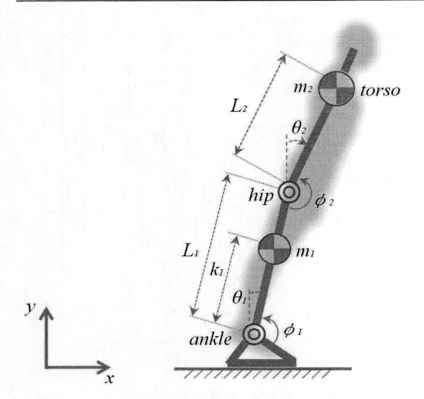

Figure 5. Double-link inverted pendulum with the ankle $\theta_1$ and hip $\theta_2$ joints [Li, 2010].

Although this model is an obvious improvement compared to the single link model, experimental investigations of the muscular electrical activity [Pinter, 2008] as well as motion analysis investigations using infrared cameras and markers [Stockwell, 1981; Wei-Li-Hsu, 2008] have shown that while maintaining a static erect posture several other joints besides the hip and the ankle are in continuous motion, suggesting that models incorporating more segments connected by more joints, and hence having more degrees of freedom, could even more accurately represent the actual human body. For this reason, models with 3 joints [Hemami and Jaswa, 1978] and then 4 joints [Stockwell, 1981] have been introduced. In particular, the 4-joints models consist of five rigid bodies (feet, legs, thighs, torso and upper extremities, head) represented by four rigid segments (the feet are constrained to the support surface and therefore not considered) connected by four rotational joints (ankle, knee, hip and neck) as illustrated in Figure 6.

Even the equations for a double inverted pendulum are quite complicated and difficult to be studied in closed form. When more joints are present, solving the equations in closed form is almost impossible. Hence for these models once the equations for each segment are obtained, the model is usually solved numerically. In general, it is quite easy to obtain the equations governing a n-segments model. Considering two-dimensional models, each segments has three degrees of freedom consisting of two translations and one rotation. The model is therefore represented by 3n equations and every segment is subjected to forces and torques representing the inertial effects, the reaction or joint forces exchanged with the neighboring segments, the internal and external perturbations, and the muscular activity necessary to maintain the posture.

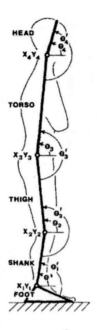

Figure 6. Four-link inverted pendulum with the ankle $\theta_1$, knee $\theta_2$, hip $\theta_3$, and neck $\theta_4$ joints [modified from Stockwell 1981].

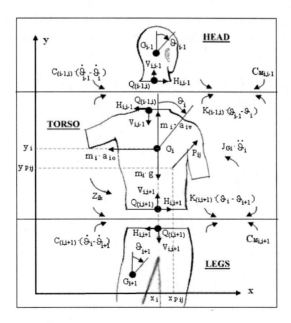

Figure 7. Schematic representation of the geometry, forces and moments acting on each body segment[Pascolo, 2009].

## Table 1. Nomenclature used in the n-segmental model equations

| SYMBOL | DESCRIPTION |
|---|---|
| $\theta_i$ | angular displacement of (i) segment, clockwise from vertical ax |
| $l_i$ | (i) segment lenght |
| $G_i$ | (i) segment COM |
| $l_{gi}$ | distance between joint (i) and (i) segment COM |
| $x_i, y_i$ | (i) segment COM coordinates |
| $a_{io}, a_{iv}$ | (i) segment COM horizontal and vertical acceleration |
| $W_i = m_i \cdot g$ | weight of (i) segment |
| $J_{Gi}$ | Inertial moment of (i) segment |
| $P_{i,j}$ | j-th perturbation force on (i) segment |
| $x_{P_{ij}}, y_{P_{ij}}$ | j-th perturbation force on (i) segment coordinates |
| $Z_{i,j}$ | j-th perturbation torque on (i) segment |
| $Q_{i,i\pm 1}$ | joint position between (i) and (i±1) segments |
| $H_{i,i\pm 1}$ | horizontal force between (i) and (i±1) segments |
| $V_{i,i\pm 1}$ | vertical force between (i) and (i±1) segments |
| $T_{i,i\pm 1}$ | muscular torque between (i) and (i±1) segments |
| $K_{i,i\pm 1} \cdot (\theta_i - \theta_{i\pm 1})$ | torque due to elasticity between (i) and (i±1) segments |
| $C_{i,i\pm 1} \cdot (\dot{\theta}_i - \dot{\theta}_{i\pm 1})$ | torque due to viscosity between (i) and (i±1) segments |

In general, considering the coordinate system adopted in Figure 7, each segment *i* is connected to the segments *(i-1)* and *(i+1)* by two rotational joints. According to the nomenclature reported in Table 1, the equilibrium equations for each segments are as follows:

Horizontal translation:

$$-m_i \cdot a_{i,h} + \sum_{j=1}^{m} P_{ij,h} + H_{(i,i+1)} \tag{8}$$

Vertical translation:

$$-W_i - m_i \cdot a_{i,v} + \sum_{j=1}^{m} P_{ij,v} + V_{(i,i+1)} \tag{9}$$

Rotation:

$$J_{Gi} \cdot \ddot{\theta}_i + m_i \cdot a_{i,h} \cdot y_i + m_i \cdot a_{i,v} \cdot x_i +$$

*(inertial contribution)*

$$+ \sum_{k=1}^{o} Z_{ij} + \sum_{j=1}^{m} (-P_{ij,h} \cdot y_{Pij} + P_{ij,v} \cdot x_{Pij}) - m_i \cdot g \cdot x_i +$$

(perturbation +self weight)

$$+V_{i,i+1} \cdot x_{Q(i,i+1)} - V_{i-1,i} \cdot x_{Q(i-1,i)} +$$

(vertical reaction to the joints)

$$+H_{i,i+1} \cdot y_{Q(i,i+1)} - H_{i-1,i} \cdot y_{Q(i-1}$$
(10)

(horizontal reaction to the joints)

$$+K_{i,i+1} \cdot (\theta_i - \theta_{i+1}) - K_{i-1,i} \cdot (\theta_{i-1} - \theta_i) +$$

(torque due to the elasticity)

$$+C_{i,i+1} \cdot (\dot{\theta}_i - \dot{\theta}_{i+1}) - C_{i-1,i} \cdot (\dot{\theta}_{i-1} - \dot{\theta}_i) +$$

(torque due to the viscosity)

$$+T_{i-1,i} - T_{i,i+1}$$

(torque due to muscular activity)

When Equations (8), (9), and (10) are solved simultaneously for each segment i, it is possible to calculate the overall torque $C_a$ applied to the ankle joint, as the sum of all the torques applied to each joint. Therefore, it is possible to obtain the movement of the COP with respect to the movement of the COM (see Figure 8).

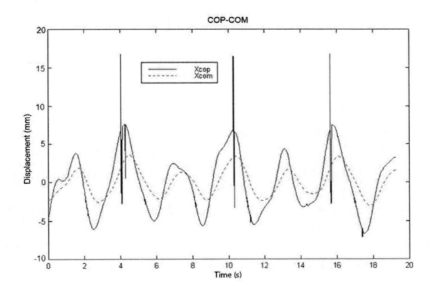

Figure 8. Anterior-posterior COP-COM plot for the four-link inverted pendulum model[Roiatti, 2003].

The results obtained using multi-link inverted pendulum models (with 4 or 5 degrees of freedoms [Stockwell, 1981; Pascolo and Roiatti, 2003]) qualitatively resemble much more the experimental results compared to what is obtained using more simple models. And using 4-5 segments as well as linearizing the equations does not preclude the possibility of including the major movement control strategies used by the human neuro-muscular system.

Considering the movement of the COP in the anterior-posterior plane (Figure 8) and in the mediolateral plane (Figure 9), and introducing an optimum feedback control mechanism based on the minimization of the energy, the oscillations obtained from the model are similar to those measured experimentally:

- A-P model: ≈13mm of harmonic oscillation at a frequency <0.5Hz
- M-L model: ≈10mm of biharmonic oscillation at a frequency <1.2Hz

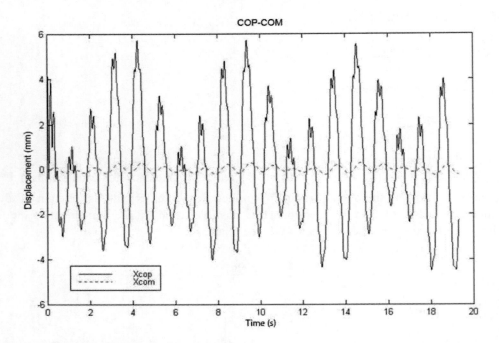

Figure 9.Medio-lateral COP-COM plot for the four-link inverted pendulum model[Roiatti, 2003].

The behavior of the COP-COM plots are quite repetitive, lacking the pseudo-randomness found in the experimental results: this can be explained considering that the internal perturbations $P_{i,j}$ used in the model to simulate the breathing and the cardiac contractions are by definition repetitive.

The major limitations of the dynamic of these models, which are highly unstable is which control mechanism is used and how it is implemented. Therefore their biofidelity is limited. Moreover the models are by definition bi-dimensional, thus the behavior in the anterior-posterior and in the medio-lateral planes can only be simulated one at a time. This is a serious limitation as in reality the oscillations in the two planes are coupled. Furthermore, it is not possible for these models to build the statokinesiogram (SKG), i.e. the representation of the path followed by the COP on the support surface as seen from above.

## Coupled 2d Multi-Link Inverted Pendulum Model

The intrinsic limitations of the bi-dimensional models are overcome by considering models that couple two 2D multi-link inverted pendulum models, one in the sagittal and one in the frontal plane respectively. Figure 10 shows one of such models [Roiatti, 2003] where the sagittal model has four degrees of freedom, and the frontal has three.

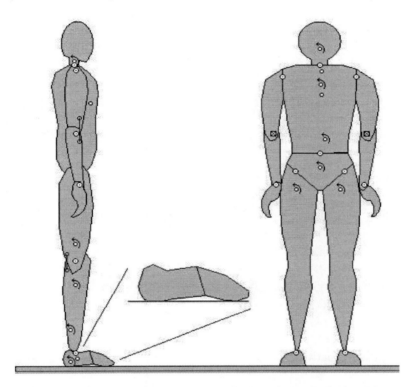

Figure 10. 2D coupled model: anterior-posterior and medio-lateral view[Roiatti, 2003].

Since certain movements such as the forward motion of the head and trunk produce lateral adjustments of the erect posture in order to maintain the equilibrium, it becomes paramount to define the interactions between the torques applied to the two models, since they are not indeed independent. This approach, known as pseudo-modal, allows to partially simulate some of the 3D aspects of the neuromuscular control system.

The reaction forces and angular displacements between each segment of the model, as well as the effects of the internal and external perturbations, are usually calculated using non-linear differential equations solved using algorithms such as the Newton-Rapson, whereas once the control mechanism, based on feedback mechanisms, is introduced in the equations, these are linearized to have a mathematical stable solution of the problem. This can be done, since the equations are solved around the equilibrium point, therefore $sin\theta \approx \theta \; e \; cos\theta \approx 1; \dot{\theta} \cdot \theta \approx 0$ for small angles of rotation and for low oscillation frequencies.

Considering Equation (10) and using the nomenclature defined in Table 1, the sagittal model of Figure 10, comprising the head, trunk, thighs and shanks, can be described mathematically using four differential equations. Considering first the equilibrium of the shanks (segment 1) around the ankle joints (Figure 11), the equation becomes:

$$J_{G1} \cdot \ddot{\theta}_1 = m_1 \cdot a_{1,h} \cdot l_{g1} \cdot \cos\varphi_1 + m_1 \cdot a_{1,v} \cdot l_{g1} \cdot \sin\varphi_1 +$$

(inertial contribution)

$$-m_1 \cdot g \cdot l_{g1} \cdot \sin\varphi_1 +$$

(self weight)

$$V_{1,2} \cdot l_1 \cdot \sin\varphi_1 + H_{1,2} \cdot l_1 \cdot \cos\varphi_1 \qquad (11)$$

(vertical and horizontal reaction to the joints)

$$-K_{1,2} \cdot (\theta_1 - \theta_2) + K_{0,1} \cdot (\theta_1) +$$

(torque due to the elasticity)

$$-C_{1,2} \cdot (\dot{\theta}_1 - \dot{\theta}_2) + C_{0,1} \cdot (\dot{\theta}_1) +$$

(torque due to the viscosity)

$$+T_1 - T_2$$

(torque due to muscular activity)

Considering only small movements around the equilibrium point, it is possible to linearize Equation (11):

$$[J_{G1} + l_{g1}^2 \cdot m_1 + l_1^2 \cdot (m_2 + m_3 + m_4)] \cdot \frac{d^2\varphi_1}{dt^2} =$$
$$= g[l_{g1} \cdot m_1 + l_1 \cdot (m_2 + m_3 + m_4)] \cdot \varphi_1 + T_1 - T_2 +$$
$$-l_1 \cdot \frac{d^2\varphi_2}{dt^2} \cdot [l_{g2} \cdot m_2 + l_2 \cdot (m_3 + m_4)] - l_1 \cdot \frac{d^2\varphi_3}{dt^2} \qquad (12)$$
$$\cdot (m_3 \cdot l_{g3} + m_4 \cdot l_3) - l_1 \cdot \frac{d^2\varphi_4}{dt^2} \cdot l_{g4} \cdot m_4 - K_{0,1} \cdot \varphi_1 +$$
$$-C_{0,1} \cdot \frac{d\varphi_1}{dt} - K_{1,2} \cdot (\varphi_1 - \varphi_2) - C_{1,2} \left(\frac{d\varphi_1}{dt} - \frac{d\varphi_2}{dt}\right)$$

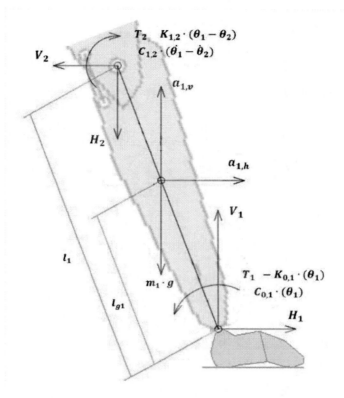

Figure 11. Forces and torques applied to segment 1, the shank [Roiatti, 2003].

Similarly, considering the equilibrium of the thighs (segment 2), trunk (segment 3) and head (segment 4), the linearized equations become respectively:

$$[J_{G2} + l_{g2}^2 \cdot m_2 + l_2^2 \cdot (m_3 + m_4)] \cdot \frac{d^2\varphi_2}{dt^2} =$$
$$= g[l_{g2} \cdot m_2 + l_2 \cdot (m_3 + m_4)] \cdot \varphi_2 + T_2 - T_3 +$$
$$- l_1 \cdot \frac{d^2\varphi_1}{dt^2} \cdot [l_{g2} \cdot m_2 + (m_3 + m_4) \cdot l_2] - l_2 \cdot \frac{d}{i} \quad (13)$$

$$(m_3 \cdot l_{g3} + m_4 \cdot l_3) - l_2 \cdot \frac{d^2\varphi_4}{dt^2} \cdot l_{g4} \cdot m_4 + K_{1,2} \cdot (\varphi_1 - \varphi_2) +$$
$$+ C_{1,2} \cdot \left(\frac{d\varphi_1}{dt} - \frac{d\varphi_2}{dt}\right) - K_{2,3} \cdot (\varphi_2 - \varphi_3) - C_{2,3}\left(\frac{d\varphi_2}{dt} - \frac{d\varphi_3}{dt}\right)$$

$$[J_{G3} + l_{g3}^2 \cdot m_3 + l_3^2 \cdot m_4] \cdot \frac{d^2\varphi_3}{dt^2} =$$
$$= g[l_{g3} \cdot m_3 + l_3 \cdot m_4] \cdot \varphi_3 + T_3 - T_4 +$$
$$- l_1 \cdot \frac{d^2\varphi_1}{dt^2} \cdot [l_{g3} \cdot m_3 + m_4 \cdot l_3] - l_2 \cdot \frac{d}{t} \quad (14)$$

$$(m_3 \cdot l_{g3} + m_4 \cdot l_3) - l_3 \cdot \frac{d^2\varphi_4}{dt^2} \cdot l_{g4} \cdot m_4 + K_{2,3} \cdot (\varphi_2 - \varphi_3) +$$

$$+C_{2,3} \cdot \left(\frac{d\varphi_2}{dt} - \frac{d\varphi_3}{dt}\right) - K_{3,4} \cdot (\varphi_3 - \varphi_4) - C_{3,4} \cdot \left(\frac{d\varphi_3}{dt} - \frac{d\varphi_4}{dt}\right)$$

$$[J_{G4} + l_{g4}^2 \cdot m_4] \cdot \frac{d^2\varphi_4}{dt^2} =$$

$$= g \cdot l_{g4} \cdot m_4 \cdot \varphi_4 + M_4 +$$

$$-l_1 \cdot \frac{d^2\varphi_1}{dt^2} \cdot l_{g4} \cdot m_4 - l_2 \cdot \frac{d}{t} \quad (15)$$

$$\cdot m_4 \cdot l_{g4} - l_3 \cdot \frac{d^2\varphi_3}{dt^2} \cdot l_{g4} \cdot m_4 + K_{3,4} \cdot (\varphi_3 - \varphi_4) +$$

$$+C_{3,4} \cdot \left(\frac{d\varphi_3}{dt} - \frac{d\varphi_4}{dt}\right)$$

where the subscripts *0*, *1*, *2*, *3*, and *4* represent respectively the different segments, with the feet being segment 0.

Similarly, the frontal model of Figure 10, comprising the head, trunk and legs, can be described mathematically using three linearized differential equations:

$$[J_{G1} + l_{g1}^2 \cdot m_1 + l_1^2 \cdot (m_2 + m_3)] \cdot \frac{d^2\varphi_1}{dt^2} =$$

$$= g[l_{g1} \cdot m_1 + l_1 \cdot (m_2 + m_3)] \cdot \varphi_1 + T_1 - T_2 +$$

$$-l_1 \cdot \frac{d^2\varphi_2}{dt^2} \cdot [l_{g2} \cdot m_2 + l_2 \cdot m_3] - l_2 \cdot \frac{d}{t} \quad (16)$$

$$\cdot (m_3 \cdot l_{g3}) - K_{0,1} \cdot \varphi_1 +$$

$$-C_{0,1} \cdot \frac{d\varphi_1}{dt} - K_{1,2} \cdot (\varphi_1 - \varphi_2) - C_{1,2} \cdot \left(\frac{d\varphi_1}{dt} - \frac{d\varphi_2}{dt}\right)$$

$$[J_{G2} + l_{g2}^2 \cdot m_2 + l_2^2 \cdot m_3] \cdot \frac{d^2\varphi_2}{dt^2} =$$

$$= g[l_{g2} \cdot m_2 + l_2 \cdot m_3] \cdot \varphi_2 + T_2 - T_3 +$$

$$-l_1 \cdot \frac{d^2\varphi_1}{dt^2} \cdot [l_{g2} \cdot m_2 + m_3 \cdot l_2] - l_2 \cdot \frac{d}{t} \quad (17)$$

$$(m_3 \cdot l_{g3}) + K_{1,2} \cdot (\varphi_1 - \varphi_2) +$$

$$+C_{1,2} \cdot \left(\frac{d\varphi_1}{dt} - \frac{d\varphi_2}{dt}\right) - K_{2,3} \cdot (\varphi_2 - \varphi_3) - C_{2,3} \cdot \left(\frac{d\varphi_2}{dt} - \frac{d\varphi_3}{dt}\right)$$

$$[J_{G3} + l_{g3}^2 \cdot m_3] \cdot \frac{d^2\varphi_3}{dt^2} =$$

$$= g \cdot l_{g3} \cdot m_3 \cdot \varphi_3 + T_3 +$$

$$-l_1 \cdot \frac{d^2\varphi_1}{dt^2} \cdot l_{g3} \cdot m_3 - l_2 \cdot \frac{d}{t} \quad (18)$$

$$(m_3 \cdot l_{g3}) + K_{2,3} \cdot (\varphi_2 - \varphi_3) +$$

$$+C_{2,3} \cdot \left(\frac{d\varphi_2}{dt} - \frac{d\varphi_3}{dt}\right)$$

where the subscripts *0*, *1*, *2*, and *3* represent respectively the different segments, with the feet being segment 0, the legs segment 1, the trunk segment 2, and the head segment 3.

Using a matrix formulation, Equations (12-15) and Equations (16-18) can be written as:

$$\underline{a_s} \cdot \underline{\ddot{\varphi}} = \underline{b_s} \cdot \underline{\varphi} + \underline{c_s} \cdot \underline{M} \quad \text{(Sagittal model)} \tag{19}$$

$$\underline{a_f} \cdot \underline{\ddot{\varphi}} = \underline{b_f} \cdot \underline{\varphi} + \underline{c_f} \cdot \underline{M} \quad \text{(Frontal model)} \tag{20}$$

where $\underline{a}$ is the mass matrix (diagonal), $\underline{b}$ is the stiffness matrix (also diagonal), is the load matrix, and , , and are the vectors representing the angular accelerations, angular displacements and torques applied to the model respectively.

When considering the coupling of the two models, the matrices can be combined into one:

$$\underline{a_t} = \begin{bmatrix} \underline{a_s} & \underline{Z}_{(4\times3)} \\ \underline{Z}_{(3\times4)} & \underline{a_f} \end{bmatrix} \tag{21}$$

$$\underline{b_t} = \begin{bmatrix} & & & & c_{15} & c_{16} & c_{17} \\ & \underline{b_s} & & & c_{25} & c_{26} & c_{27} \\ & & & & c_{35} & c_{36} & c_{37} \\ & & & & c_{45} & c_{46} & c_{47} \\ c_{51} & c_{52} & c_{53} & c_{54} & & & \\ c_{61} & c_{62} & c_{63} & c_{64} & & \underline{b_f} & \\ c_{71} & c_{72} & c_{73} & c_{74} & & & \end{bmatrix}$$
(22)

$$\underline{c_t} = \begin{bmatrix} \underline{c_s} & \underline{Z}_{(4\times3)} \\ \underline{Z}_{(3\times4)} & \underline{c_f} \end{bmatrix} \tag{23}$$

where $\underline{Z}_{(i\times j)}$ represent a matrix of zeros, those dimension is $(i\times j)$. In the matrix $\underline{b_t}$, the coefficients $c_{ij}$ allow to define the interactions between the two models, usually determined with a lot of trial and error comparing the results of the model with those obtained experimentally.

Therefore the entire behavior of the coupled model can be expressed as:

$$\underline{a_t} \cdot \underline{\ddot{\varphi}} = \underline{b_t} \cdot \underline{\varphi} + \underline{c_t} \cdot \underline{M} \tag{24}$$

These equations can then be coupled with an optimal control mechanism that calculates the best strategy to maintain the erect posture and a straight head position (equivalent to staring right ahead) [Pascolo, 2003]. An example of control mechanism strategy that could be used with this coupled model is minimizing the energy, assuming that in rest conditions and for static posture, the human body tries to minimize the energy expenditure to maintain equilibrium [PascoloandSaccavini, 2004].

When considering the advantages of the coupled model with respect to the previously discussed models, it is evident that when combining the movement in two planes, the statokinesiogram can be defined: the movement of the COP obtained using the coupled model (Figure 12) is very similar to that obtained experimentally (Figure 13 – acquired using a custom designed platform and digitized using National Instruments BNC2090 - Biobench), although it can be easily appreciated how the experimental result appears to have much higher frequency movements. These however are not always real, but rather in most situations, as in this case, are artifacts caused by the noise of the instrumentation (force platform) used. This can be appreciated by comparing the results with those obtained using a different instrument (Figure 14), instrument designed specifically to measure the postural stability of a subject [CAPS™ Professional, Vestibular Technologies, LLC. – Cheyenne WY, U.S.A.].

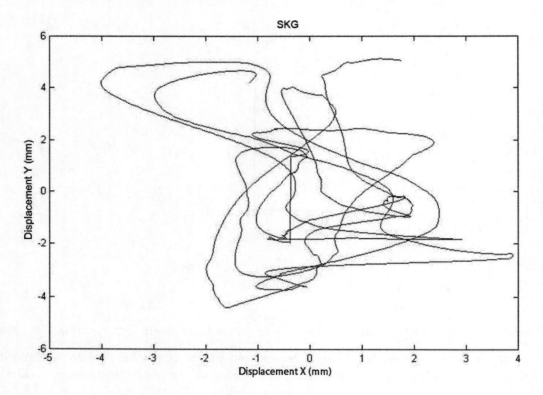

Figure 12.Statokinesiogram of the 2D coupled model [Pascolo –and Roiatti, 2003].

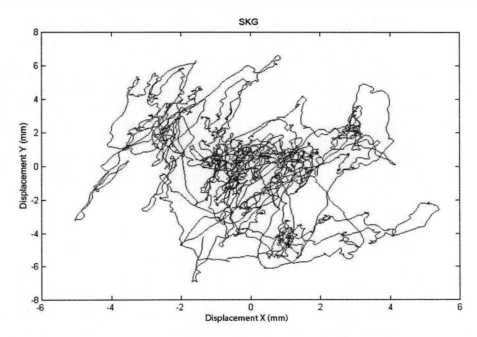

Figure 13. Statokinesiogram measured experimentally for an healthy subjectusing a custom designed platform and digitized using National Instruments BNC2090 – Biobench.

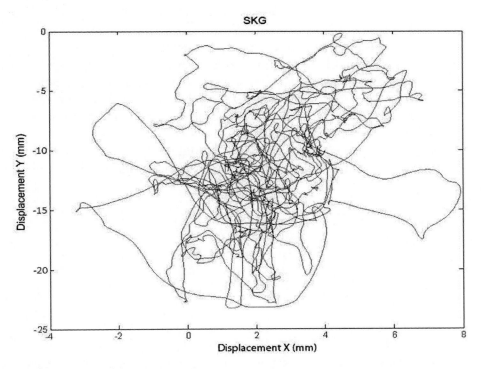

Figure 14. Statokinesiogram measured experimentally for an healthy subject using a dedicated platform[CAPS™ Professional, Vestibular technologies, LLC – Cheyenne WY, U.S.A.].

Even more so than in the simplified models, the strategy used by the control mechanism, as well as the mechanical properties associated with each joint in the model are paramount in the coupled models to guarantee a good approximation of the experimental results.

From a mechanical point of view, the limitations of the coupled models are mainly having neglected certain coupled movements of the legs (such as the torsional movements of the ankle and hip joints, and the independent knee movements). These movements produce a rotation of the pelvic structure around a vertical axis that, although minimal, cannot be neglected to guarantee a physiological simulation of the erect posture.

Therefore, the coupled models allow to verify the interaction between the oscillations in the anterior-posterior and medio-lateral planes, but require a lot of trial and error to obtain the best coupling coefficients.

## 3d Model

The availability of software applications that allow sophisticated 3D modeling of the human body has allowed the development of models for simulating the erect posture [Pittini, 2005; Winter, 2003; Losan, 2005], models that are more complex and with higher biofidelity levels than those obtained using 2D or coupled 2D techniques.

This 3D approach allows in fact not only to consider one rotation (or two in the case of the coupled 2D model), but all three physiological rotations present in certain human joints such as the ankle, the hip and the neck. Therefore, the model can include also the small, but, as said before, significant rotations around a vertical axis that help maintaining the equilibrium while quietly standing. Furthermore, the movements of the knees can be independent, with consequent introduction of the pelvic rotation.

Furthermore, the 3D model allows for greater biofidelity in the description of the internal perturbations, such as the breathing and the cardiac activity, and their distribution and points of application, as well as in the description of the resultant force and pressure applied under the foot, the boundary condition of the model and what is usually used to validate the model by comparing it with experimental results.

Considering one example of these 3D models [Pittini, 2005], the model (Figure 15) comprises sixteen rigid bodies, each with its own mass and inertial properties. Their geometry is defined as:

- cylinders (neck, upper arms and feet)
- frustum (thighs, shanks and arms)
- ellipsoid (head)
- plates (hands, support surfaces of the feet)
- plates (abdomen, thorax and hands)

These rigid bodies are connected by joints (Figure 16) defined as:

- 3D or spherical (wrists, ankles, hips, shoulders, and the joints between abdomen and thorax, thorax and neck, and neck and head)
- 2D or rotoidal (knees, shanks and arms)

Note that in this model the feet are considered as a single rigid body constrained to the ground.

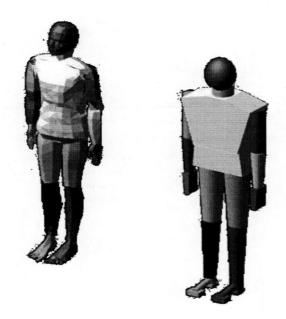

Figure 15. 3D multi-body model[Pittini, 2005].

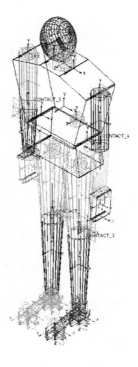

Figure 16. Joints in the 3D multi-body model[Pittini, 2005].

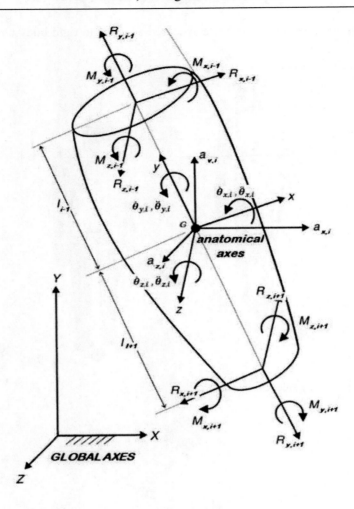

Figure 17. Forces and moments acting on the 3D *i-th*bodyXYZ are the global coordinate system; xyz the local coordinate system [modified from Winter, 1990].

The first major improvement compared to the previously discussed models is the representation of the trunk as two bodies, the abdomen and the thorax, connected by a spherical joint that allows the rotation of the thorax with respect to the abdomen along all three axes. Thus, part of the flexibility of the trunk due to the presence of the spinal joints can be incorporated in the model as can be the effects of the contraction of the trunk muscles.

From an analytical point of view, the model comprises n rigid bodies, and each rigid body has 6 degrees of freedom, three translations and three rotations, and is under the effect of a system of forces and moments due to the weight and inertia of the body itself, the contact forces and moments between adjacent bodies, internal and external perturbations, as well as muscular activities necessary to maintain the upright posture. Figure 17 and Table 2 contain the nomenclature used for a generic i-th body.

## Table 2. Nomenclature used in the 3D *i-th* body equations

| SYMBOL | DESCRIPTION |
|---|---|
| x, y, z | local axes system |
| X, Y, Z | global axes system |
| $G_i$ | (*i*) body center of mass (COM) |
| $\vec{v}_{x,y,z_i}$ | COM x,y,z velocity |
| $\vec{a}_{x,y,z_i}$ | COM x,y,z acceleration |
| $\dot{\theta}_{x,y,z_i}$ | angular x, y, z velocity of (*i*) body |
| $\ddot{\theta}_{x,y,z_i}$ | angular x, y, z acceleration of (*i*) body |
| $l_{i\pm1}$ | distance between joint ($i\pm1$) and (*i*) body COM (G) |
| $\vec{W}_i = m_i \cdot g$ | weight of (*i*) body |
| $\bar{J}_{Gi}$ | inertia tensor of (*i*) body |
| $J_{G,x,y,z_i}$ | x, y, z principal moment of inertia |
| $\vec{P}_{j,i}$ | *j-th* perturbation force on (*i*) body |
| $\vec{Z}_{j,i}$ | *j-th* perturbation torque on (*i*) body |
| $\vec{R}_{j,i\pm1}$ | force between (*i*) and ($i\pm1$) body |
| $\vec{M}_{i\pm1}$ | torque between (*i*) and ($i\pm$) body due to muscular activity $\vec{T}_{i\pm1}, \vec{K}_{i\pm1}, \vec{C}_{i\pm1}$, external and internal perturbations $\vec{Z}_{j,i\pm1}$ and $\vec{P}_{j,i\pm1}$ |
| $\vec{T}_{i\pm1}$ | muscular torque between (*i*) and ($i\pm1$) body |
| $\vec{K}_{i,i\pm1} \times (\theta_i - \theta_{i\pm1})$ | torque due to elasticity between (*i*) and ($i\pm1$) body |
| $\vec{C}_{i,i\pm1} \times (\dot{\theta}_i - \dot{\theta}_{i\pm1})$ | torque due to viscosity between (*i*) and ($i\pm1$) body |

Considering the first equilibrium equation of the model in the global coordinate system:

$$m_i \cdot \vec{a}_i = \sum_{j=1}^{m} \vec{R}_{j,i+1} + \sum_{j=1}^{m} \vec{R}_{j,i-1} + \sum_{j=1}^{m} \vec{P}_{j,i} + \vec{W}_i \qquad (25)$$

it is possible to obtain the translation equations along the Cartesian axes for the i-th body:

– Translation along the x axis:

$$-m_i \cdot a_{X,i} + \sum_{j=1}^{m} R_{X_{j,i+1}} + \sum_{j=1}^{m} R_{X_{j,i-1}} + \sum_{j=1}^{m} P_{Y_{j,i}} = 0 \qquad (26)$$

– Translation along the y axis:

$$-W_i - m_i \cdot a_{Y,i} + \sum_{j=1}^{m} R_{Y_{j,i+1}} + \sum_{j=1}^{m} R_{Y_{j,i-1}} + \sum_{j=1}^{m} P_{Y_{j,i}} = 0 \qquad (27)$$

– Translation along the z axis:

$$-m_i \cdot a_{Z,i} + \sum_{j=1}^{m} R_{Z_{j,i+1}} + \sum_{j=1}^{m} R_{Z_{j,i-1}} + \sum_{j=1}^{m} P_{Z_{j,i}} = 0 \qquad (28)$$

The second equilibrium equation of the model (using for simplicity the local coordinate system centered in the center of mass of the i-th body) can be written as:

$$\frac{d}{dt} \cdot \left[ l_{i-1} \times m_i \cdot \vec{v}_{Gi} + \bar{J}_{Gi} \cdot \dot{\vec{\theta}}_i \right] + \vec{v}(G_i) \times m_i \cdot \vec{v}_{Gi} =$$

(inertial contribution)

$$= \vec{Z}_{j,i} + \sum_{j=1}^{m} l_{i-1} \times \vec{P}_{j,i-1} + \sum_{j=1}^{m} l_{i+1} \times \vec{P}_{j,i+1} +$$

(perturbation)

$$+ \quad \sum_{j=1}^{m} l_{i-1} \times \bar{R}_{j,i-1} + \sum_{j=1}^{m} l_{i+1} \times \bar{R}_+ \qquad (29)$$

(reaction to the joints)

$$+ \bar{K}_{i,i+1} \times (\vec{\theta}_i - \vec{\theta}_{i+1}) - \bar{K}_{i-1,i} \times (\vec{\theta}_{i-1} - \vec{\theta}_i) +$$

(torque due to the elasticity)

$$+ \vec{C}_{i,i+1} \times (\dot{\vec{\theta}}_i - \dot{\vec{\theta}}_{i+1}) - \vec{C}_{i-1,i} \times (\dot{\vec{\theta}}_{i-1} - \dot{\vec{\theta}}_i) +$$

(torque due to the viscosity)

$$+ \quad \vec{T}_{(i,i-1)} - \vec{T}_{(i)}$$

(torque due to muscular activity)

But since $\vec{v}_{Gi} = 0$, only $\frac{d}{dt} \cdot \left[ \bar{J}_{Gi} \cdot \dot{\vec{\theta}}_i \right]$ remains in the first term of Equation (29), and using the local coordinate system defined in the center of mass, the rotational matrix $\bar{J}_{Gi}$ becomes constant over time. Therefore the rotational equations along the Cartesian axes for the i-th body become:

Rotation along the x axis:

$$J_{Gx_i} \cdot \ddot{\theta}_{x_i} + (J_{Gz_i} - J_{Gy_i}) \cdot \dot{\theta}_{y_i} \cdot \dot{\theta}_{z_i} =$$

(inertial contribution)

$$= Z_{xj,i} + \sum_{j=1}^{m} l_{i-1} \cdot P_{zj,i-1} + \sum_{j=1}^{m} l_{i+1} \cdot P_{zj,i+1} +$$

(perturbation)

$$+ \quad \sum_{j=1}^{m} l_{i-1} \cdot R_{zj,i-1} + \sum_{j=1}^{m} l_{i+1} \cdot R_{z_+} \tag{30}$$

(reaction to the joints)

$$-K_{i,i+1} \cdot (\theta_{x_i} - \theta_{x_{i+1}}) + K_{i-1,i} \cdot (\theta_{x_{i-1}} - \theta_{x_i}) +$$

(torque due to the elasticity)

$$-C_{i,i+1} \cdot (\dot{\theta}_{x_i} - \dot{\theta}_{x_{i+1}}) + \vec{C}_{i-1,i} \cdot (\dot{\theta}_{x_{i-1}} - \dot{\theta}_{x_i}) +$$

(torque due to the viscosity)

$$+T_{x(i,i-1)} - T_{x(i,i+1)}$$

(torque due to muscular activity)

Rotation along the y axis:

$$J_{Gy_i} \cdot \ddot{\theta}_{y_i} + (J_{Gx_i} - J_{Gz_i}) \cdot \dot{\theta}_{x_i} \cdot \dot{\theta}_{z_i} =$$

(inertial contribution)

$$= Z_y \tag{31}$$

(perturbation)

$$-K_{i,i+1} \cdot (\theta_{y_i} - \theta_{y_{i+1}}) + K_{i-1,i} \cdot (\theta_{y_{i-1}} - \theta_{y_i}) +$$

(torque due to the elasticity)

$$-C_{i,i+1} \cdot (\dot{\theta}_{y_i} - \dot{\theta}_{y_{i+1}}) + \vec{C}_{i-1,i} \cdot (\dot{\theta}_{y_{i-1}} - \dot{\theta}_{y_i}) +$$

(torque due to the viscosity)

$$+ T_{y_{(i,i-1)}} - T_{y_{(i,i+1)}}$$

(torque due to muscular activity)

Rotation along the z axis:
$$J_{Gz_i} \cdot \ddot{\theta}_{z_i} + (J_{Gy_i} - J_{Gx_i}) \cdot \dot{\theta}_{x_i} \cdot \dot{\theta}_{y_i} =$$

(inertial contribution)

$$= Z_{zj,i} + \sum_{j=1}^{m} l_{i-1} \cdot P_{xj,i-1} + \sum_{j=1}^{m} l_{i+1} \cdot P_{xj,i+1} +$$

(perturbation)

$$+ \quad \sum_{j=1}^{m} l_{i-1} \cdot R_{xj,i-1} + \sum_{j=1}^{m} l_{i+1} \cdot R_{x_+} \tag{32}$$

(reaction to the joints)

$$-K_{i,i+1} \cdot (\theta_{z_i} - \theta_{z_{i+1}}) + K_{i-1,i} \cdot (\theta_{z_{i-1}} - \theta_{z_i}) +$$

(torque due to the elasticity)

$$-\bar{C}_{i,i+1} \cdot (\dot{\theta}_{z_i} - \dot{\theta}_{z_{i+1}}) + \bar{C}_{i-1,i} \cdot (\dot{\theta}_{z_{i-1}} - \dot{\theta}_{z_i}) +$$

(torque due to the viscosity)

$$+ \quad T_{z(i,i-1)} - T_{z(i}$$

(torque due to muscular activity)

The model of Figure 16 is represented by a system of 16x6 non-linear, differential equations that can be solved to obtain the stability of the model. When including a control mechanism based on the minimization of the angular displacements in the various joints, it is possible to appreciate the importance of using spherical versus rotoidal joints for simulating the ankle and hip, even when a feedback control mechanism is not included in the model (Figures 18 and 19).

Comparing these results with experimental data, it is apparent that using spherical joints (Figure 19) provides a better simulation for the oscillations in the sagittal plane (displacements along the z axis), thus the model has better biofidelity.

As for the coupled 2D multi-link inverted pendulum model, the stabilization of the model can be achieved by introducing an external biofeedback control system based on the minimization of the energy.

Further improvement of the biofidelity of the model can be achieved by adding the following:

- two torques applied to each joint, to simulate the combined effect of the agonistic and antagonistic muscles acting on the specific joint

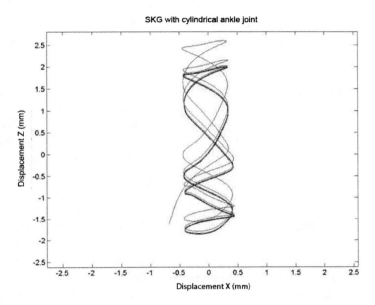

Figure 18.Statokinesiogram of the 3D model without feedback control(mechanical impedence), and a revolute ankle joint [Pittini, 2005].

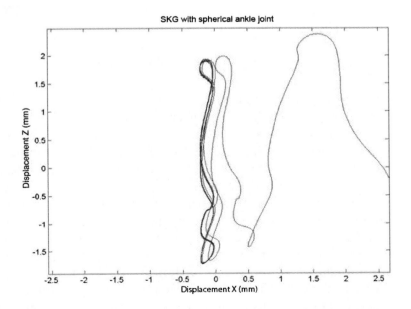

Figure 19.Statokinesiogram of the 3D model without feedback control(mechanical impedence), and a spherical ankle joint [Pittini, 2005].

- muscles described using a modified-Hill model [Pascoloet al., 2005a]: each muscle is simulated as a spring-damper actuator, with a non-linear characteristic for the spring stiffness to better simulate the different mechanical properties of the physiological muscle when is actively contracted and when it is elastically stretched.

Furthermore, it is possible to modify the control mechanism so that, like in the human nervous system, there are delays in the feedback loop: when introducing two of such types of delays, it is possible to simulate the involuntary, fast muscular reaction based on local and spinal reflexes, as well as conscious, slower muscular contraction mediated by the brain [Zatsiorsky and Duarte, 2000].

Using a 3D multi-body approach allows to have better consistency of the numerical results with the experimental data. Even simulating the multi-segmental spine (and associated intervertebral joints) with only one spherical joint (thus removing secondary degrees of freedom of the trunk) gives good results, without the mathematical complexity associated with a more sophisticated model of the trunk. Improvements of the model include modelingthe flexible spine (and deformabletrunk structure) and simulating the intrinsic perturbation due to the breathing and the cardiac output using bodies capable of changing their volume (to account for the expansion and contraction of the thoracic cavity during the breathing cycle) and their mass distribution (to account for the heart contraction and blood ejection). These latter improvements would be better approximation of the real system than the fictitious external forces applied to the model to simulate the same phenomena.

However, adding these improvements might not produce better results and improve the biofidelity of the model since the model could become unstable due to numerical reasons (ill-conditioning of the problem when solving the non-linear differential equations). Better results could also be achieved by improving the description and characteristics of the biofeedback control mechanism rather than by increasing the degrees of freedom and the complexity of the geometrical model.

## VALIDATION OF THE MODELS

As the goal of any model is to be used in simulations of real systems, the only way to validate them is to compare the results of experiments conducted on the real physical system with those obtained from the simulations under the same conditions. In case of models of human stability, this means comparing results of the SKG as well as other posturographic measures such as the average velocity of the COP path, the area of the path described by the COP movement and any of several other measures of postural stability developed over the several decades of research in this field [Chaudhry, 2005;Rougier, 2008]. Of course in doing so it is necessary to consider how the experimental results could be affected by undesired factors such as the resolution, accuracy and noise of the instrumentation used to collect such data, as well as eventual unknown presence of conditions affecting the experimental results of specific individuals (from whom the data are collected) such as undiagnosed pathological conditions. Fortunately, these effects can often be compensated for by considering, at least in the model validation process, the data obtained from a variety of individuals reduced by means of statistical aggregation. On the other hand, compensating for instrumentation issues is much more difficult as these can be considered systemic in nature. For instance, many force platforms (to detect the ground reaction forces and the COP path) as well as motion analysis systems (to detect the kinematics) have been originally designed for gait analysis or sport related experiments where forces and range of movement are much larger than those encountered when considering human equilibrium and posture. Although many investigators have used these instruments for their balance experiments and still do [Clark et al., 2010], the instruments' resolution, accuracy and noise are often not adequate and tend to cover the phenomena they are suppose to detect and quantify [Pagnaccoet al., 2011]. Refer to Figures 13 and 14 to appreciate the difference between the two groups of instruments.

Since in creating the model, certain assumptions (either implicit or explicit) have been made, it is paramount that the experiments used to validate the model reflect these assumptions. For instance, if the model is a 2D single inverted pendulum which has the inherent assumption that the only strategy used to maintain the equilibrium is the ankle strategy, it is more appropriate to validate the model using results from experiments where the subjects are instructed to only use an ankle strategy and avoid as much as possible movements of any other joints. This does not preclude the possibility of then comparing the results with experiments obtained under more "natural" and "unconstrained" conditions but this would have the objective of investigating the biofidelity of the model rather than its validation.

In certain situations, especially with more complex models both in terms of geometry and of control systems, it is possible and advisable to validate them not just under unperturbed static erect postural conditions, but also in the presence of external perturbations. These can be perturbation of the support surface: for instance, using platforms that move in one or more directions suddenly or more slowly [EquiTest®, NeuroCom International, Inc. – Clackamas OR, U.S.A.], using platforms that tilt in one or more directions either freely under the movement of the subject [Stabilomètre, SATEL – Blagnac, France; Delos Equilibrium Board, DELOS S.r.l. – Turin, Italy] or in a controlled way imposed by the device [Balance Quest, FRAMIRAL® – Cannes, France], or even using foam cushions that decouple the perturbation under each foot and randomize the perturbation itself [CAPS™ Professional, Vestibular Technologies, LLC. – Cheyenne WY, U.S.A.; VSR™, NeuroCom International, Inc. – Clackamas OR, U.S.A.]. It is also possible to use perturbation of the system that are different from those associated with the base of support: for instance, using known force impulses applied to any part of the body to simulate destabilizing impact forces to see how the model in general and the control mechanism in particular react to those perturbations [Pascolo, 2008].

## BIOFIDELITY OF THE MODELS

Biofidelity of the model is a complex issue. For a model to be useful it needs not only to reproduce as close as possible experimental observations, but it has to do so while at the same time providing as close a representation as possible of the underlying physical system it is designed to represent, both in terms of geometry and of its mechanical and control characteristics. On the other hand, one of the useful characteristics of the models is that they are a much simpler and more understandable system to work with than the physical entity they want to represent. In other words, models are created by making simplifying assumptions that allow to deal with the reality of complex systems in a feasible way. Therefore, there is always a trade off when creating a model: on one side, it should be as a close representation of the real system as possible, while on the other hand be as simple and manageable as it can be for the purpose of the desired investigation. As such, a model might have good biofidelity for certain aspects while being poorly biofidelic in others.

For instance, two dimensional single link inverted pendulum models obviously present very little biofidelity in general, except when simulating the ankle strategy. On the other hand, they are simple and easy to implement and give an overall first approximation of the standing human. Multi-segmental two dimensional models add complexity but also biofidelity as they allow to contemplate more complicated postural control strategies including the interaction between different parts of the body. Similarly, coupled 2D multi-link models allow for considering at least some of the interactions occurring between the sagittal and coronal planes, whereas full 3D models allow much more realistic modeling of the complex 3D interactions between various parts of the body while maintaining a static posture.

Although three dimensional models appear to be a great improvement in biofidelity, they still suffer from several limitations as to an accurate representation of a standing human. For instance, joint geometry is often simplified (consider the complex geometry of the rotoidal joint of the knee compared to its usual mathematical representation as a simple cylindrical joint), and the change in mass distribution of the soft tissues caused by the movement or the muscular contraction is neglected. Similarly, models still neglect the movement of various parts of the body including the internal organs. Whereas the most sophisticated models include somehow the effects of cardiac contractions as a cyclic perturbing force, other perturbations to balance such as involuntary muscular contractions of the digestive system, gastric movements, and changes in the geometry and distribution of masses caused by respiration, swallowing, digestion, and muscular contractions, are still not considered, sometimes for the simple reason that measuring experimentally their magnitude and characteristics is still impractical.

Even more difficult appears to be the modeling of the neuromuscular control system and especially the role of the central nervous system. For instance, it is unknown, and therefore it is impossible nowadays to model, why a subject tends to unconsciously sway away from an obnoxious or perceived dangerous noise, but tends to sway toward a pleasant or interesting sound [Blouin et al., 2006; Agaeva et al., 2006]. Similarly, although it is most often assumed that the overall control criterion in maintaining posture is the minimization of the overall energy expenditure, it is in everyone experience the fact that in some situations this is not the case, for instance when standing on unstable or slippery surfaces like ice, or in situations of perceived danger. Another aspect is that most likely the postural control mechanisms have as a goal the stabilization (and when this is impossible, the protection) of the head, whereas most models are designed to maintain stability of the various body segments. In other words, they often consider a goal (the stabilization of the various body parts) what is most likely the mean to achieve the stabilization of the head.

The biofidelity of the models becomes even more important when considering the possibility of using the mathematical models to better understand not only the physiological aspect of the standing posture, but also the effects of certain pathologies, thus helping the clinician to better understand the underlying pathology. For instance, if the control mechanism contemplates the presence of time delays in the feedback loop, it is possible to simulate the effect of multiple sclerosis which is known to cause delays in the neuro-signal transmission. Similarly, if the model includes a complex muscle model, it is possible to superimpose the effect of debilitating conditions such as muscular fatigue or weaknesses, or if the model includes complex joint geometry, it is possible to simulate the effect of joint damage [Tagaw, 2000].

## CONCLUSIONS

Over the years models of increasing complexity have been developed to better understand how humans maintain the upright posture. Although with increased complexity usually comes an increased biofidelity, at this time models are more accurate in describing the biomechanics than the neuromuscular system and therefore are not yet sufficiently biofidelic to allow an in-depth study of human standing and in particular to investigate the effects of pathologies that might affect balance. On the other hand, they are already sufficient to provide insight in regards to the cinematic and kinetic aspects of balance and locomotion [Hurmuzlu, 2004; Johansson, 2009].

For these reasons anddue the opportunity offered by mathematical tools, e.g. [Pascolo, 2006] experimental (i. e., posturographic) rather than simulation studies are still the preferred way to investigate the effects of pathologies such as Parkinson's disease [Schieppati, 1999; Pascolo, 2005b; Ganesan, 2010], or diabetes [Uccioli, 1995] or the effects of rehabilitation [Baydal-Bertomeuet al., 2010] as well as the general psychophysical conditions [Pascolo, 2009; Nieschalket al., 1999].

## REFERENCES

Agaeva M.Y. et al. (2006), Effects of a sound source moving in a vertical plane on postural responses in humans. *Neurosci. Behav. Physiol.* 36:7, 773-80.

Alexandrov A. V. et al. (2005) Feedback equilibrium control during human standing, *Biol.Cybern.,*93, 309–322.

Allum J. H. J. et al. (2002) Differences between trunk sway characteristics on a foam support surface and on the Equitest® ankle-sway-referenced support surface. *Gait and posture*, 16, 264-270.

Andres, R.O. (1979) A postural measurement system for induced body sway assessment, Ph.D. Dissertation, University of Michigan, Ann Arbor, MI.

Andres, R.O. and Anderson D.J. (1980) Designing a better postural measurement system. *Am. J. Otolaryngol.*1:3, 197-206.

Aramaki Y. et al. (2001) Reciprocal angular acceleration of the ankle and hip joints during quiet standing in humans. *Exp. Brain Res.* 136, 463-73.

Baker, S.P. and Harvey, A.H. (1985) Fall injuries in elderly. *Clin. Geriat. Med.*1, 501-512.

Baydal-Bertomeu, J.M et al. (2010) Study of the efficacy and reliability of a posturography system compared with the scale of Berg, Rehabilitacion44, 304-310.

Bhattacharya, A., Morgan, R., Shukla, R., Ramakrishanan, H.K., Wang, L. (1987) Non-invasive estimation of afferent inputs for postural stability under low levels of alcohol. *Ann. Biomed. Engng.*15, 533-550.

Blouin J.S. et al. (2006) Startle responses elicited by whiplash perturbations. *J. Physiol.* 573:Pt 3, 857-67.

Bottaro, A., Casadio, M., Morasso, P., and Sanguineti, V. (2005) Body sway during quiet standing: Is it the residual chattering of an intermittent stabilization process? *Human Movement Science*, 24, 588–615.

Brocklehurst, J.C., Robertson, D. and James-Groom, P. (1982) Clinical correlates of sway in old age-sensory modalities. *Age Agng.*11, 1-10.

Cavanagh, P.R. (1980) A technique for averaging center of pressure paths from a force platform. *J. Biomech.*13, 397-406.

Chandler, J.M., Duncan P.W., Studenki, S.A. (1990) Balance performance on the postural stress test: comparison of joung adults, healthy elderly, and fallers. *Physical Therapy*70:7,410-415.

Chaudhry, H. et al. (2005) Postural stability index is a more valid measure of stability than equilibrium score. *Journal of Rehabilitation Research and Development*, 42, 547-555.

Cordo, P.J. and Nasher L.M. (1982) Properties of postural adjustments associated with rapid arm movements. *J. Neurophys.*47:2, 287-302.

Creath R. et al. (2005) A unified view of quiet and perturbed stance: simultaneous co-existing excitable modes, *Neuroscience Letters,*377, 75-80.

Cybulski G.R. and Jaeger R.J. (1986) Standing performance of persons with paraplegia. *Arch.Phys. Med.Rehabil.* 67, 103-108

Elftman, H. (1934) A cinematic study of the distribution of the center of pressure in the human foot. *Anatomical Rec.*59, 481-491.

Era, P. and Heikkinen, E. (1985) Postural sway during standing and unexpected disturbance of balance in random samples of men of differen ages. *J. Geront.*40, 287-295.

Frank, J.S., Patla, A.E., Winter, D.A. (1989) Some observations on the use of center of pressure signal for assessment of balance. Proc. 19th Conf. of the Int.Soc. of Biomechanics, Los Angeles, June 1989.

Fregly, A.R. (1974) Vestibular ataxia and its measurement in man. Handbook of Sensory Physiology, Springer Publishing Co., Berlin, 321-360.

Friendli, W.G., Hallet, M., Simon, S.R. (1984) Postrural adjustments associated with rapid voluntary arm movements. *J. Neurol. Neurosurg. and Psychiatry*47, 611-622.

Ganesan M., Pal P.K., Gupta A. and Sathyaprabha, T.N. (2010) Dynamic posturography in evaluation of balance in patients of Parkinson's disease with normal pull test: Concept of a diagonal pull test. *Parkinsonism and Related Disorders*, 16, 595-599.

Goldie, P.A., Bach, T.M., Evans,O.M. (1989) Force platform measures for evaluating postural control: reliability and validity. *Arch. Phys. Med. Rehabil.*70, 510-517.

Gurfinkel E.V. (1973) Physical foundations of stabilography. *Agressologie*14, 9-14.

Gurfinkel V.S. and Osovets, S.M. (1972) Dynamics of equilibrium of the vertical posture in man. *Biophysics*, 17, 496-506.

Harris, G.F. (1986) Overview: postural stability. In Kondraske and Robinson (Eds.): Proceedings of the 8th Annual Conference of the IEEE/EMBS, 243-257.

Hasan, S.S., Goldner, D.N., Lichtenstein, M.J., Wood, A.J.J. and Shiavi, R.G (1990) Selecting a suitable biomechanics platform measure of sway. *Proc. IEEE EMBS*12, 2105-2106.

Hasan, S.S., Lichtenstein, M.J. and Shiavi, R.G (1990) Effect of loss of balance on biomechanics platform measures of sway: influence of stance and a method for adjustment. *J. Bimech.* 23:8, 783-789.

Hasselkus, B.R. and Shambes, G.M. (1975) Aging and postural sway in women. *J.Geront.*30, 661- 667.

Hemami H. and Jaswa V. (1978) On a three-link model of the dynamics of standing up and sitting down. IEEE Trans. On Systems, Man, and Cybernetics, 8, 115–120.

Hemami H. et al. (1978) Biped stability considerations with vestibular models. *IEEE Trans Autom Control*,AC-23, 1074-1079.

Hunter I. W. and Kearney R. E. (1981) Respiratory components of human postural sway. Neuroscience Letters, 25, 155-159.

Hurmuzlu Y., Genot F. and Brogliato B. (2004) Modeling, stability and control of biped robots--a general framework, Automatica, 40, 1647-1664.

Imms, F.J. and Edholm,O.G. (1981) Studies of gait and mobility in the elderly. *Age Agng.*10, 147-156.

Jarret, M.O.(1976) A television computer system for human locomotion. *Ph.D. Dissertation*, University of Strathclyde, Glasgow, Scotland.

Johansson, R. and Magnusson, M. (1991) Human postural dynamics. *CRC Crit. Rev. Biomed. Engng.*18:6, 413-437.

Johansson R., Fransson P. and Magnusson M. (2009) Optimal coordination and control of posturenext term and movements. *Journal of Physiology-Paris*, 103, 159-177

Kapteyn, T.S., Bles, W., Njiokiktjien, C.J., Kodde, L., Massen, C.H., et al. (1983) Standardization in platform stabilometry being a part of posturography. *Agressologie*24, 321-326.

Koozekanani, S.H., Stockwell, C.W., McGhee, R.B., Firoozmand, F. (1980) on the role of dynamic models in quantitative posturography. *IEEE Trans. Biomed. Engng.*27, 605-609.

Li Y. (2010) An optimal control model for human postural regulation, Ph.D. Dissertation, University of Maryland, College park, MD.

Lichtenstein, M.J., Shields, S.L., Shiavi, R.G. and Burger, M.C. (1988) Clinical determinants of biomechanics platform measures of balance in aged women. *J. Am. Geriat. Soc.*36, 996-1002.

Loram, I.D. and Lakie, M. (2002) Human balancing of an inverted pendulum: Position control by small, ballistic-like, throw and catch movements. *J. Physiology*, 540, 1111-1124.

Loram, I.D., Maganaris, C.N. and Lakie, M. (2005) Active, non-spring-like muscle movements in human postural sway: How might paradoxical changes in muscle length be produced? *J. Physiology*, 564, 281-293.

Miller, C.W. (1978) Survival and ambulation following hip fracture. *J. Bone Jt. Surg.*60A, 930-934.

Morasso, P. and Sanguineti, V. (2002) Ankle stiffness alone cannot stabilize upright standing. *J. Neurophysiology*, 88, 2157–2162.

Murray, M.P., Seireg, A.A. and Scholz, R.C. (1967) Center of gravity, center of pressure, and supportive forces during human activities. *J. Appl. Physiol.*23,831-838.

Murray, M.P., Wood, Seireg, A.A. and Sepic, S.B. (1975) Normal postural stability and steadyness: quantitative assessment. *J. Bone Jt Surg.* 57A, 510-516.

Nashner, L.M. and Woollacott, M. (1979) The organization of rapid postural adjustments of standing humans: an experimental-conceptual model. In Talbot and Humphrey (Eds.) Posture and movement, Raven Press, New York, 243-257.

Nieschalk M. et al. (1999) Effects-of-alcohol-on-body-sway-patterns-in-human-subjects. *Int.J. Leg. Med.*, 112, 253-260.

Overstall, P.W, Exton-Smith, A.N., Imms, F.J. and Johnson, A.L. (1977) Falls in the elderly related to postural imbalance.*Br. Med.* J.1, 261-264.

Pascolo P., Roiatti S., De Bortoli L. and Saccavini M. (2003) L'attività muscolare nella statica eretta (Controllo ottimo sulla base del costo energetico). Workshop su handicap: ricerca, assistenza ed integrazione, 48-54, Pavia, 2003 - ed. Università di Pavia, Italy.

Pascolo P. and Saccavini M. (2004) The stabilometric evaluation of the erect stance (energy-based optimal control in a numerical model). *Europa Medicophysica*, 40, 59-65.

Pascolo P., Colautti F., Antonutto G. (2005a) Un modello a elementi discreti del muscolo scheletrico, Sistemi di Ingegneria Biomedica, 97 - 104, Milano- ed. Biosys-ANIPLA.

Pascolo P., Marini A, Carniel R and Barazza F (2005b). Posture as a chaotic system and an application to the Parkinson's disease. *Chaos, Solitons and Fractals*24, 1343-1346.

Pascolo P., Barazza F and Carniel R (2006). Considerations on the application of the chaos paradigm to describe the postural sway. *Chaos, Solitons and Fractals*27, 1339-1346.

Pascolo P., Vangi D. (2008). Human cervical spine behaviour in the rear-end impact: influence of guard level. Atti del Congresso Nazionale di Bioingegneria, 425-426, Pisa, Italy.

Pascolo P., Carniel R and Pinese P (2009). Human stability in the erect stance: Alcohol effects and audio-visual perturbations. *Journal of Biomechanics*42, 504-509.

Patla, A.E., Winter, D.A., Frank, J.S. Walt, S.E., Prasad, S. (1989) Identification of age-related changes in the balance-control system. Proc. *APTA Symposium on Balance*, 43-56.

Peterka, R. J. (2002) Sensorimotor integration in human postural control. *J. Neurophysiology*, 88, 1097–1118.

Pinter I. J., Van Swigchem R., Van Soest K. A. J. and Rozendaal L. A. (2008) The dynamics of postural sway cannot be captured using a one-segment inverted pendulum model: a PCS on segment rotations during unperturbed stance.*J. Neurophysiology*, 100, 3197-3208.

Pittini C. (2005) Indagine sulla postura (simulazioni e confronti con rilievi sperimentali), M.D. Thesis, University of Udine, Udine, Italy.

Riley, P.O., Mann, R.W., Hodge, W.A. (1990) Modelling of the biomechanics of posture and balance. *J. Biomech.*23, 503-506.

Ring, C., Nayak, U.S.L. and Isaacs, B. (1988) Balance function in elderly people who have and who have not fallen. *Arch. phys. Med. Rehabil.*69, 261-264.

Robin, D.W., Hasan, S.S., Lichtenstein, M.J., Shiavi and R.G Wood, A.J.J. (1991) Dose-related effect of triazolam on postural sway. *Clin. Pharmacol. Ther.*44, 581-588.

Roiatti S. (2001) Indagine teorico sperimentale sull'attività ottimale delle fibre muscolari nella stazione eretta (stabilometria e statokinesigramma), M.D. Thesis, University of Udine, Udine, Italy.

Romberg, M.H. (1853) Manual of nervous disorders of man. Sydenham Society, London, 395-401.

Rougier P. R. (2008) What insights can be gained when analysing the resultant centre of pressure trajectory?, *Neurophysiologie Clinique/Clinical Neurophysiology*, 38, 363-373.

Ruder, G.K., MacKinnon, C.D., Winter, D.A. (1989) COP vs COG changes during quiet stance and voluntary sway in the frontal and sagittal planes. Proc. 19th Conf. of the Int.Soc. of Biomechanics, Los Angeles, June 1989.

Schenkman, M. (1989) Interrelationship of neurological and mechanical factors in balance control. *Proc. APTA Symposium on Balance*, 29-42.

Schieppati, M. et al. (1999) Subjective perception of body sway. Journal of Neurology Neurosurgery and Psychiatry, 66. 313-322.

Sheldon, J.H. (1963) The effects of age on the control of sway. *Geront. clin.* 5, 129-138.

Shimba, T. (1984) An estimation of center of gravity from force platform data. *J. Biomech.*17:1, 53-60.

Smith, J.W. (1957) The forces operating at the human ankle joint during standing. *J. Anatomy*, 91, 545-564.

Soutas-Little, R.W. (1990) Center of pressure plots for clinical uses. Biomechanics of Normal and Prosthetic GaitASME, BED-Vol. 4, DSC-Vol.7, 69-75.

Soutas-Little, R.W., Andary, M.T. and Soutas-Little, P. (1991) Role of ground reaction torque in postural stability. *Proc. IEEE EMBS13*, 2002-2003.

Spaepan, A.J., Vranken, M. and Willems, E.J. (1977) Comparison of the movements of the center of gravity and of the center of pressure in stabilometric studies. *Agressologie*18, 109-113.

Stockwell C. W. Koozekanani, S.H. and Barin, K. (1981) A physical model of human postural dynamics. Annals of the New York Academy of Sciences374, 722-730.

Tagaw Y., Shiba N., Matsuo S. and Yamashita T. (2000) Analysis of human abnormal walking using a multi-body model: Joint models for abnormal walking and walking aids to reduce compensatory action. *Journal of Biomechanics*. 33, 1405-1414.

Uccioli, L., et al. (1995) Body sway in diabetic neuropathy. *Diabetes Care*, 18, 339-344.

Valk Fai, T (1973) Analysis of the dynamical behaviour of the body whilst 'standing still'. *Agressologie*14, 21-25.

Wei-Li Hsu, (2008). Multi-joint coordination underlies upright postural control, Ph.D. Dissertation, University of Delaware, Newark, DE.

Weiss, N.S., Liff, J.M., Ure, C.L., Ballard, J.H., Abbott, G.H. and Daling, J.R. (1983) Mortality in women following hip fracture. *J. chron. Dis.*36, 879-882.

Welch, T.D.J. and Ting, L.H. (2008) A feedback model reproduces muscle activity during human postural responses to support-surface translations. *J. Neurophysiology*, 99, 1032-1038.

Winter, D.A. (1987) Sagittal plane balance and posture in human walking. IEEE Engng. *Med. Biol. Mag.Sept.* 1987, 8-11.

Winter, D.A. (1990) Biomechanics of motor control and human movement, 2nd ed., Wiley-Interscience, New York.

Winter, D.A., Patla A.E. and Frank, J.S. (1990) Assessment of balance control in humans. *Med. Prog. Technol.*16,31-51.

Winter D. A. et al., (1998) Stiffnes control of balance in quiet standing. *J. Neurophysiol*, 80:1211-1221.

Winter D. A., Aftab E. Patla, MiladIshac, William H. Gage (2003) Motor mechanisms of balance during quiet standing, *Journal of Electromyography and Kinesiology*, 13, 49-56,

Woollacott, M., Bonnet, M. and Yabe, K. (1984) Preparatory process for anticipatory postural adjustment: modulation of leg reflex pathways during preparation for arm movements in standing man. *Exp. Brain Res.* 55, 63-271.

Zatsiorsky V. Duarte M. (2000) Rambling and trembling in quiet standing. *Motor. Control*, 4, 185-200.

In: Posture: Types, Assessment and Control
Editors: A. Wright and S. Rothenberg, pp. 137-154
ISBN 978-1-61324-107-3
© 2011 Nova Science Publishers, Inc.

*Chapter 5*

# THE RELATIONSHIP BETWEEN MUSCLE-TENDON UNIT STIFFNESS, JOINT STABILITY AND POSTURE, THE RISK OF INJURY, PERFORMANCE, RESONANCE AND ENERGY EXPENDITURE

*Aurélio Faria,*[\*,1] *Ronaldo Gabriel,*[2]
*João Abrantes,*[3] *Helena Moreira,*[4]
*Paola Wood*[5]*, and Tanya Camacho*[5]

[1]Department of Sport Science / CIDESD / University of Beira Interior, Covilhã, Portugal;
[2]Department of Sport Sciences, Exercise and Health / CITAB /
University of Trás-os-Montes and Alto Douro, Vila Real, Portugal;
[3]MovLab / CICANT / Universidade Lusófona de Humanidades e Tecnologias
Lisboa, Portugal;
[4]Department of Sport Sciences, Exercise and Health / CIDESD / University of Trás-os-Montes and Alto Douro, Vila Real, Portugal
[5]Department of Biokinetics, Sport and Leisure Sciences /
University of Pretoria, Pretoria, South Africa

## ABSTRACT

The predominant role that the musculoskeletal system and, more specifically, the muscle tendon unit play in human motion performance and rehabilitation has been questioned in recent investigations. An attempt to deepen the understanding of how the muscle-tendon unit may contribute to improve human motion performance and rehabilitation has been undertaken by various researchers however this understanding is still limited. The biomechanical properties of the muscle tendon unit and their association to joint stability and posture, the risk of injury, performance, resonance and energy expenditure as well as possible differences between sexes needs to be a source of

---

[\*] Corresponding Author: Aurélio Faria, Department of Sports Science, University of Beira Interior Rua Marquês D´Ávila e Bolama 6201-001 Covilhã, Portugal Tel. +351275329153/Fax. +351275329157 Email: afaria@ubi.pt.

constant enquiry to ensure a better understanding of this topic and thereby assisting in the application of this knowledge into the fields of sport performance, clinical decision making and rehabilitation. With the purpose to provide an update of the muscle-tendon unit stiffness literature this review includes relevant information for the assessment and comprehension of this biomechanical property and its relationship with joint stability and posture, the risk of injury, performance, resonance and energy expenditure. More specifically the following topics are reviewed: (1) Definition of stiffness and methods used in stiffness evaluation; (2) Stiffness, stability and posture; (3) Stiffness, resonance and energy expenditure; (4) Stiffness and performance; (4) Stiffness and the risk of injury. Finally some directions for future work are proposed. This review will contribute to increase the knowledge of the musculoskeletal system and provide a stronger basis for the development of future works and intervention programs in the fields of sport performance, clinical decision making and rehabilitation.

## INTRODUCTION

Muscle-tendon unit (MTU) stiffness is considered an important factor in the musculoskeletal system. The three main reasons for this, which are highlighted in published research (Wilson et al., 1991, Winter et al., 2001, Granata et al., 2002a, Butler et al., 2003, Williams III et al., 2004, Edwards, 2007), are related to joint stability and posture, the risk of injury, and performance. Other reasons have been postulated (Hoyt and Taylor, 1981, Bach et al., 1983, Shorten, 1987) to be related to resonance and energy expenditure. The control of stability and posture involves the modulation of stiffness through the spring-like behavior provided by the muscle-tendon unit whose stiffness or resistance to stretch, can be modified dynamically by the level of muscular activation. This indicates that it may be possible to regulate stability and posture through stiffness modulation. Some studies (Butler et al., 2003, Faria et al., 2009) have shown that an increased stiffness may be beneficial to performance while excessive or insufficient stiffness increases the risk of bone and soft tissue injuries, respectively. It seems that an optimal level of stiffness in the muscle-tendon unit may contribute to improved human motion performance. The resonance frequency can be accomplished by selecting movement frequencies that coincide with the natural frequency of the massspring system, while stiffness can play a role in regulation of movement frequencies (Farley et al., 1991, Granata et al., 2002a). Furthermore, the stride frequency and speed, usually used in gaits by different animals, are those where storage and recovery of elastic strain energy is maximized. The motor system can take advantage of resonance and in so doing it can minimize effort or maximize performance (Shorten, 1987).

Therefore, the purpose of this chapter is to provide an update of the literature on muscle-tendon unit stiffness and its relationship with joint stability and posture, the risk of injury, performance, resonance and energy expenditure. Furthermore this review also includes relevant information for the assessment and comprehension of the muscletendon unit stiffness and the differences that may exist between the sexes. It is our hope that this chapter will provide some insight into the current thought of the role of muscletendon unit stiffness in the areas mentioned above.

## DEFINITION OF STIFFNESS AND METHODS USED IN STIFFNESS EVALUATION

Studies of the biomechanical properties of muscles and tendons are more prevalent in the literature as researchers try to deepen the understanding of the complexities of the biomechanics of human movement. Viscoelastic characteristics of the muscle-tendon unit play an important role in the life of living beings, particularly in human life by enhancing the effectiveness and efficiency of human performance. Of special importance is the ability of these tissues to store energy when deformed (stretched) through force and to recoil after being stretched (Shorten, 1987, Fukashiro et al., 2001). In physics, as part of Hooke's Law, the elastic behavior (stiffness (k)) may be described by the relationship between the deformation of an elastic object and the force applied to it ($F = k.x$). Objects that observe this law should be deformable bodies, considering that their shape is not permanently changed, with the ability to store and return elastic energy. For an ideal linear spring, the force that deforms (stretches) the spring is in direct proportion to the amount of deformation. An ideal spring moves only Definition of stiffness and methods used in stiffness evaluation

Studies of the biomechanical properties of muscles and tendons are more prevalent in the literature as researchers try to deepen the understanding of the complexities of the biomechanics of human movement. Viscoelastic characteristics of the muscle-tendon unit play an important role in the life of living beings, particularly in human life by enhancing the effectiveness and efficiency of human performance. Of special importance is the ability of these tissues to store energy when deformed (stretched) through force and to recoil after being stretched (Shorten, 1987, Fukashiro et al., 2001). In physics, as part of Hooke's Law, the elastic behavior (stiffness (k)) may be described by the relationship between the deformation of an elastic object and the force applied to it ($F = k.x$). Objects that observe this law should be deformable bodies, considering that their shape is not permanently changed, with the ability to store and return elastic energy. For an ideal linear spring, the force that deforms (stretches) the spring is in direct proportion to the amount of deformation. An ideal spring moves only in one direction, is massless and has a stiffness that is independent of time, length and velocity. In addition, it is also assumed that the mass of the system is concentrated at a point at one end of the spring. However the joints of the human body don't behave exactly like a spring. According to Latash and Zatsiorsky (1993) an accurate model should include all the elements that contribute to stiffness. The overall stiffness of the human body depends, not only on elements such as muscles and tendons, elements like bones, cartilage and ligaments must also be considered. Further on, the role of the central nervous system, the viscosity and the time delays of the muscle reflex have to be incorporated. Additionally, the model must be able to accommodate the dependence of time, length and velocity when assessing stiffness and encompass various parallel elastic components (PEC) and series elastic components (SEC), several degrees of freedom at joints and be controlled by more than two muscles some of which are biarticular, (Latash and Zatsiorsky, 1993, Zatsiorsky, 2002, Butler et al., 2003). A measurement that covers all of these elements is currently still very complex. This may explain why many published investigations still employ the mass-spring model in their procedures. However as this measure does not account for the behavior of all the components described above Latash and Zatsiorsky (1993) designated it as ''quasistiffness''.

The two main methods used to measure the stiffness of isolated muscles and tendons onsists of the a method (Morgan, 1977) and the null-point method (Rack and Westbury, 1984). However, in order to study the biomechanical properties of muscles and tendons "in vivo" other methods have been developed. These include the impulse response or free vibration/oscillation technique (Cavagna, 1970, Hunter and Kearney, 1982, Hunter and Kearney, 1983, Aruin and Zatsiorsky, 1984, Shorten, 1987, Lafortune et al., 1996, Hunter and Spriggs, 2000, Fukashiro et al., 2001, Babic and Lenarcic, 2004, Faria et al., 2009), the quick release method (Pousson et al., 1990, Fukashiro et al., 1995a), the ultrasound method

Fukashiro et al., 1995b, Levinson et al., 1995, Maganaris and Paul, 1999, Kubo et al., 2001, Magnusson et al., 2001, Maganaris and Paul, 2002, Reeves et al., 2003, Lichtwark and Wilson, 2008, Kay and Blazevich, 2009) and the magnetic resonance method (Kruse et al., 2000, Heers et al., 2003, Jenkyn et al., 2003, Uffmann et al., 2004, Bensamoun et al., 2006). A review and explanation of other methods is also found in Butler et al. (2003). More specifically Butler et al. (2003) demonstrates how vertical stiffness, leg stiffness and torsional stiffness can be assessed. Like all methods the ones discussed above also have some limitations that should be considered when assessing the biomechanical properties of muscles and tendons. The limitations of the impulse response or free vibration/oscillation technique include the following: Most of the times muscles and tendons are assumed the main contributors to Stiffness, stability and posture

The concept of posture refers to the orientation of the body segments to each other and is usually applied to static or quasi-static positions such as sitting and standing (Watkins, 2010). On the other hand the concept of stability from a biomechanical and motor control point of view can be considered as the ability of a system to return to its original condition following a disturbance (Wagner and Blickhan, 1999) whilst joint stability can be defined as the joint's ability to hold a certain joint position according to a given motor pathway (Gabriel et al., 2008). The stiffness seems to somehow be related with the capacity of those structures to resist perturbations and in this way contribute to stability and posture. The biomechanical properties of MTU provide some kind of spring-like behavior to these structures, whose stiffness or resistance to stretch, can be modified dynamically by the level of muscular activation. Granata et al. (2004) stated that musculoskeletal stiffness is a main component of stability and neuromotor function, with various studies showing the relevance of dynamic stiffness adjustments to the maintenance of stability during different motor tasks and situations. For example, Duan et al. (1997) reported that nonlinear joint stiffness can be incorporated into gait models to overcome stability problems. The non-linear muscle force-stiffness relationship was shown to greatly alter the individual stabilizing potential of the muscle throughout its progression of force development. It was suggested that this knowledge should be incorporated into stability models to assist in recognizing unstable events that lead to injuries (Brown and McGill, 2005). In another study ankle instability was assessed by measuring the electromechanical delay of the peroneal muscles (Isabelle et al., 2003) and it was reported that electromechanical delay was significantly higher in subjects with functional ankle instability suggesting that a lower ankle musculo-tendinous stiffness may contribute to the ankle instability. Carpenter et al. (2001), in a study on the influence of postural threat on the control of upright stance, reported an enhancement of ankle stiffness as a strategy to maintain a tighter control of upright posture when standing under conditions of increased postural threat. The effects of joint stiffness on standing stability was investigated by Edwards (2007) who showed that ankle stability decreases with the increase in body mass index.

According to this author ankle stiffness should be increased to compensate for a higher body mass index in order to improve postural stability. An increase in triceps surae MTU stiffness attributed to obesity was also reported in postmenopausal females and linked to reasons of stability and posture (Faria et al., 2009). When increased forces are applied to the body, greater resistance to movement is required to produce controlled movements (Butler et al, 2003). Considering that obese subjects show greater inertia this suggests that they develop a set of adaptations and/or strategies that might lead to higher values of MTU stiffness. The concept that muscle stiffness during quiet standing controls balance was introduced by Winter et al. (1998). These authors argued that as the body sways about some desired position the center-of-mass (COM) tends to move in phase with the center-of-pressure (COP) due to the action of spring-like muscles. Similarly it was reported that, in response to sudden horizontal displacements of the support surface, a considerable decrease in the rate of forward velocity of the COM occurs due to the increase in MTU stiffness. However, some criticism of the methods used in that study were presented by Morasso and Schieppati (1999) who reported model and empiric consistency inadequacies. For these authors the in-phase relation between the trajectories of the COP and the COM is not determined by control patterns but rather by the physics. Furthermore they argued that the stiffness of the ankle muscles was insufficient to stabilize the body's "inverted pendulum". Referring to the same issue Winter et al. (2001) published a new study refuting the criticism presented by Morasso and Schieppati (1999) and reinforcing the idea that stiffness characteristics of the ankle plantar flexors provide a simple and stable operating point for control of upright posture. Meanwhile Morasso and Schieppati (2002) published another study again stating that ankle muscle stiffness alone cannot stabilize balance during quiet standing. Similarly, in response to the claim made by Winter et al. (1998, 2001) that stability cannot be maintained unless the intrinsic ankle stiffness is greater than the gravitational spring, Loram and Lakie (2002) reported that their results do not support these assertions because even at ankle torques higher than those encountered in quiet standing the intrinsic stiffness is too low and indicated that stability of the COM can be maintained with low intrinsic ankle stiffness if there is an alternative neural mechanism for modulating ankle torque. For these authors the body's COM is controlled by anticipatory modulation of the proximal offset position of the weak spring which is the Achilles' tendon. The paper presented by Casadio et al. (2005) also seems to consubstantiate and complement the work performed by Loram and Lakie (2002). Although various studies have reported conflicting results, some relationship between stiffness, stability and posture seem to exist. Additional studies are needed to improve the knowledge about these issues.

Another confounding factor in understanding the relationship between MTU and stability and posture is the differences that may exist between males and females. With active stiffness contributing, in some degree, to dynamic joint stability and because research has identified lower structural musculotendinous stiffness in females than in males it was suggested that potential sex differences in joint stability may exist (Blackburn et al., 2006). Differences in active stiffness across sex were observed for the total leg (Granata et al., 2002a, Padua et al., 2005), triceps surae (Blackburn et al., 2006, Gabriel et al., 2008) and knee flexors (Granata et al., 2002b, Blackburn et al., 2004).

Foure et al. (2009) studied the active part of the plantar flexors and also reported greater joint stiffness in men compared to women. In relation to passive stiffness the men were found to have greater stiffness than women at 10° of ankle dorsiflexion during a slow dynamic (movement) stretch of the calf muscle-tendon unit (Riemann et al., 2001a, Gajdosik et al.,

2006). Greater passive stiffness has also been reported for the knee joint complex (Oatis, 1993) in men compared to women as for the knee flexors (Gajdosik et al., 1990, Blackburn et al., 2004), ankle plantar flexors (Foure et al., 2009) and elbow flexors (Chleboun et al., 1997). Generally, women tend to show lower musculotendinous flexibility when compared to men and it was hypothesized that these differences may be attributed to geometrical factors (Blackburn et al., 2004). Foure et al. (2009) studied the passive and the active part of the plantar flexors and suggested that the gender differences in active stiffness can result from geometrical and/or intrinsic mechanical properties of the muscle–tendon unit structures. For these authors the differences in geometry and intrinsic mechanical properties may be attributed to the greater stress applied on the muscle–tendon unit by men and to hormonal characteristics. Chleboun et al.(1997) found a positive relationship between volume and stiffness and reported that 84% and 62% of stiffness variance was attributable to muscle volume in the shoulder flexed and extended position, respectively. While, Gajdosik et al. (1990) suggested that lower passive hamstring stiffness in females was attributable to lower muscle mass, and Oatis (1993) reported that the differences in passive knee joint stiffness between sexes may be attributed to mass discrepancies of the limb.

## STIFFNESS, RESONANCE AND ENERGY EXPENDITURE

The natural frequency of oscillation is the frequency at which a "pendulum-like" system oscillates as it comes to rest whilst the resonance frequency is the buildup of large amplitude oscillations that takes place when a structure is excited at its natural frequency. When a cyclic load is applied to a damped mass-spring system the amplitude response of the system results from the relationship established between the frequency at which the cyclic load is applied and the natural frequency of the system. When these two frequencies coincide with each other the amplitude of the mass-spring system tends to its highest, and the system is said to resonate. In other words the magnitude of force needed to achieve a given amplitude of movement in the system is at its lowest at the resonant frequency (Shorten, 1987). A common and revealing example of this phenomenon is a playground swing. In this situation if a person is pushed in time with the natural interval of the swing this will make the swing go increasingly higher until maximum amplitude is achieved. However if the attempts to push the swing are performed out of phase with the swing oscillating frequency a decrease in swing amplitude will result, due to the reduction of some of the swing energy by the opposing forces of the pushes.

In a study (Hoyt and Taylor, 1981) on gait and the energetics of locomotion in horses it was shown that quadrupeds choose the most economical (i.e. lowest metabolic energy consumed) speeds within each gait, furthermore moving a given distance at lower or higher speeds will considerably increase the energy cost. The authors also observed that the minimum cost was similar for each gait (walk, trot and gallop) and indicated that the natural gait at any speed entails the smallest possible energy expenditure. Similarly it was suggested (Taylor, 1985) that some sort of tuned mechanical system, operating at its optimal efficiency, may play a role in this process. Studies about hopping kangaroos (Dawson and Taylor, 1973) and galloping quadrupeds (Heglund et al., 1974) were also highlighted (Taylor, 1985) as proof of this tuned mechanism since these animals tend to use similar stride frequencies at two- to three-fold range of speeds. Furthermore Taylor (1985) quoting McMahon (1975) reported that these frequencies are the resonant frequencies of the body, as galloping frequency changes with body mass and body dimensions in a manner that is consistent with the changes in resonant frequency predicted by the multi-jointed spring model used by McMahon (1975). As with hopping kangaroos and galloping horses, hopping subjects use a nearly constant frequency over a wide range of speeds reinforcing the idea that hopping-galloping frequency is a tuned resonant frequency of a "whole body spring" (Taylor, 1985). Taylor (1985) suggested that the stride frequency and speed that animals usually use in their gaits are those where storage and recovery of elastic strain energy is maximized. This author also reported that when animals change their gait from a trot to a gallop the peak muscle stresses are reduced which reflects a redistribution of force over time, and the recruitment of a larger, more compliant spring system. He also mentioned that during steady-state running, galloping and hopping, the major muscle groups regularly use the stretch-shorten cycle (SSC) during stride, which enables them to operate in concert with their tendons as spring systems. In order to operate these muscle-tendon spring systems during locomotion, it is necessary that they be alternately turned on and off during each stride cycle. Furthermore both the energetic cost of locomotion and the cost of generating force during locomotion appear to be directly proportional to the frequency at which the muscles are turned on and off (Taylor, 1985).

Other authors reported (Bach et al., 1983, Shorten, 1987) that the motor system can take advantage of resonance and by doing so it can minimize effort or maximize performance. Bach et al. (1983) studied the resonance of the human body during voluntary oscillations around the ankle joint and accounted that motor systems can take advantage of resonance by selecting movement frequencies that coincide with the natural frequency of the mass-spring system. The adjustments of movement frequencies can be achieved by different ways. For instance, Farley and Gonzalez (1996) reported that the stiffness of leg spring increased between the lowest and highest stride frequencies and concluded that the most important body spring system adjustment to accommodate higher stride frequencies arise from a stiffer leg spring. A mass-springdamper model was used by Derrick et al. (2000) in running activities to simulate the vertical ground reaction force as stride length changes. In this study two springs in series with a mass were used. The first one simulated the behavior of body structures that produce the active portion of the ground reaction force and the second one the behavior of the components that cause the impact portion of the ground reaction force.

The increase of the stride length was associated with a 50% decrease in the active spring stiffness and a 20% increase in the impact spring. Based on these results it was suggested that the stiffness during the impact may contribute towards preventing the collapse of the supporting leg. This is due to the increased contact velocities seen in the longer strides. Studies about hop in place also reported that leg stiffness increased with hoping frequency (Farley et al., 1991, Granata et al., 2002a). In an earlier study by McMahon and Greene (1979) both ground contact time and step length where shown to increase on very compliant surfaces and as a result running speeds were moderately reduced. Bach et al. (1983) reported that one subject in the non-fatigued state at a stride frequency of 1.66 strides/s had a frequency during ankle extension of 4.40 Hz and in the fatigued state at a stride frequency of 1.52 strides/s the ankle extension frequency was disproportionately lower at 3.68 Hz. The authors suggested that this decrease indicated changes in the overall mechanics of the stride so that the frequency in fatigue is much closer to the resonant frequency (3.06 Hz) for a one legged model.

These investigators conjectured that in the fatigued state the body may swop from a speed optimizing strategy to an energy optimizing strategy, and adjust gait to take advantage of mechanical characteristics offered by the system.

Ahlborn and Blake (2002) used a theoretical pendulum model to evaluate resonance at walking, walk-run transition and running. The model centers on forced harmonic motion at resonance, and relates running speed, body mass, impact force and limb length. It also exploits a quantitative value for the transition speed from walking to running. According to these authors biomechanical energy can be briefly stored by human beings in elastic oscillations in different body parts and in pendulum-like oscillations. By doing that humans and other living beings may be able to reduce energy consumption. Nevertheless this energy saving only occurs if these oscillations are tuned to the leg propagation frequency (Ahlborn and Blake, 2002). Based on a comparison of the model equations for walking and running with experimental data, it was suggested, that humans and animals tend to adopt a motion where the propagation frequency is tuned into the elastic and the pendulum frequencies of their legs (Ahlborn and Blake, 2002). This ensures that the locomotion system work at the lowest power input of a forced harmonic motion system. Supporting this is the study performed by Ferris et al. (1998) that investigated what happened with leg stiffness during running if subjects ran on surfaces of different elasticity. These authors (Ferris et al., 1998) found that runners adjust their leg stiffness to accommodate changes in surface stiffness and by doing that the total stiffness remained constant. As runner's legs tend to be stiffer and compress less when running on a compliant surface than in a hard non-compliant surface, during this process some energy is stored in elastic deformation according to the stiffness of the track. Similarly, Farley et al. (1998) reported that it is important to perform adjustments in joint stiffness and limb geometry to adjust leg stiffness and allow similar hopping on different surfaces. It is also important to note that energy will be stored and returned in each step by the compliant elastic surface thus reducing the work performed by the muscles (Ferris et al., 1998). However, if the elastic frequency is not in tuned with the leg frequency, the energy stored will be greatly wasted (Ahlborn and Blake, 2002).

Takeshita et al. (2006) investigated the resonance in the human medial gastrocnemius muscle during cyclic ankle bending exercise at eight different frequencies. They showed that both the amplitude ratio and phase difference between the fascicle and MTU lengths were dependent on the movement frequency. The results also showed that, at higher frequencies, the fascicle lengths varied out of phase with the MTU length whereas at lower frequencies they varied almost in phase. Additionally, at intermediate frequencies the amplitude of the fascicle became very small compared with that of the MTU, which was considered to be resonance. These authors (Takeshita et al., 2006) suggested that the resonant effect owing to the viscoelasticity of tendinous tissue, may be one of the reasons for the existence of the energetically optimal speed in walking. In their conclusion they reported that the behavior of the muscle-tendon unit is highly dependent on the movement frequency due the viscoelasticity of the muscle-tendon unit. Some investigations on resonance of the upper extremities have also been performed. In a study on the storage and utilization of elastic energy in musculature, Denoth (1985) reported that only when the effective frequency of the contractile component activity matches the natural frequency of the SEC can optimal performance occur in a throwing movement. Wilson et al. (1991) studied the optimal stiffness of a SEC in a stretch-shorten cycle activity. They showed that the optimal maximal stiffness of the SEC during the rebound bench press lift is towards the compliant end of the elasticity.

ontinuum, indicating that this may need to occur within the parameters of achieving equivalence between the natural and movement frequencies. According to this interpretation they concluded that the optimal stiffness may be a resonant-compliant SEC. Further reports related with resonance of the upper extremity can be found in the following studies (Joyce et al., 1974, Lakie et al., 1984, Amis et al., 1987, Walsh and Wright, 1987).

## STIFFNESS AND PERFORMANCE

Research investigating the relationship between MTU stiffness and performance has been done in recent years and the results seems to indicate that some degree of stiffness is needed for optimal utilization of the SSC, specifically for efficient utilization of the elastic energy stored in the musculoskeletal system that occurs during the loading portion of movement (Latash and Zatsiorsky, 1993, Butler et al., 2003). One of the advantages of the SSC muscle action related to efficiency is that the MTU can store elastic energy during the eccentric (braking) phase of SSC, which can then be recoiled in the subsequent concentric (push-off) phase, thus saving metabolic energy (Kuitunen et al., 2007). The SSC can be defined as a pattern of eccentric contraction followed, without a pause, by concentric contraction (Komi, 2003, Watkins, 2010). According to Watkins (2010) if concentric contraction takes place without prestretch, the initial phase of contraction is used to remove the slack in the SEC and only after the slack has been taken up can the force, produced by the muscle, be transmitted to the skeleton. Taking up this slack before force can be transmitted to the skeleton consumes energy and is therefore not efficient. With age, this slack might increase and/or the behavior of the SEC may change. Some studies (Narici and Maganaris, 2006, Narici et al., 2008) reported that old tendons are more compliant (less stiffness) when compared with younger tendons. Similarly older tendons will take a longer time to be stretched and are less capable than younger ones to transmit fast forces from muscles to bones, taking longer to then effectively react in order to avoid slipping or tripping. Wilson et al (1994) argued that a stiffer muscle-tendon unit would enhance isometric or concentric force production compared with a more compliant system, not only because of a decrease of the shortening velocity of the contractile component but also due to a relatively longer length of the contractile component throughout the contraction. Moreover a stiffer MTU may be beneficial and facilitate the transmission of force from the contractile component to the skeletal structures. The strong relationship between the MTU stiffness and isometric and concentric performance may have huge applications in different activities (e.g. boxing, cycling) that involve a rapid development of force in an isometric or concentric muscular contraction (Wilson et al., 1994). Despite the relationship formerly mentioned been operative during the concentric phase of an SSC activity in such movements the elastic characteristics of the muscle-tendon unit could also have a large effect on the use of elastic strain energy (Wilson et al., 1994). For instance it was observed (Wilson et al., 1992) that the SSC performance was enhanced in a heavily loaded bench press movement by a reduction of the muscle-tendon unit stiffness, whilst in a similar bench press movement the elastic energy was maximized by an highly compliant elastic system (Wilson et al., 1991). According to this findings, Wilson et al. (1994) suggested that the improvement in the use of elastic energy, that results from reducing the muscle-tendon unit stiffness, outweighs the performance augmentation to the concentric phase of movement associated with a stiff musculotendinous unit, in at least some SSC movements. However these authors (Wilson et al., 1994) also highlighted that those activities where a rapid development of force is very important (e.g. running) a stiffer MTU might be more valuable. Several published research have analyzed the relationship between stiffness and performance during hopping. From these hopping in place studies (Farley et al., 1991, Granata et al., 2002a, Rapoport et al., 2003, Dalleau et al., 2004, Chang et al., 2008, Hobara et al., 2008, Hobara et al., 2010) it was reported that leg stiffness increased as hopping frequency increased. Furthermore this is usually associated with a decrease in ground contact time (Farley et al., 1991, Ferris and Farley, 1997, Granata et al., 2002a, Rapoport et al., 2003, Chang et al., 2008, Hobara et al., 2008, Hobara et al., 2010). Granata et al. (2002a) also observed that not only leg stiffness increased when hopping frequency increased but males showed significantly greater leg stiffness than females at each hopping frequency studied.

Hobara et al. (2008) examined the determinants of the difference in leg stiffness between endurance- and power-trained athletes during two-legged hopping at two different frequencies. The power-trained athletes showed significantly higher leg stiffness than the distance runners at both hopping frequencies. The knee stiffness was also significantly greater in the power-trained athletes than in the distance runners at 1.5 Hz and in ankle stiffness at 3.0 Hz. Additionally, Farley et al. (1991) suggested that an increase in the stiffness of the leg or the hopping height result in order to accommodate hopping frequency at a given frequency. During running (Luhtanen and Komi, 1980, Mero and Komi, 1986, Arampatzis et al., 1999, Seyfarth et al., 2002) and sprinting (Stefanyshyn and Nigg, 1998, Kuitunen et al., 2002) leg stiffness was also reported to increase as speed increases. However some studies have suggested that leg stiffness is independent of running (He et al., 1991, Farley et al., 1993) and sprinting speed (Morin et al., 2006). Most of these studies suggest that as the physical demands of the activity increase, stiffness also increases, perhaps to resist collapse of the lower extremity during the early phase of landing and allow for maximum energy return during the propulsive phase (Stefanyshyn and Nigg, 1998, Arampatzis et al., 1999, 2001a, 2001b, Granata et al., 2002a, Seyfarth et al., 2002, Butler et al., 2003). Published research has also shown some relationship between stiffness and stride parameters (McMahon et al., 1987,

Farley and Gonzalez, 1996, Derrick et al., 2000). The overall results suggest a decrease in stiffness when the stride length increases. McMahon et al. (1987) , tested the normal and Groucho running (exaggerated knee flexion) on a treadmill. The authors showed a similar cadence between normal and Groucho running at the same speed; a decrease in the vertical stiffness with a concomitant increase in step length with Groucho running; a decrease in the transmission of mechanical shock from the foot to the skull with a required 50% increase in the rate of O2 consumption. In a review by Butler et al. (2003), discussing the implications of lower extremity stiffness for performance and injury, also reported that running economy as measured by oxygen consumption is related to stiffness. More specifically it was mentioned that an increased stiffness is associated with economy. Derrick et al. (2000) simulated the vertical ground reaction forces for a human runner during stride length changes and reported that subjects increased their stride length while the stiffness of the active spring decreased by 51%. Farley and Gonzalez (1996) tested human subjects running on a treadmill-mounted force platform while using a range of stride frequencies. The authors reported that when the stride length increased the stride frequencies decreased to accommodate the stiffness of the leg spring. The authors also attributed the increase in vertical stiffness observed at higher stride frequencies to the leg spring stiffness. However Butler et al. (2003) advised that caution be exercised when considering these results, as although the increase in the runner's stride length may be beneficial for performance this alteration may negatively affect the velocity due to the decrease in stiffness.

## STIFFNESS AND THE RISK OF INJURY

Due to the lack of prospective studies, no direct link has been established between MTU stiffness and the risk of injury. Nevertheless, some studies suggest that too much or too little stiffness may play a role in the occurrence of injuries. The explanation is that insufficient MTU stiffness may be related to excessive joint motion and instability leading to soft tissue injuries (Granata et al., 2002a, Butler et al., 2003, Faria et al., 2009). An overload of structures associated with force attenuation may occur (Williams et al., 2004) if a system becomes too compliant (little stiffness). On the contrary, too much stiffness may be related to bone injuries, the reason being that increased leg stiffness is usually associated with reduced lower extremity excursions and increased peak forces. The association between these factors typically leads to increased loading rates which have been linked to increased shock having to be absorbed by the lower extremity (Hennig and Lafortune, 1991, Butler et al., 2003). The increased risk of bone injury, such as knee osteoarthritis and stress fractures, may result from increased peak forces, loading rates, and shocks (Burr et al., 1985, Grimston et al.,

1991, Butler et al., 2003). Additionally, plantar fasciitis and midfoot arthritis may also be linked to MTU stiffness (Faria et al., 2009).

## CONCLUSION AND PROPOSED DIRECTIONS FOR FUTURE WORK

There are currently several methods available to evaluate the biomechanical properties of muscles and tendons. All methods have limitations and should therefore be used with caution and in accordance with the objectives of the intended research.

Despite this, recent methods like the ultrasound and magnetic resonance seem to have overcome some of the limitations of the previous methods, thus making them a better choice.

It was suggested that musculoskeletal stiffness is a main component of stability and neuromotor function -specifically dynamic stiffness adjustments, as it seems to be relevant to the maintenance of stability during different motor tasks and situations.

Some research reported that instability may be overcome by increasing musculotendinous stiffness and others indicated that an enhancement of ankle stiffness can be used as a strategy to maintain a tighter control of upright posture. Nevertheless conflicting results have been reported. Further studies are required to enhance the knowledge about these issues.

The human motor system seems to be able to capitalize on the resonance frequency and therefore minimize effort or maximize performance. This is done by selecting movement frequencies that coincide with the natural frequency of the massspring system. One way to achieve this may be through the regulation of stiffness to accommodate the stride frequencies requested. Although some studies about resonance frequency have been performed only a few have analyzed the implications of the resonance frequency in human activities, creating a vast field for future research.

In relation to performance, literature suggests that increased stiffness is associated with increased hopping frequency, hopping height, velocity and economy.

One of the explanations for these results may be related with the ability of the motor system to resist the collapse of the lower extremity during locomotion and be capable to efficiently use the elastic energy during the propulsive phase.

It has been suggested in retrospective studies that excessive or insufficient stiffness comport a risk factor for injuries. In particular higher values of stiffness have been associated to bone injuries while soft tissue injuries have been linked to lower values of stiffness.. However, due to the lack of prospective studies no direct link has been established between stiffness and the risk of injury. Therefore future research is needed to substantiate these findings.

## REFERENCES

Ahlborn, B. K. and Blake, R. W. 2002. Walking and running at resonance. *Zoology,* 105, 165-174.

Amis, A., Prochazka, A., Short, D., Trend, P. and Ward, A. 1987. Relative displacements in muscle and tendon during human arm movements. *Journal of Physiology*, 389, 37.

Arampatzis, A., Brüggemann, G. and Klapsing, G. 2001a. Leg stiffness and mechanical energetic processes during jumping on a sprung surface. *Medicine and Science in Sports and Exercise*, 33, 923-931.

Arampatzis, A., Brüggemann, G. and Metzler, V. 1999. The effect of speed on leg stiffness and joint kinetics in human running. *Journal of Biomechanics,* 32, 1349-1353.

Arampatzis, A., Schade, F., Walsh, M. and Brüggemann, G. 2001b. Influence of leg stiffness and its effect on myodynamic jumping performance. *Journal of Electromyography and Kinesiology*, 11, 355-364.

Aruin, A. S. and Zatsiorsky, V. M. 1984. Biomechanical characteristics of human ankle-joint muscles. *European Journal of Applied Physiology and Occupational Physiology*, 52, 400-406.

Babic, J. and Lenarcic, J. 2004. In vivo determination of triceps surae muscletendon complex viscoelastic properties. *European Journal of Applied Physiology*, 92, 477-484.

Bach, T., Chapman, A. and Calvert, T. 1983. Mechanical resonance of the human body during voluntary oscillations about the ankle joint. *Journal of Biomechanics*, 16, 85-90.

Bensamoun, S. F., Ringleb, S. I., Littrell, L., Chen, Q., Brennan, M., Ehman, R. L. And An, K.-N. 2006. Determination Of Thigh Muscle Stiffness Using magnetic resonance elastography. *Journal of Magnetic Resonance Imaging*, 23, 242-247.

Blackburn, J. T., Padua, D. A., Weinhold, P. S. and Guskiewicz, K. M. 2006. Comparison of triceps surae structural stiffness and material modulus across sex. Clinical Biomechanics, 21, 159-167.

Blackburn, J. T., Riemann, B. L., Padua, D. A. and Guskiewicz, K. M. 2004. Sex comparison of extensibility, passive, and active stiffness of the knee flexors. *Clinical Biomechanics*, 19, 36-43.

Brown, S. H. M. and Mcgill, S. M. 2005. Muscle force-stiffness characteristics influence joint stability: A spine example. *Clinical Biomechanics*, 20, 917-922.

Burr, D., Martin, R., Schaffler, M. and RADIN, E. 1985. Bone remodeling in response to in vivo fatigue microdamage. *Journal of Biomechanics*, 18, 189-200.

Butler, R. J., Crowell Iii, H. P. and Davis, I. M. 2003. Lower extremity stiffness: implications for performance and injury. *Clinical Biomechanics* 18, 511-517.

Carpenter, M., Frank, J., Silcher, C. and Peysar, G. 2001. The influence of postural threat on the control of upright stance. *Experimental Brain Research*, 138, 210-218.

Casadio, M., Morasso, P. G. And Sanguineti, V. 2005. Direct measurement of ankle stiffness during quiet standing: implications for control modelling and clinical application. *Gait and Posture*, 21, 410-24.

Cavagna, G. A. 1970. Elastic bounce of the body. *Journal of Applied Physiology*, 29, 279-282.

Chang, Y.-H., Roiz, R. A. and Auyang, A. G. 2008. Intralimb compensation strategy depends on the nature of joint perturbation in human hopping. *Journal of Biomechanics*, 41, 1832-1839.

Chleboun, G. S., Howell, J. N., Conatser, R. R. and Giesey, J. J. 1997. The relationship between elbow flexor volume and angular stiffness at the elbow. *Clinical Biomechanics*, 12, 383-392.

Dalleau, G., Belli, A., Viale, F., Lacour, J. and Bourdin, M. 2004. A simple method for field measurements of leg stiffness in hopping. *International Journal of Sports Medicine*, 25, 170-176.

Dawson, T. J. and Taylor, C. R. 1973. Energetic Cost of Locomotion in Kangaroos. *Nature*, 246, 313-314.

Denoth, J. Year. Storage And Utilisation of Elastic Energy In Musculature. In: Winter, D. A., Norman, R. W., Wells, R. P., Hayes, K. C. And Patla, A. E., eds. Biomechanics IX-B (International series on biomechanics), 1985. Human Kinetics Publishers, Champaign, IL, 65-70.

Derrick, T., Caldwell, G. and Hamill, J. 2000. Modeling the Stiffness Characteristics of the Human Body While Running With Various Stride Lengths. *Journal of Applied Biomechanics*, 16, 36-51.

Duan, X., Allen, R. and Sun, J. 1997. A stiffness-varying model of human gait. *Medical Engineering and Physics*, 19, 518-524.

Edwards, W. T. 2007. Effect of joint stiffness on standing stability. *Gait and Posture*, 25, 432-439.

Faria, A., Gabriel, R., Abrantes, J., Brás, R. and Moreira, H. 2009. Triceps-surae musculotendinous stiffness: Relative differences between obese and non-obese postmenopausal women. *Clinical Biomechanics*, 24, 866–871.

Faria, A., Gabriel, R., Abrantes, J., Brás, R. and Moreira, H. 2010. The relationship of body mass index, age and triceps-surae musculotendinous stiffness with the foot arch structure of postmenopausal women. *Clinical Biomechanics*, 25, 588-593.

Farley, C., Glasheen, J. and Mcmahon, T. 1993. Running springs: speed and animal size. *The Journal of Experimental Biology*, 185, 71-86.

Farley, C. and Gonzalez, O. 1996. Leg stiffness and stride frequency in human running. *Journal of Biomechanics*, 29, 181-186.

Farley, C. T., Blickhan, R., Saito, J. And Taylor, C. R. 1991. Hopping frequency in humans: a test of how springs set stride frequency in bouncing gaits. *Journal of Applied Physiology*, 71, 2127-2132.

Farley, C. T., Houdijk, H. H., Van Strien, C. And Louie, M. 1998. Mechanism of leg stiffness adjustment for hopping on surfaces of different stiffnesses. *Journal of Applied Physiology*, 85, 1044-1055.

Ferris, D. P. and Farley, C. T. 1997. Interaction of leg stiffness and surface stiffness during human hopping. *Journal of Applied Physiology*, 82, 15-22.

Ferris, D. P., Louie, M. and Farley, C. T. 1998. Running in the real world: adjusting leg stiffness for different surfaces. Proceedings of the Royal Society of London. Series B, *Biological Sciences*, 265, 989-994.

Foure, A., Nordez, A. and Cornu, C. 2009. Gender differences in the passive and active parts of plantar flexors series elastic component stiffness. *Computer Methods in Biomechanics and Biomedical Engineering*, 12, 109-110.

Fukashiro, S., Noda, M. and Shibayama, A. 2001. In vivo determination of muscle viscoelasticity in the human leg. *Acta physiologica Scandinavica*, 172, 241-248.

Fukashiro, S., Okada, J. and Fukunaga, T. Year. Contribution Of Series Elastic component in elbow flexion using stretch-shortening cycle. In: Hakkinen, K., Keskinen, K. L., Komi, P. V. And Mero, A., eds. The XVth congress of the ISB, book of abstracts, 1995a Jyvaskyla, Finland. Gummerus Kirjapaino, 292– 293.

Fukashiro, S., Rob, M., Ichinose, Y., Kawakami, Y. And Fukunaga, T. 1995b. Ultrasonography gives directly but noninvasively elastic characteristic of human tendon in vivo. *European Journal of Applied Physiology*, 71, 555-557.

Gabriel, R., Abrantes, J., Granata, K., Bulas-Cruz, J., Melo-Pinto, P. and Filipe, V. 2008. Dynamic joint stiffness of the ankle during walking: Gender-related differences. *Physical Therapy in Sport*, 9, 16-24.

Gajdosik, R., Lentz, D., Mcfarley, D., Meyer, K. and Riggin, T. 2006. Dynamic elastic and static viscoelastic stress-relaxation properties of the calf muscle-tendon unit of men and women. *Isokinetics and Exercise Science*, 14, 33-44.

Gajdosik, R. L., Giuliani, C. A. And Bohannon, R. W. 1990. Passive compliance and length of the hamstring muscles of healthy men anc women. *Clinical Biomechanics,* 5, 23-29.

Granata, K. P., Padua, D. A. and Wilson, S. E. 2002a. Gender differences in active musculoskeletal stiffness. Part II. Quantification of leg stiffness during functional hopping tasks. *Journal of Electromyography and Kinesiology*, 12, 127-135.

Granata, K. P., Wilson, S. E., Massimini, A. K. and Gabriel, R. 2004. Active stiffness of the ankle in response to inertial and elastic loads. *Journal of Electromyography and Kinesiology,* 14, 599-609.

Granata, K. P., Wilson, S. E. and Padua, D. A. 2002b. Gender differences in active musculoskeletal stiffness. Part I. Quantification in controlled measurements of knee joint dynamics. *Journal of Electromyography and Kinesiology*, 12, 119-26.

Grimston, S., Engsberg, J., Kloiber, R. and Hanley, D. 1991. Bone mass, external loads, and stress fracture in female runners. *Journal of Applied Biomechanics*, 7, 293-302.

He, J. P., Kram, R. and Mcmahon, T. A. 1991. Mechanics of running under simulated low gravity. *Journal of Applied Physiology*, 71, 863-870.

Heers, G., Jenkyn, T., Alex Dresner, M., Klein, M.-O., R Basford, J., R Kaufman, K., L Ehman, R. and An, K.-N. 2003. Measurement of muscle activity with magnetic resonance elastography. *Clinical Biomechanics*, 18, 537 542.

Heglund, N., Taylor, C. and Mcmahon, T. 1974. Scaling stride frequency and gait to animal size: mice to horses. *Science*, 186, 1112.

Hennig, E. and Lafortune, M. 1991. Relationships between ground reaction force and tibial bone acceleration parameters. *International Journal of Sport Biomechanics*, 7, 303-309.

Hobara, H., Inoue, K., Muraoka, T., Omuro, K., Sakamoto, M. and Kanosue, K. 2010. Leg stiffness adjustment for a range of hopping frequencies in humans. *Journal of Biomechanics*, 43, 506-511.

Hobara, H., Kimura, K., Omuro, K., Gomi, K., Muraoka, T., Iso, S. and Kanosue, K. 2008. Determinants of difference in leg stiffness between endurance- and power-trained athletes. *Journal of Biomechanics*, 41, 506-14.

Hoyt, D. F. and Taylor, C. R. 1981. Gait and the energetics of locomotion in horses. *Nature*, 292, 239-240.

Hunter, D. G. and Spriggs, J. 2000. Investigation into the relationship between the passive flexibility and active stiffness of the ankle plantar-flexor muscles. *Clinical Biomechanics*, 15, 600-606.

Hunter, I. and Kearney, R. 1982. Dynamics of human ankle stiffness: variation with mean ankle torque. *Journal of Biomechanics*, 15, 747-752.

Hunter, I. W. and Kearney, R. E. 1983. Invariance of ankle dynamic stiffness during fatiguing muscle contractions. *Journal of Biomechanics*, 16, 985-991.

Isabelle, M., Sylvie, Q. and Chantal, P. 2003. Electromechanical assessment of ankle stability. *European Journal of Applied Physiology*, 88, 558-564.

Jenkyn, T. R., Ehman, R. L. and An, K.-N. 2003. Noninvasive muscle tension measurement using the novel technique of magnetic resonance elastography (MRE). *Journal of Biomechanics*, 36, 1917-1921.

Joyce, G. C., Rack, P. M. H. and Ross, H. F. 1974. The forces generated at the human elbow joint in response to imposed sinusoidal movements of the forearm. *Journal of Physiology*, 240, 351-374.

Kay, A. D. and Blazevich, A. J. 2009. Isometric contractions reduce plantar flexor moment, Achilles tendon stiffness, and neuromuscular activity but remove the subsequent effects of stretch. *Journal of Applied Physiology*, 107, 1181-1189.

Komi, P. 2003. Stretch-shortening cycle. Strength and power in sport. 2nd ed.: Blackwell.

Kruse, S., Smith, J., Lawrence, A., Dresner, M., Manduca, A., Greenleaf, J. and Ehman, R. 2000. Tissue characterization using magnetic resonance elastography: preliminary results*. *Physics in Medicine and Biology*, 45, 1579-1590.

Kubo, K., Kanehisa, H. and Fukunaga, T. 2001. Effects of different duration isometric contractions on tendon elasticity in human quadriceps muscles. *Journal of Physiology*, 536, 649-655.

Kuitunen, S., Komi, P. and Kyröläinen, H. 2002. Knee and ankle joint stiffness in sprint running. *Medicine and Science in Sports and Exercise*, 34, 166-173.

Kuitunen, S., Kyrolainen, H., Avela, J. and Komi, P. 2007. Leg stiffness modulation during exhaustive stretch-shortening cycle exercise. *Scandinavian Journal of Medicine and Science in Sports*, 17, 67-75.

Lafortune, M. A., Hennig, E. M. and Lake, M. J. 1996. Dominant role of interface over knee angle for cushioning impact loading and regulating initial leg stiffness. *Journal of Biomechanics*, 29, 1523-1529.

Lakie, M., Walsh, E. and Wright, G. 1984. Resonance at the wrist demonstrated by the use of a torque motor: an instrumental analysis of muscle tone in man. *Journal of Physiology*, 353, 265-285.

Latash, M. L. and Zatsiorsky, V. M. 1993. Joint stiffness: Myth or reality? *Human Movement Science*, 12, 653-692.

Levinson, S. F., Shinagawa, M. and Sato, T. 1995. Sonoelastic determination of human skeletal muscle elasticity. *Journal of Biomechanics*, 28, 1145-1154.

Lichtwark, G. A. and Wilson, A. M. 2008. Optimal muscle fascicle length and tendon stiffness for maximising gastrocnemius efficiency during human walking and running. *Journal of Theoretical Biology*, 252, 662-673.

Loram, I. and Lakie, M. 2002. Direct measurement of human ankle stiffness during quiet standing: the intrinsic mechanical stiffness is insufficient for stability. *Journal of Physiology*, 545, 1041-1053.

Luhtanen, P. and Komi, P. V. 1980. Force-, power-, and elasticity-velocity relationships in walking, running, and jumping. *European Journal of Applied Physiology*, 44, 279-289.

Maganaris, C. and Paul, J. 2002. Tensile properties of the in vivo human astrocnemius tendon. *Journal of Biomechanics*, 35, 1639-1646.

Maganaris, C. N. and Paul, J. P. 1999. In vivo human tendon mechanical properties. *Journal of Physiology*, 521, 307-313.

Magnusson, S., Aagaard, P., Rosager, S., Dyhre-Poulsen, P. And Kjaer, M. 2001. Load–displacement properties of the human triceps surae aponeurosis in vivo. *Journal of Physiology*, 531, 277-288.

Mcmahon, T., Valiant, G. and Frederick, E. 1987. Groucho running. *Journal of Applied Physiology,* 62, 2326-2337.

Mcmahon, T. A. 1975. Using body size to understand the structural design of animals: quadrupedal locomotion. *Journal of Applied Physiology,* 39, 619-627.

Mcmahon, T. A. and Greene, P. R. 1979. The influence of track compliance on running. *Journal of Biomechanics*, 12, 893-904.

Mero, A. and Komi, P. 1986. Force-, EMG-, and elasticity-velocity relationships at submaximal, maximal and supramaximal running speeds in sprinters. *European Journal of Applied Physiology and Occupational Physiology*, 55, 553-561.

Morasso, P. and Schieppati, M. 1999. Can muscle stiffness alone stabilize upright standing? *Journal of Neurophysiology,* 82, 1622-1626.

Morasso, P. G. and Sanguineti, V. 2002. Ankle muscle stiffness alone cannot stabilize balance during quiet standing. *Journal of Neurophysiology*, 88, 2157 62.

Morgan, D. L. 1977. Separation of active and passive components of short-range stiffness of muscle. *American Journal of Physiology - Cell Physiology*, 232, C45-49.

Morin, J., Jeannin, T., Chevallier, B. and Belli, A. 2006. Spring-mass model characteristics during sprint running: correlation with performance and fatigueinduced changes. *International Journal of Sports Medicine*, 27, 158-165.

Narici, M., Maffulli, N. and Maganaris, C. 2008. Ageing of human muscles and tendons. Disability and Rehabilitation, 30, 1548-1554.

Narici, M. V. and Maganaris, C. N. 2006. Adaptability of elderly human muscles and tendons to increased loading. *Journal of Anatomy*, 208, 433-443.

Oatis, C. A. 1993. The use of a mechanical model to describe the stiffness and damping characteristics of the knee joint in healthy adults. *Physical Therapy*, 73, 740-749.

Padua, D., Carcia, C., Arnold, B. and Granata, K. 2005. Gender differences in leg stiffness and stiffness recruitment strategy during two-legged hopping. *Journal of Motor Behavior*, 37, 111-126.

Pousson, M., Van Hoecke, J. and Goubel, F. 1990. Changes in elastic characteristics of human muscle induced by eccentric exercise. *Journal of Biomechanics*, 23, 343-488.

Rack, P. and Westbury, D. 1984. Elastic properties of the cat soleus tendon and their functional importance. *Journal of Physiology,* 347, 479-495.

Rapoport, S., Mizrahi, J., Kimmel, E., Verbitsky, O. and Isakov, E. 2003. Constant and variable stiffness and damping of the leg joints in human hopping. *Journal of Biomechanical Engineering*, 125, 507.

Reeves, N., Maganaris, C. and Narici, M. 2003. Effect of strength training on human patella tendon mechanical properties of older individuals. *Journal of Physiology*, 548, 971-981.

Riemann, B., Demont, R., Ryu, K. and Lephart, S. 2001a. The effects of sex, joint angle, and the gastrocnemius muscle on passive ankle joint complex stiffness.

Riemann, B. L., Demont, R. G., Ryu, K. and Lephart, S. M. 2001b. The Effects of Sex, Joint Angle, and the Gastrocnemius Muscle on Passive Ankle Joint Complex Stiffness. *Journal of Athletic Training*, 36, 369-375.

Seyfarth, A., Geyer, H., Günther, M. and Blickhan, R. 2002. A movement criterion for running. *Journal of Biomechanics,* 35, 649-655.

Shorten, M. R. 1987. Muscle Elasticity and Human Performance. Current Research In Sports Biomechanics. *Medicine and Sport Science*, 25, 1-18.

Stefanyshyn, D. and Nigg, B. 1998. Dynamic Angular Stiffness Of The Ankle Joint during running and sprinting. *Journal of Applied Biomechanics*, 14, 292-299.

Takeshita, D., Shibayama, A., Muraoka, T., Muramatsu, T.Nagano, A., Fukunaga, T. and Fukashiro, S. 2006. Resonance in the human medial gastrocnemius muscle during cyclic ankle bending exercise. *Journal of Applied Physiology*, 101, 111-118.

Taylor, C. 1985. Force development during sustained locomotion: a determinant of gait, speed and metabolic power. *The Journal of Experimental Biology*, 115, 253-262.

Uffmann, K., Maderwald, S., Ajaj, W., Galban, C., Mateiescu, S., Quick, H. And Ladd, M. 2004. In vivo elasticity measurements of extremity skeletal muscle with MR elastography. *NMR in Biomedicine*, 17, 181-190.

Wagner, H. and Blickhan, R. 1999. Stabilizing function of skeletal muscles: an analytical investigation. *Journal of Theoretical Biology*, 199, 163-179.

Walsh, E. and Wright, G. 1987. Inertia, resonant frequency, stiffness and kinetic energy of the human forearm. *Experimental Physiology*, 72, 161-170.

Watkins, J. 2010. Structure and Function of the Musculoskeletal System, Human Kinetics.

Williams Iii, D. S., Davis, I. M., Scholz, J. P., Hamill, J. And Buchanan, T. S. 2004. High-arched runners exhibit increased leg stiffness compared to lowarched runners. *Gait and Posture*, 19, 263-269.

Wilson, G., Wood, G. and Elliott, B. 1991. Optimal stiffness of series elastic component in a stretch-shorten cycle activity. *Journal of Applied Physiology*, 70, 825-833.

Wilson, G. J., Elliott, B. C. and Wood, G. A. 1992. Stretch shorten cycle performance enhancement through flexibility training. *Medicine and Science in Sports and Exercise,* 24, 116-23.

Wilson, G. J., Murphy, A. J. and Pryor, J. F. 1994. Musculotendinous stiffness: its relationship to eccentric, isometric, and concentric performance. *Journal of Applied Physiology*, 76, 14-9.

Winter, D. A., Patla, A. E., Prince, F., Ishac, M. and Gielo-Perczak, K. 1998. Stiffness control of balance in quiet standing. *Journal of Neurophysiology*, 80, 1211-1221.

Winter, D. A., Patla, A. E., Rietdyk, S. and Ishac, M. G. 2001. Ankle Muscle Stiffness in the Control of Balance During Quiet Standing. *Journal of Neurophysiology*, 85, 2630-2633.

Zatsiorsky, V. M. 2002. Kinetics of Human Motion, Human Kinetics.

In: Posture: Types, Assessment and Control
Editors: A. Wright and S. Rothenberg, pp. 155-174
ISBN 978-1-61324-107-3
© 2011 Nova Science Publishers, Inc.

*Chapter 6*

# H-REFLEX ASSESSMENT AS A TOOL FOR UNDERSTANDING MOTOR FUNCTIONS IN POSTURAL CONTROL

### *Yung-Sheng Chen and Shi Zhou*[*]

School of Health and Human Science, Southern Cross University, Australia

## ABSTRACT

The Hoffmann reflex (H-reflex) has been extensively used to investigate spinal reflexive function in clinical and human movement studies. The H-reflex is induced by applying an electrical stimulation on a peripheral nerve branch and recording EMG from a muscle innervated by this nerve. The response of the α-motoneuron pool to the stimulation, as indicated by the peak-to-peak amplitude of H-reflex, reflects inhibitory and excitatory modulation of the spinal motoneuron pool during a motor task. Recently, the H-reflex modulation in relation to postural control has been addressed in a number of laboratory-based investigations. There has been evidence that the modulation of H-reflex is task-dependent. Specificity of the H-reflex in adaptation to exercise intervention has also been revealed. This chapter provides a discussion on the H-reflex modulation during a variety of postural tasks and its adaptation to exercise training. The soleus (SOL) H-reflex is the focus because this muscle plays a critical role in maintaining an upright standing posture and the studies on SOL H-reflex modulation may help us to understand the neural mechanisms in postural control.

## 1. INTRODUCTION

The Hoffmann reflex (H-reflex) is an electrical stimulation induced monosynaptic reflex that is used to investigate the effect of group Ia excitatory inputs on spinal α-motoneuron activation in clinical and human movement studies. The H-reflex response has been reported

---

[*] Corresponding Author: Professor Shi Zhou, School of Health and Human Sciences, Southern Cross University, Lismore, NSW 2480, Australia, Tel: + 61 2 66203991, Fax: + 61 2 66269583, E-mail: shi.zhou@scu.edu.au.

to vary with changes in body position (Angulo-Kinzler, Mynark, and Koceja, 1998; Chalmers and Knutzen, 2002; Knikou and Rymer, 2003), joint movement (Alrowayeh, Sabbahi, and Etnyre, 2005; Chen et al., 2010; Hwang, 2002) and different phases of walking (Capaday and Stein, 1987; Simonsen and Dyhre-Poulsen, 1999) and drop jump (Dyhre-Poulsen, Simonsen, and Voigt, 1991; Taube et al., 2008). Recently, it has been shown that the H-reflex modulation is related to the phase and direction of postural sway and postural stability (Tokuno, Carpenter, Thorstensson, Garland, and Cresswell, 2007; Tokuno, Garland, Carpenter, Thorstensson, and Cresswell, 2008). The relationship of the H-reflex modulation and the ability to control upright posture has also been examined in relation to acute (Trimble and Koceja, 1994, 2001) and short-term balance training (Schubert et al., 2008; Taube, Gruber, et al., 2007; Taube, Kullmann, et al., 2007). It appears that the H-reflex modulation has phase- and task-dependent specificity in respect to the postural conditions.

The aim of this chapter is to provide an analysis of current literature with a focus on the soleus (SOL) H-reflex modulation in relation to control of upright posture.

## 2. PHYSIOLOGY OF H-REFLEX

### 2.1. The H-Reflex Pathway

The physiological pathway of H-reflex is similar to a muscle stretch reflex (Voerman, Gregoric, and Hermens, 2005). The stretch reflex is initiated from the receptors in muscle spindles while the H-reflex is elicited by applying a single percutaneous electrical pulse to a peripheral nerve branch which has a mixture of sensory and motor nerve fibres (Zehr, 2002). In both the stretch reflex and H-reflex, ascending signals are mainly conducted by the group Ia fibres to the spinal cord and descending signals are conducted by the same axons from the spinal α-motoneurons. When an electrical stimulation is delivered to the nerve branch, two sets of evoked membrane action potentials, as recorded by an electromyograph (EMG), can be observed from the muscles that are innervated by the stimulated nerve (Palmieri, Ingersoll, and Hoffman, 2004). The first evoked potential (a complex EMG waveform) is recorded after a short latency of approximately 10 ms, and is referred to as the M-wave. The second waveform is recorded after a longer latency (~ 30ms) and is referred to as the H-wave.

The M-wave is caused by the evoked potential on the nerve branch that travels from the location of the electrical stimulation to the target muscle. The size of M-wave reflects the number of motor nerve fibres being activated simultaneously (Tucker, Tuncer, and Turker, 2005). In contrast, the H-wave is a result of group Ia afferent inputs in response to the electrical stimulation (Palmieri, et al., 2004; Tucker, et al., 2005). The reflex arc includes the group Ia afferent fibres from the location of the electrical stimulation (ascending portion) to the spinal cord where synaptic transmission occurs between the afferent fibres and motor neurones, and efferent fibres from the motor neurones (descending portion) to the muscles they innervate. At the synapses the Ia afferent fibres release neurotransmitters onto the α-motoneurons and induce excitatory postsynaptic potentials (EPSP). When the EPSP reaches excitation threshold an action potential is produced and travels along efferent (motor) fibres to the target muscle. Consequently, the H-wave can be recorded and a twitch response is produced by the muscle. The amplitude of the H-wave (normally noted as the H-reflex) reflects the summed effects of monosynaptic Ia afferent projections on the spinal α-motoneuron pool (Zehr, 2002). The Ia afferent to motoneuron synaptic transmission and the excitability of the α-motoneuron can be potentially influenced by any presynaptic or postsynaptic neural activities at the spinal level (Misiaszek, 2003).

In general, the diameter of the sensory Ia fibres is relatively large and the excitation threshold of these fibres is relatively low. In contrast, the axon diameter of the motor fibres is smaller and the threshold level of α-motoneuron axons is higher (Bostock and Rothwell, 1997). Therefore, when electrical stimulation intensity increases from low to high levels, H-reflex response is elicited at lower intensities before the M-wave can be evoked. When the stimulation intensity is adjusted to an appropriate level, both of the H- and M-waves can be induced simultaneously. As illustrated in Figure 1, low stimulation intensity only elicits action potential on the sensory Ia afferent axon (response 2). The response 2 (action potential) travels to the spinal cord and then induces an EPSP on the synaptic-connected α-motoneuron. Subsequently, an action potential (response 3) is generated by the motoneuron and then propagates to the target muscle (H-reflex). The action potential generated on the α-motoneuron axons propagates to both the target muscle and the spinal cord. The descending volley reaches the muscle via transmission at the neuromuscular junction and induces the M-wave. The ascending volley travels along the α-motoneurons axon that may collide with the action potential generated by the motoneuron. The collision may result in partial or complete cancellation of the H-wave, depending upon the stimulation intensity (Aagaard, Simonsen, Andersen, Magnusson, and Dyhre-Poulsen, 2002b). With progressively increased stimulation intensities, a recruitment curve for the H-wave and M-wave, respectively, can be established (Figure 2). It has been suggested that the optimal stimulation intensity to be used in H-reflex studies is at the level that induces the maximal H-wave ($H_{max}$) or an H-wave that is accompanied by an M-wave which has the size of 10-25% of the maximal M-wave ($M_{max}$) throughout the experiment (Zehr, 2002).

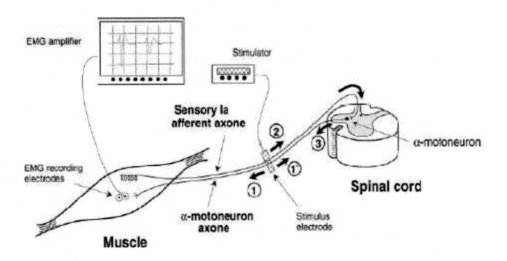

Figure 1. Simplified illustration of the H-reflex pathway [adapted from Aagaard, et al., (2002b) with permission].

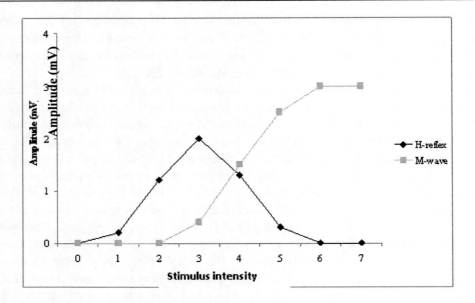

Figure 2. Exemplified H-reflex and M-wave recruitment curve. The stimulation intensity is gradually increased from 1 (weakest intensity) to 7 (strongest intensity). In health humans, the H-reflex (black line) appears first with absence of the M-wave at lower intensities (intensities 1 and 2). The $H_{max}$ that occurs at intensity 3 is usually accompanied with a small M-wave. As the stimulation intensity progressively increases, the size of M-wave (grey line) increases and the size of H-reflex decreases accordingly (from intensity 3 to intensity 5). When the $M_{max}$ is reached, the H-reflex ultimately vanishes (intensity 6 and 7) [adapted from Palmieri, et al., (2004) with permission].

## 2.2. Influence of the Supraspinal Inputs

The neural inputs from the supraspinal pathways have ultimate influence on the H-reflex (Figure 3) (Hultborn, 2006). The pathway from a pyramidal fibre to a spinal α-motoneuron or interneuron is a monosynaptic connection (Petersen, Pyndt, and Nielsen, 2003). The descending drives affect the H-reflex modulation via either direct regulation of the motoneuron membrane potential, or indirect regulation of interneuronal circuitry that may result in selective activation of the spinal motoneurons through various mechanisms such as presynaptic inhibition (Iles, 1996; Nielsen and Petersen, 1994), recurrent inhibition (Mazzocchio, Rossi, and Rothwell, 1994) and reciprocal inhibition (Iles and Pisini, 1992), etc. (Figure 3).

Transcranial magnetic stimulation (TMS) has been used in combination with the H-reflex test to investigate the influence of corticospinal projection on spinal motoneuron excitability [for details, see review by Taube et al. (2008)]. TMS can activate specific groups of neurons in the primary motor cortex via a transient magnetic field change (Nielsen and Petersen, 1994, 1995; Nielsen, Petersen, Deuschl, and Ballegaard, 1993; Nozaki et al., 2003). The general method is to apply a TMS 2-4 ms after a peripheral nerve stimulation for the conditioning H-reflex test. Due to the fact that the latency of the motor evoked potentials (MEPs) induced by the TMS is few milliseconds shorter that the latency of the H-reflex, the descending signals arrive to the α-motoneurons earlier than the ascending Ia inputs (Carroll, Riek, and Carson, 2001).

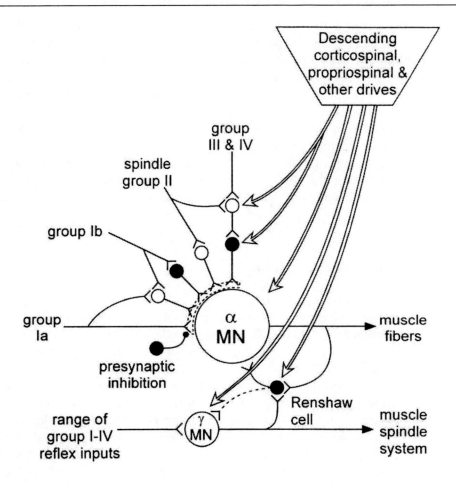

Figure 3. A schematic diagram of spinal networks [cited from Gandevia(2001) with permission]. Open circles represent excitatory interneurons, whereas the filled circles represent inhibitory interneurons. Sensory inputs from the group I, II, III, and IV afferent fibres converge toward the α-motoneurons. These inhibitory and excitatory interneurons mediate the release of neurotransmitters of the α-motoneurons. Factors that limit the excitation of α-motoneurons also include motor drives from descending pathways and inhibitory adjustment from the Renshaw cells. Descending inputs can directly or indirectly influence the inhibitory and excitatory interneurons, α and γ motoneurons, and Renshaw cells in the spinal circuitry. Descending inputs may selectively recruit a particular population of interneurons and motoneurons, depending upon the state of movement.

Therefore, the descending inputs have affected the α-motoneuron by inducing a conditioning effect before the ascending inputs arrive. Because the descending inputs are affected by the excitability of the motor cortex and the projection between the motor cortex and α-motoneurons is monosynaptic, any change in size of the H-reflex after the conditioning TMS is considered as an alternation of neuronal excitability at the cortical level.

Nielsen and colleagues (1993) reported that the amplitude of H-reflex conditioned with TMS did not change during rest, whereas the amplitude increased during voluntary contraction of the upper and lower limb muscles, indicating the influence of corticospinal drive on the spinal motoneuron pool. These authors also reported that the corticospinal descending signal elicited by TMS increased the size of SOL H-reflex during plantarflexion but depressed the size of SOL H-reflex during co-contraction of the calf and tibialis anterior (TA) muscles. It is possible that the corticospinal drive activated antagonist motoneurons and inhibitory interneurons during co-contraction that resulted in suppression of the agonists' activation. Following this study, Nielsen and Petersen (1995) extended their early work by an investigation on the modulation of conditioned SOL H-reflex during dynamic muscle contractions. The size of conditioned SOL H-reflex increased at the onset of a dynamic ramp-and-hold plantarflexion. In addition, the facilitation effect on the SOL H-reflex was greater during rapid dynamic contraction (increased by 57% of the control reflex size) than that during slow dynamic contractions (increased by 30% during 300 ms of ramp duration and by 8% during 600 ms of ramp duration). Therefore, the level of cortical motoneuron activation appears to affect the excitability of spinal motoneurons differently in execution of different motor tasks.

## 2.3. Influence of the Peripheral Inputs

The proprioceptive, cutaneous, visual and other types of sensory receptors are responsible for detecting environmental changes. When the receptors are stimulated, action potentials are generated on the sensory nerve fibres. The action potentials propagate to the spinal cord and supraspinal regions, causing corresponding sensations and eliciting reflexes and motor responses (Brooke and Zehr, 2006).

There has been evidence that sensory afferents may affect the H-reflex modulation. For example, a conditioning stimulation applied to the metatarsal region had an inhibitory effect on the SOL H-reflex, whereas a conditioning stimulation delivered to the heel region facilitated the SOL H-reflex response (Sayenko et al., 2009). It has also been shown that the visual feedback contributes to the H-reflex modulation. The SOL H-reflex is depressed during standing when eyes closed compared to that in eyes open condition (Earles, Koceja, and Shively, 2000). Moreover, the vestibular input is also a sensory source that may affect the H-reflex modulation. For example, Lowrey and Bent (2009) utilised a bipolar binaural galvanic vestibular stimulation (GVS) 100 ms prior to elicitation of the SOL H-reflex. The result showed that the SOL H-reflex conditioned by GVS was ~20% greater than that without GVS.

## 2.4. Assessment of the H-Reflex

The methodology and technical considerations for measurement of the H-reflex have been discussed in detail elsewhere (Chen and Zhou, 2011). To obtain quality data in the assessment, several aspects should be carefully considered, including the configuration and placement of the stimulation electrodes, stimulation parameters, configuration and placement of EMG electrodes, potential influence from joint angle and intensity of muscle contraction, etc.

In general, the H-reflex test has a high test-retest reliability for a static motor task (Chen, et al., 2010; Christie, Inglis, Boucher, and Gabriel, 2005; Clark, Cook, and Ploutz-Snyder, 2007). However, reliability of the H-reflex test for a dynamic motor task has not yet been reported in the literature. In term of the peak-to-peak amplitude of H-reflex, high intraclass correlation coefficients (ICC) have been reported for repeated measurements of the upper limb muscles over three consecutive days (0.99 in the flexor carpi radialis and 0.94 in the extensor carpi radialis longus) (Stowe, Hughes-Zahner, Stylianou, Schindler-Ivens, and Quaney, 2008). For the thigh muscles, the H-reflex of the vastus medialis demonstrated test-retest ICCs in the range from 0.73 to 0.98 during standing with the knee joint angle positioned at 0, 30, 45, and 60 degrees from full extension (Alrowayeh and Sabbahi, 2006). For the leg muscles, ICC values for the $H_{max}$ in a prone position over two consecutive days were reported to be 0.99 in the SOL, 0.99 in the peroneal, and 0.86 in the TA muscles (Palmieri, Hoffman, and Ingersoll, 2002).

High reliability of the SOL H-reflex has also been reported for measurements in lying, sitting, and standing positions (Ali and Sabbahi, 2001; Handcock, Williams, and Sullivan, 2001; Hopkins, Ingersoll, Cordova, and Edwards, 2000; Mynark, 2005). The gastrocnemius muscle showed an ICC from 0.58 to 0.94 during lying and standing at various ankle joint positions (Alrowayeh and Sabbahi, 2009). Furthermore, reliable measurements of the H-reflex were reported for the abductor brevis hallucis muscle, with ICC of 0.68 for the $H_{max}$, 0.82 for the latency of $H_{max}$, and 0.79 for the $H_{max}/M_{max}$ ratio (Versino, et al., 2007). A high level of test-retest reliability of the SOL H-reflex has been found in a prone (ICC = 0.97) (Ali and Sabbahi, 2001), supine (ICC = 0.94) (Hopkins, et al., 2000), or sitting (ICC = 0.92) (Chen, et al., 2010) position. During standing, the degree of test-retest reliability of the SOL H-reflex appears to slightly affected but the ICC value is still high (ICC = 0.80) (Hopkins, et al., 2000).

In addition, high levels of reliability have been reported for repeated measurements of the SOL H-reflex during submaximal voluntary muscle contractions. In a recent observation in our laboratory (Chen, et al., 2010), high ICC values of the SOL $H_{max}$ were found during isometric contractions at 10% of the maximal voluntary contraction (MVC) level at three different ankle joint positions (neutral 0°: ICC = 0.92, plantarflexion 20°: 0.93, and dorsiflexion 20°: 0.95). However, varied ICC values, range from 0.62 to 0.97, were found during contractions at 30% and 50 % MVC at these ankle joint positions.

A standard method used in interpretation of the H-reflex test results is to normalise the peak-to-peak amplitude of recorded H-reflex to the peak-to-peak amplitude of $M_{max}$ (Palmieri, et al., 2004). The $H_{max}/M_{max}$ ratio is commonly used to assess the proportion of entire motoneuron pool activated by the Ia afferent inputs (Zehr, 2002). The H-reflex size may be affected by factors in either the spinal cord or peripheral nerve and muscle, while the size of M-wave is not affected by the spinal motoneuron excitability. Therefore to record the amplitude of $M_{max}$ and to normalise the H-reflex amplitude to the $M_{max}$ may help in determining the effects of peripheral factors and prevention of misinterpretation of the excitatory or inhibitory effect of the reflex modulation under a given testing condition (Tucker and Turker, 2007).

Recording background EMG prior to the delivery of stimulation is another consideration in the H-reflex test. The reason for recording background EMG is to normalise the H-reflex responses in repeated trials that may be affected by the baseline EMG (Zehr, 2002). For example, the ratio of H-reflex amplitude to background EMG can be used to estimate the contribution of Ia afferent inputs to motoneuron activation via the Ia-motoneuron-spinal loop during execution of motor tasks (Capaday, 1997).

It should be noted that the H-reflex test is not a robust measurement. The spinal cord circuitry is oligosynaptic, therefore, neural inputs from both the ascending and descending pathways can potentially affect the H-reflex modulation (Zehr, 2002). Moreover, the H-reflex response reflects the neural activity at the spinal level. The mechanisms involving in motor output regulation at the supraspinal levels, such as cortical inhibition, may not be studies by the means of the H-reflex test.

Furthermore, the H-reflex may not be elicited successfully in a small portion of healthy populations under some testing conditions. An unpublished observation in our laboratory found that the SOL H-reflex response was present during passive shortening movement but was absent during passive lengthening movement in a small number of older adults. The neural mechanisms for the absence of H-reflex response during lengthening plantarflexors muscle activity are unclear, but it is speculated to be related to quiescence of muscle spindle activity (Burke, Hagbarth, and Lofstedt, 1978). It has been suggested that the failure of H-reflex elicitation in some older adults might be due to age-related spinal stenosis (Egli et al., 2007).

## 3. H-Reflex Modulation During Postural Tasks

### 3.1. Upright Standing

The major role of reflex regulation in postural control is autogenic adjustment of muscle tone in the postural muscles (Loram, Maganaris, and Lakie, 2005). The regulation of muscle tone in the agonist and antagonist muscles of the ankle joint is essential to postural stability during upright standing (Nardone, Giordano, Corrà, and Schieppati, 1990). Assessment of the H-reflex modulation in the ankle muscles provides an indication of neural control changes during standing (Tokuno, et al., 2007; Tokuno, et al., 2008). For examples, some studies that employed the centre of pressure (COP) measurement have shown a reciprocal relationship between the amplitude of SOL H-reflex and postural control performance during quiet standing under different sensory conditions (Earles, et al., 2000; Huang, Cherng, Yang, Chen, and Hwang, 2009; Koceja, Markus, and Trimble, 1995; Taube, Leukel, and Gollhofer, 2008). The SOL H-reflex amplitude is larger while the COP value is smaller during standing on a stable surface than that during standing on an unstable surface. The primary neural mechanism underlying the SOL H-reflex variation during postural control is suggested to be presynaptic inhibition (Taube, Gruber, and Gollhofer, 2008). Other inhibitory mechanisms such as recurrent (Barbeau, Marchand-Pauvert, Meunier, Nicolas, and Pierrot-Deseilligny, 2000) and Ib inhibitions (Faist, et al., 2006) may also be involved in the spinal reflex regulation of postural control.

There is a difference in the H-reflex behaviour between young and older adults when the sensory condition becomes more complex during standing. Earles and colleagues (2000) investigated the effect of ageing on the SOL H-reflex modulation in static postural tasks. Twelve young and ten older participants were instructed to stand on stable or unstable surfaces with eyes open or closed. The results demonstrated that young adults showed a depression, while older adults showed a facilitation of the SOL H-reflex during standing on an unstable surface with eyes open. However, depression of the SOL H-reflex was found in both young and older groups during standing on an unstable surface with eyes closed. This finding indicates that visual inputs can affect the SOL H-reflex modulation during standing and this modulation is different between young and older adults. The results have also revealed that the SOL H-reflex of older adults was correlated to the activation of the TA muscle as indicated by background EMG during the postural tasks, but this relationship was absent in young adults.

In a clinical investigation, Hwang et al. (2004) assessed the effect of body weight loading on the SOL H-reflex modulation during standing in patients with a history of stroke in five years. The patients showed absence of the SOL H-reflex modulation during sitting and standing with 10%, 50%, and 90% of body weight shifted to the tested leg, compared to a downward regulation that was observed in the healthy participants. The practical implication of this finding is that simple movement like weight-shift might not help hemiplegic patients for improvement in balance control (Hwang, et al., 2004).

## 3.2. Postural Perturbation

When the postural condition becomes more challengeable, the supraspinal mechanisms play a major role in motor output regulation. Solopova and colleagues (2003) reported that there was a facilitation of motor cortical response in postural adjustment during standing on a rocking platform. Increase in cortical excitability was observed as the size of MEPs increased 2.2 times when the participants shifted from a stable surface to a rocking platform. Taube and colleagues (2006) investigated the roles of cortical and spinal mechanisms during postural perturbation. In their study, participants were asked to maintain an upright stance on a treadmill while a surface perturbation was rapidly induced by a backward acceleration with the velocity of 60 m/s. The H-reflex, TMS, and H-reflex conditioned with TMS were used to examine the spinal, cortical, and corticospinal excitability, respectively. In the baseline measurement, short- (SLR, first deflection of reflex response), medium- (MLR, reflex response between 65 and 80 ms) and long-latency (LLR, reflex response after 85 ms) reflex activities elicited by rapid backward perturbations were measured against background EMG. During postural perturbations, three tests were conducted: 1) the SOL H-reflex elicited at the time of peak SLR and LLR (the SOL H-reflex induced at the MLR were absent in majority of participants), 2) the SOL MEPs induced by TMS with sub-threshold intensity at the time of peak SLR, MLR, and LLR, and 3) the SOL H-reflex conditioned with TMS at sub-threshold intensity elicited at the time of peak SLR, MLR, and LLR. Under the first experimental condition, the SOL H-reflex amplitude and $H_{max}/M_{max}$ ratio were significantly facilitated at LLR, compared to that at SLR. In response to the second experimental condition, the SOL MEPs induced by TMS was greater at LLR than that at SLR and MLR. Similarly, when the SOL H-reflex response was conditioned with sub-threshold TMS, there was a significant increase of the H-reflex amplitude at LLR than that at SLR and MLR. As the LLR has been suggested to be a transcortical reflex, significant changes of the SOL H-reflex, MEPs and conditioned SOL H-reflex at around 85 ms after the onset of postural perturbation would indicate a contribution of cortical control to the SOL motoneuron activities during postural perturbation (Morita et al., 2000).

## 3.3. Body Orientation

Postural orientation refers to limb and head placements in multifarious planes in respect to the vertical axis (Horak, 2006). Vestibular inputs are the predominant sensory source to detect head movement in reference to gravity and are important to adjustment of postural muscle activity (Inglis, Shupert, Hlavacka, and Horak, 1995). The functional roles of the vestibular system are complex but generally related to facilitation of postural reflexes (Horak, Earhart, and Dietz, 2001). Any head movement can elicit vestibular signals via sensory receptors in the otoliths organ and semicircular canals. The state of vestibular sensory inputs depends upon angular velocity and direction of head movement and can influence the H-reflex modulation through the vestibulospinal pathway (Kennedy, Cresswell, Chua, and Inglis, 2004).

Knikou and Rymer (2003) investigated the SOL H-reflex modulation in response to static and dynamic changes of body tilt in forward and backward directions in the sagittal plane. The result showed that the SOL H-reflex was significantly facilitated when the body orientation was changed, compared with the baseline SOL H-reflex recorded in the supine position. These findings suggest that the vestibular system has contributed to the modulation of SOL motoneuron activation in response to static and dynamic changes in head position. However, in comparison with the control position, a depression of SOL H-reflex was observed during unsupported standing (vertical position). The possible mechanisms underlying the reduction in the SOL H-reflex response during unsupported standing is the presynaptic inhibition of Ia afferent terminals (Ali and Sabbahi, 2000) and/or postsynaptic inhibition (Fátima Goulart, Valls-Solé, and Alvarez, 2000) induced by the somatosensory inputs from the mechanoreceptors due to weight-bearing standing.

## 3.4. Isolated Joint Movement

### *Static Ankle Joint Position*

Maintenance of ankle joint position is dependent upon the efficacy of autogenic monosynaptic reflex (Allum and Mauritz, 1984). The SOL H-reflex modulation has shown position-dependency in maintaining static ankle joint positions (Chen, et al., 2010; Hwang, 2002). Hwang (2002) reported that the SOL H-reflex was depressed at the dorsiflexion and was slightly facilitated at the plantarflexion, as compared to that at the neutral ankle position. The SOL H-reflex depression at the dorsiflexion is suggested as the result of presynaptic and postsynaptic inhibitions on the SOL motoneuron. The presynaptic and postsynaptic inhibitions were induced by passive stretch of the plantarflexors and the degree of inhibitory effect was dependent upon the angle of dorsiflexion (Guissard and Duchateau, 2006). Guissard et al. (2001) reported that the presynaptic inhibitory mechanisms dominated the regulation of spinal motor output at the dorsiflexion of 10 degree as evidenced by changed SOL H-reflex amplitude and unchanged MEPs. In contrast, the postsynaptic inhibitory mechanisms played a role in reduction of motoneuron excitability at the dorsiflexion of 20 degree as evidenced by a parallel change of H-reflex and MEPs responses.

*Dynamic Ankle Joint Movement*

Alternations in muscle fibre length during dynamic ankle joint movement can affect the H-reflex modulation. It has been reported that the SOL H-reflex response decreased during passive lengthening movement, compared with that during passive shortening movement (Duclay and Martin, 2005). Similar modulation of the SOL H-reflex has also been reported during shortening and lengthening voluntary contractions imposed with submaximal (Nordlund, Thorstensson, and Cresswell, 2002) and maximal efforts (Duclay and Martin, 2005). The SOL H-reflex modulation during dynamic joint movement is mainly influenced by presynaptic inhibitory mechanisms (Duchateau and Enoka, 2008). In addition, the velocity of dynamic ankle joint movement can also influence the H-reflex modulation. Duclay et al. (2009) demonstrated that the SOL H-reflex amplitude decreased significantly when angular velocity increased during passive and active dynamic ankle movements. However, the medial gastrocnemius (MG) H-reflex modulation was not affected by variation of angle velocities in the respective dynamic action. This difference in H-reflex modulation is possibly related to different distribution of muscle fibre types in the SOL and MG muscles. The SOL is dominated by slow twitch motor units and the MG muscle consists of mainly fast twitch motor units (Tucker, et al., 2005). The motoneurons of the fast and slow twitch motor units have different activation thresholds and may respond differently according to the velocity of dynamic ankle joint movement.

## 3.5. Sit-To-Stand, Walking, and Drop Jump

The H-reflex modulation during dynamic postural tasks has not been adequately studied. This is because there are many methodological concerns (e.g. the reliability of the methods to record the H-reflex or the stimulation method) that may have limited the application of H-reflex assessment under such conditions.

*Sit-to-Stand*

To our knowledge, Goular and Valls- Solé (2001) were the only authors who have reported the H-reflex modulation of the ankle muscles during the sit-to-stand performance. Because the sit-to-stand movement is a long-duration motor task and requires descending drives from supraspinal levels, the authors utilised the TMS to investigate the MEPs in different time intervals during the motor task. The H-reflex and MEPs were recorded from the TA and SOL muscles between 0 and 1500 ms after a "go" signal was given. In the first 600 ms of movement, the TA H-reflex response increased and the SOL H-reflex deceased. Conversely, the TA H-reflex response returned to the baseline level and the SOL H-reflex increased between 700 and 1500 ms of the movement. Similar changes of the motoneuron excitability in the TA and SOL muscles were also observed in the MEPs, except the slight increase of SOL MEPs in the first 600 ms of movement. These findings suggest that the reciprocal changes of the H-reflex modulation between the TA and SOL muscles during the sit-to-stand movement are influenced by the corticospinal descending drives. However, it should be noted that the sit-to-stand task involves many lower limb and trunk muscles, therefore, further investigations are required to substantiate the reciprocal influence on other agonist and antagonists muscles.

*Walking*

The H-reflex modulation during walking has been examined (Capaday and Stein, 1987; Simonsen and Dyhre-Poulsen, 1999; Simonsen, Dyhre-Poulsen, Alkjaer, Aagaard, and Magnusson, 2002). In general, the SOL H-reflex is modulated in a phase-dependent manner and varies individually during walking. The excitatory effect of group Ia afferent inputs on the α-motoneuron activity was facilitated during the late stance phase of walking and depressed during the early stance and swing phases of walking (Capaday and Stein, 1987).

*Drop Jump*

The H-reflex modulation was found to be phase-dependent during drop jump performance (Dyhre-Poulsen, et al., 1991; Leukel, Gollhofer, Keller, and Taube, 2008; Leukel, Taube, Gruber, Hodapp, and Gollhofer, 2008; Taube, Leukel, Schubert, et al., 2008). There has been evidence that the SOL H-reflex was depressed during the takeoff and flight phases of drop jump (Dyhre-Poulsen, et al., 1991). During the landing, the SOL H-reflex was facilitated during the stance phase and was depressed before the takeoff phase (Dyhre-Poulsen, et al., 1991; Taube, Leukel, Schubert, et al., 2008). The modulation of SOL H-reflex was also affected by the falling height as it was depressed during drop-jumps from a higher falling height (76 cm) in comparison to that during drop-jumps from a low falling height (31 cm) (Leukel, Gollhofer, et al., 2008; Leukel, Taube, et al., 2008). The significant depression of the SOL H-reflex from a higher falling height is suggested as a functional strategy to reduce the muscle strain in attempt to prevent fall injuries caused by the higher load. Because the nature of drop jump is a self-initiated movement, the specific characteristics of H-reflex are related to the descending drive (Taube, Leukel, Schubert, et al., 2008).

## 3.6. Adaptations to Exercise Training Interventions

The H-reflex modulation can be used as an indication of neural adaptations to exercise training at the spinal level (Zehr, 2002). Wolpaw (2007) highlighted an important role of activity-dependent spinal plasticity. It has been described that in the early stage of human development the spinal plasticity is predominantly formed for learning locomotion and removal behaviour from external stimuli (withdrawal reflex). On the other hand, in the later stage of human development, spinal plasticity plays a pivotal role in development of novel motor skills. It is now recognised that the spinal motoneurons are responsible for not only simple reflex actions, but also has a modulatory effect on the spinal circuitry in adaptation to given training tasks (Wolpaw and Carp, 2006).

The H-reflex has shown specificity in adaptation to exercise interventions (Zehr, 2002). It has been suggested that the H-reflex response is down-regulated after a balance training (Schubert, et al., 2008; Taube, Kullmann, et al., 2007; Trimble and Koceja, 1994) and is up-regulated after a strength training (Aagaard, Simonsen, Andersen, Magnusson, and Dyhre-Poulsen, 2002a; Taube, Kullmann, et al., 2007). The adaptation of H-reflex to a given training may be attributable to the spinal mechanisms with a possible involvement of supraspinal modulation of the spinal inhibitory mechanisms (Taube, Gruber, et al., 2008). In the following discussion we use balance training and Tai Chi practice as examples to discuss the mechanisms of adaptations to exercise intervention in relation to H-reflex modulation.

It is interesting to note that downward regulation of SOL H-reflex has been consistently reported after acute (Mynark and Koceja, 2002; Trimble, Du, Brunt, and Thompson, 2000; Trimble and Koceja, 1994) or short-term (Schubert, et al., 2008; Taube, Gruber, et al., 2007; Taube, Kullmann, et al., 2007) balance training. The reduction of SOL H-reflex after balance training is associated with improvement of postural stability, as indicated by the mean displacement of COP values. This neural adaptation is suggested as a result of motor efficacy that is possibly related to training-induced alternations of the spinal inhibitory mechanisms and the supraspinal mechanisms (Taube, Gruber, et al., 2008).

Tai Chi is a Chinese martial art exercise and has been used as an exercise intervention for improvement of postural control in older adults (Verhagen, Immink, van der Meulen, and Bierma-Zeinstra, 2004). Improvement of postural control in older adults has been reported after Tai Chi training that has been suggested as a result of neural adaptation in kinematic proprioception (Tsang and Hui-Chan, 2003, 2004), vestibular function (Tsang and Hui-Chan, 2006; Tsang, Wong, Fu, and Hui-Chan, 2004), and reaction time (Fong and Ng, 2006). Recently, a study in our laboratory investigated the effect of 12 weeks Tai Chi training on the SOL H-reflex modulation and control of quiet standing in older adults. The results (unpublished) demonstrated an increase in the SOL H-reflex during standing on stable or unstable surfaces with eyes open or closed after the Tai Chi training (see Figure 4). However, the ability to control static upright posture, as indicated by the mean displacement of COP values in anterior-posterior and medial-lateral directions, did not show an improvement after the 12 weeks of training, whereas there was a significant increase in the plantarflexion muscle strength. It is speculated that the lack of improvement in postural control performance might be related to insufficient length of the training period. Previous studies have reported no significant improvement of postural stability after three months of Tai Chi training (Fong and Ng, 2006; Lelard, Doutrellot, David, and Ahmaidi, 2010), but beneficial effect on balance control was found after one or more years of Tai Chi practice (Tsang and Hui-Chan, 2004; Tsang, et al., 2004).

## 4. SUMMARY

The H-reflex response is a short-latency monosynaptic reflex which has been used to investigate the effects of group Ia afferent inputs on the spinal $\alpha$-motoneuron activation. The excitatory and inhibitory inputs from the peripheral and supraspinal neural pathways can potentially influence the H-reflex modulation via either direct regulation of the motoneuron membrane potential or indirect regulation of the spinal interneuronal circuitry.

The modulation of SOL H-reflex has been found to be correlated to the postural stability during standing. The supraspinal mechanisms are involved in the H-reflex modulation when the postural condition becomes challengeable. During the dynamic postural control, the H-reflex modulation appears to be phase- and task-dependent. Adaptive changes of the H-reflex have been reported after balance or Tai Chi training and these changes appear to be specific to the interventions.

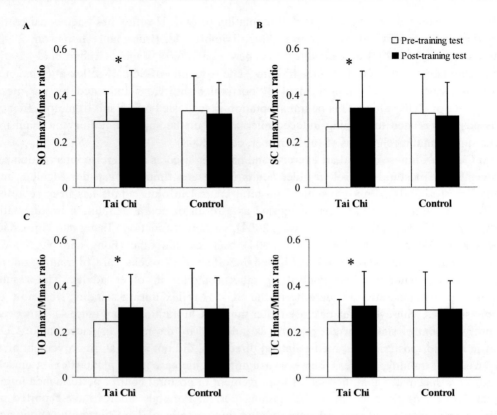

Figure 4. The SOL $H_{max}/M_{max}$ ratio before (white bars) and after (black bars) 12-week Tai Chi training in the training (N = 20; 72.9 ± 4.4 years of age) and the control group (N = 14; 72.9 ± 6.5 years of age). The SOL $H_{max}/M_{max}$ ratio is evaluated during standing with four different sensory conditions: A) stable surface with eyes open; B) stable surface with eyes closed; C) unstable surface with eyes open; D) unstable surface with eyes closed. Significant difference between the pre-and post-training tests is denoted as * ($P < 0.05$) [Unpublished observation, Chen, Y. S. (2010). Effects of ageing and Tai Chi training on soleus H-reflex in older adults, Southern Cross University, Australia]

## REFERENCES

Aagaard, P., Simonsen, E. B., Andersen, J. L., Magnusson, P., and Dyhre-Poulsen, P. (2002a). Increased rate of force development and neural drive of human skeletal muscle following resistance training. *Journal of Applied Physiology*, 93(4), 1318-1326.

Aagaard, P., Simonsen, E. B., Andersen, J. L., Magnusson, P., and Dyhre-Poulsen, P. (2002b). Neural adaptation to resistance training: changes in evoked V-wave and H-reflex responses. *Journal of Applied Physiology*, 92(6), 2309-2318.

Ali, A., and Sabbahi, M. A. (2001). Test-retest reliability of the soleus H-reflex in three different positions. *Electromyography and Clinical Neurophysiology*, 41(4), 209-214.

Ali, A. A., and Sabbahi, M. A. (2000). H-reflex changes under spinal loading and unloading conditions in normal subjects. *Clinical Neurophysiology*, 111(4), 664-670.

Allum, J. H., and Mauritz, K. H. (1984). Compensation for intrinsic muscle stiffness by short-latency reflexes in human triceps surae muscles. *Journal of Neurophysiology*, 52(5), 797-818.

Alrowayeh, H. N., and Sabbahi, M. A. (2006). Vastus medialis H-reflex reliability during standing. *Journal of Clinical Neurophysiology*, 23(1), 79-84.

Alrowayeh, H. N., and Sabbahi, M. A. (2009). Medial and lateral gastrocnemius H-reflex intersession reliability during standing and lying postures at varied foot positions in healthy participants. *Electromyography and Clinical Neurophysiology*, 49(4), 143-148.

Alrowayeh, H. N., Sabbahi, M. A., and Etnyre, B. (2005). Soleus and vastus medialis H-reflexes: similarities and differences while standing or lying during varied knee flexion angles. *Journal of Neuroscience Methods*, 144(2), 215-225.

Angulo-Kinzler, R. M., Mynark, R. G., and Koceja, D. M. (1998). Soleus H-reflex gain in elderly and young adults: modulation due to body position. *The Journals of Gerontology. Series A, Biological Sciences and Medical Sciences*, 53(2), M120-125.

Barbeau, H., Marchand-Pauvert, V., Meunier, S., Nicolas, G., and Pierrot-Deseilligny, E. (2000). Posture-related changes in heteronymous recurrent inhibition from quadriceps to ankle muscles in humans. *Experimental Brain Research*, 130(3), 345-361.

Bostock, H., and Rothwell, J. C. (1997). Latent addition in motor and sensory fibres of human peripheral nerve. *The Journal of Physiology*, 498 ( Pt 1), 277-294.

Brooke, J. D., and Zehr, E. P. (2006). Limits to fast-conducting somatosensory feedback in movement control. *Exercise and Sport Sciences Reviews*, 34(1), 22-28.

Burke, D., Hagbarth, K. E., and Lofstedt, L. (1978). Muscle spindle activity in man during shortening and lengthening contractions. *The Journal of Physiology*, 277, 131-142.

Capaday, C. (1997). Neurophysiological methods for studies of the motor system in freely moving human subjects. *Journal of Neuroscience Methods*, 74(2), 201-218.

Capaday, C., and Stein, R. B. (1987). Difference in the amplitude of the human soleus H reflex during walking and running. *Journal of Physiology*, 392, 513-522.

Carroll, T. J., Riek, S., and Carson, R. G. (2001). Corticospinal responses to motor training revealed by transcranial magnetic stimulation. *Exercise and Sport Sciences Reviews*, 29(2), 54-59.

Chalmers, G. R., and Knutzen, K. M. (2002). Soleus H-reflex gain in healthy elderly and young adults when lying, standing, and balancing. *The Journals of Gerontology. Series A, Biological Sciences and Medical Sciences*, 57(8), B321-329.

Chen, Y.-S., Zhou, S., Cartwright, C., Crowley, Z., Baglin, R., and Wang, F. (2010). Test-retest reliability of the soleus H-reflex is affected by joint positions and muscle force levels. *Journal of Electromyography and Kinesiology*, 20(5), 980-987.

Chen, Y. S., and Zhou, S. (2011). Soleus H-reflex and its relation to static postural control. Gait and Posture, 33, 169-178.

Christie, A. D., Inglis, J. G., Boucher, J. P., and Gabriel, D. A. (2005). Reliability of the FCR H-reflex. *Journal of Clinical Neurophysiology*, 22(3), 204-209.

Clark, B. C., Cook, S. B., and Ploutz-Snyder, L. L. (2007). Reliability of techniques to assess human neuromuscular function in vivo. *Journal of Electromyography and Kinesiology*, 17(1), 90-101.

Duchateau, J., and Enoka, R. M. (2008). Neural control of shortening and lengthening contractions: influence of task constraints. *The Journal of Physiology*, 586(24), 5853-5864.

Duclay, J., and Martin, A. (2005). Evoked H-reflex and V-wave responses during maximal isometric, concentric, and eccentric muscle contraction. *Journal of Neurophysiology*, 94(5), 3555-3562.

Duclay, J., Robbe, A., Pousson, M., and Martin, A. (2009). Effect of angular velocity on soleus and medial gastrocnemius H-reflex during maximal concentric and eccentric muscle contraction. *Journal of Electromyography and Kinesiology*, 19(5), 948-956.

Dyhre-Poulsen, P., Simonsen, E. B., and Voigt, M. (1991). Dynamic control of muscle stiffness and H reflex modulation during hopping and jumping in man. *The Journal of Physiology*, 437(1), 287-304.

Earles, D. R., Koceja, D. M., and Shively, C. W. (2000). Environmental changes in soleus H-reflex excitability in young and elderly subjects. *The International Journal of Neuroscience*, 105(1-4), 1-13.

Egli, D., Hausmann, O., Schmid, M., Boos, N., Dietz, V., and Curt, A. (2007). Lumbar spinal stenosis: assessment of cauda equina involvement by electrophysiological recordings. *Journal of Neurology*, 254(6), 741-750.

Faist, M., Hoefer, C., Hodapp, M., Dietz, V., Berger, W., and Duysens, J. (2006). In humans Ib facilitation depends on locomotion while suppression of Ib inhibition requires loading. *Brain Research*, 1076(1), 87-92.

Fong, S. M., and Ng, G. Y. (2006). The effects on sensorimotor performance and balance with Tai Chi training. *Archives of Physical Medicine and Rehabilitation*, 87(1), 82-87.

Gandevia, S. C. (2001). Spinal and supraspinal factors in human muscle fatigue. *Physiological Reviews*, 81(4), 1725-1789.

Goulart, F., and Valls-Solé, J. (2001). Reciprocal changes of excitability between tibialis anterior and soleus during the sit-to-stand movement. *Experimental Brain Research*, 139(4), 391-397.

Goulart, F., Valls-Solé, J., and Alvarez, R. (2000). Posture-related changes of soleus H-reflex excitability. *Muscle and Nerve,* 23(6), 925-932.

Guissard, N., and Duchateau, J. (2006). Neural aspects of muscle stretching. *Exercise and Sport Sciences Reviews,* 34(4), 154-158.

Guissard, N., Duchateau, J., and Hainaut, K. (2001). Mechanisms of decreased motoneurone excitation during passive muscle stretching. *Experimental Brain Research,* 137(2), 163-169.

Handcock, P. J., Williams, L. R., and Sullivan, S. J. (2001). The reliability of H-reflex recordings in standing subjects. *Electromyography and Clinical Neurophysiology,* 41(1), 9-15.

Hopkins, J. T., Ingersoll, C. D., Cordova, M. L., and Edwards, J. E. (2000). Intrasession and intersession reliability of the soleus H-reflex in supine and standing positions. *Electromyography and Clinical Neurophysiology,* 40(2), 89-94.

Horak, F. B. (2006). Postural orientation and equilibrium: what do we need to know about neural control of balance to prevent falls? *Age and Ageing*, 35(S2), ii7-ii11.

Horak, F. B., Earhart, G. M., and Dietz, V. (2001). Postural responses to combinations of head and body displacements: vestibular-somatosensory interactions. *Experimental Brain Research*, 141(3), 410-414.

Huang, C. Y., Cherng, R. J., Yang, Z. R., Chen, Y. T., and Hwang, I. S. (2009). Modulation of soleus H reflex due to stance pattern and haptic stabilization of posture. *Journal of Electromyography and Kinesiology*, 19(3), 492-499.

Hultborn, H. (2006). Spinal reflexes, mechanisms and concepts: from Eccles to Lundberg and beyond. *Progress in Neurobiology*, 78(3-5), 215-232.

Hwang, I. S. (2002). Assessment of soleus motoneuronal excitability using the joint angle dependent H reflex in humans. *Journal of Electromyography and Kinesiology*, 12(5), 361-366.

Hwang, I. S., Lin, C. F., Tung, L. C., and Wang, C. H. (2004). Responsiveness of the H reflex to loading and posture in patients following stroke. *Journal of Electromyography and Kinesiology*, 14(6), 653-659.

Iles, J. F. (1996). Evidence for cutaneous and corticospinal modulation of presynaptic inhibition of Ia afferents from the human lower limb. *The Journal of Physiology*, 491 (1), 197-207.

Iles, J. F., and Pisini, J. V. (1992). Cortical modulation of transmission in spinal reflex pathways of man. *The Journal of Physiology*, 455 (1), 425-446.

Inglis, J. T., Shupert, C. L., Hlavacka, F., and Horak, F. B. (1995). Effect of galvanic vestibular stimulation on human postural responses during support surface translations. *Journal of Neurophysiology*, 73(2), 896-901.

Kennedy, P. M., Cresswell, A. G., Chua, R., and Inglis, J. T. (2004). Vestibulospinal influences on lower limb motoneurons. *Canadian Journal of Physiology and Pharmacology*, 82(8-9), 675-681.

Knikou, M., and Rymer, W. Z. (2003). Static and dynamic changes in body orientation modulate spinal reflex excitability in humans. *Experimental Brain Research,* 152(4), 466-475.

Koceja, D. M., Markus, C. A., and Trimble, M. H. (1995). Postural modulation of the soleus H reflex in young and old subjects. *Electroencephalography and Clinical Neurophysiology* 97(6), 387-393.

Lelard, T., Doutrellot, P. L., David, P., and Ahmaidi, S. (2010). Effects of a 12-week Tai Chi Chuan program versus a balance training program on postural control and walking ability in older people. *Archives of Physical Medicine and Rehabilitation* 91(1), 9-14.

Leukel, C., Gollhofer, A., Keller, M., and Taube, W. (2008). Phase- and task-specific modulation of soleus H-reflexes during drop-jumps and landings. *Experimental Brain Research,* 190(1), 71-79.

Leukel, C., Taube, W., Gruber, M., Hodapp, M., and Gollhofer, A. (2008). Influence of falling height on the excitability of the soleus H-reflex during drop-jumps. *Acta Physiologica*, 192(4), 569-576.

Loram, I. D., Maganaris, C. N., and Lakie, M. (2005). Human postural sway results from frequent, ballistic bias impulses by soleus and gastrocnemius. *The Journal of Physiology*, 564(1), 295-311.

Lowrey, C. R., and Bent, L. R. (2009). Modulation of the soleus H-reflex following galvanic vestibular stimulation and cutaneous stimulation in prone human subjects. *Muscle and Nerve*, 40(2), 213-220.

Mazzocchio, R., Rossi, A., and Rothwell, J. C. (1994). Depression of Renshaw recurrent inhibition by activation of corticospinal fibres in human upper and lower limb. *The Journal of Physiology*, 481 (2), 487-498.

Misiaszek, J. E. (2003). The H-reflex as a tool in neurophysiology: its limitations and uses in understanding nervous system function. *Muscle and Nerve*, 28(2), 144-160.

Morita, Olivier, Baumgarten, Petersen, Christensen, Nielsen, et al. (2000). Differential changes in corticospinal and Ia input to tibialis anterior and soleus motor neurones during voluntary contraction in man. *Acta Physiologica Scandinavica,* 170(1).

Mynark, R. G. (2005). Reliability of the soleus H-reflex from supine to standing in young and elderly. *Clinical Neurophysiology,* 116(6), 1400-1404.

Mynark, R. G., and Koceja, D. M. (2002). Down training of the elderly soleus H reflex with the use of a spinally induced balance perturbation. *Journal of Applied Physiology,* 93(1), 127-133.

Nardone, A., Giordano, A., Corrà, T., and Schieppati, M. (1990). Responses of leg muscles in humans displaced while standing. Effects of types of perturbation and of postural set. *Brain,* 113(Pt 1), 65-84.

Nielsen, J., and Petersen, N. (1994). Is presynaptic inhibition distributed to corticospinal fibres in man? *The Journal of Physiology,* 477 (1)(1), 47-58.

Nielsen, J., and Petersen, N. (1995). Changes in the effect of magnetic brain stimulation accompanying voluntary dynamic contraction in man. *The Journal of Physiology,* 484 (3), 777-789.

Nielsen, J., Petersen, N., Deuschl, G., and Ballegaard, M. (1993). Task-related changes in the effect of magnetic brain stimulation on spinal neurones in man. *The Journal of Physiology,* 471 (1), 223-243.

Nordlund, M. M., Thorstensson, A., and Cresswell, A. G. (2002). Variations in the soleus H-reflex as a function of activation during controlled lengthening and shortening actions. *Brain Research,* 952(2), 301-307.

Nozaki, D., Kawashima, N., Aramaki, Y., Akai, M., Nakazawa, K., Nakajima, Y., et al. (2003). Sustained muscle contractions maintained by autonomous neuronal activity within the human spinal cord. *Journal of Neurophysiology,* 90(4), 2090-2097.

Palmieri, R. M., Hoffman, M. A., and Ingersoll, C. D. (2002). Intersession reliability for H-reflex measurements arising from the soleus, peroneal, and tibialis anterior musculature. *The International Journal of Neuroscience,* 112(7), 841-850.

Palmieri, R. M., Ingersoll, C. D., and Hoffman, M. A. (2004). The Hoffmann reflex: methodologic considerations and applications for use in sports medicine and athletic training research. *Journal of Athletic Training,* 39(3), 268-277.

Petersen, N. T., Pyndt, H. S., and Nielsen, J. B. (2003). Investigating human motor control by transcranial magnetic stimulation. *Experimental Brain Research,* 152(1), 1-16.

Sayenko, D. G., Vette, A. H., Obata, H., Alekhina, M. I., Akai, M., and Nakazawa, K. (2009). Differential effects of plantar cutaneous afferent excitation on soleus stretch and H-reflex. *Muscle and Nerve,* 39(6), 761-769.

Schubert, M., Beck, S., Taube, W., Amtage, F., Faist, M., and Gruber, M. (2008). Balance training and ballistic strength training are associated with task-specific corticospinal adaptations. *European Journal of Neuroscience,* 27(8), 2007-2018.

Simonsen, E. B., and Dyhre-Poulsen, P. (1999). Amplitude of the human soleus H reflex during walking and running. *The Journal of Physiology,* 515 ( Pt 3), 929-939.

Simonsen, E. B., Dyhre-Poulsen, P., Alkjaer, T., Aagaard, P., and Magnusson, S. P. (2002). Interindividual differences in H reflex modulation during normal walking. *Experimental Brain Research,* 142(1), 108-115.

Solopova, I. A., Kazennikov, O. V., Deniskina, N. B., Levik, Y. S., and Ivanenko, Y. P. (2003). Postural instability enhances motor responses to transcranial magnetic stimulation in humans. *Neuroscience Letters*, 337(1), 25-28.

Stowe, A. M., Hughes-Zahner, L., Stylianou, A. P., Schindler-Ivens, S., and Quaney, B. M. (2008). Between-day reliability of upper extremity H-reflexes. *Journal of Neuroscience Methods*, 170(2), 317-323.

Taube, W., Gruber, M., Beck, S., Faist, M., Gollhofer, A., and Schubert, M. (2007). Cortical and spinal adaptations induced by balance training: correlation between stance stability and corticospinal activation. *Acta Physiologica,* 189(4), 347-358.

Taube, W., Gruber, M., and Gollhofer, A. (2008). Spinal and supraspinal adaptations associated with balance training and their functional relevance. *Acta Physiologica,* 193(2), 101-116.

Taube, W., Kullmann, N., Leukel, C., Kurz, O., Amtage, F., and Gollhofer, A. (2007). Differential Reflex Adaptations Following Sensorimotor and Strength Training in Young Elite Athletes. *International Journal of Sports Medicine,* 28(12), 999-1005.

Taube, W., Leukel, C., and Gollhofer, A. (2008). Influence of enhanced visual feedback on postural control and spinal reflex modulation during stance. *Experimental Brain Research*, 188(3), 353-361.

Taube, W., Leukel, C., Schubert, M., Gruber, M., Rantalainen, T., and Gollhofer, A. (2008). Differential modulation of spinal and corticospinal excitability during drop jumps. *Journal of Neurophysiology,* 99(3), 1243-1252.

Taube, W., Schubert, M., Gruber, M., Beck, S., Faist, M., and Gollhofer, A. (2006). Direct corticospinal pathways contribute to neuromuscular control of perturbed stance. *Journal of Applied Physiology*, 101(2), 420-429.

Tokuno, C. D., Carpenter, M. G., Thorstensson, A., Garland, S. J., and Cresswell, A. G. (2007). Control of the triceps surae during the postural sway of quiet standing. *Acta Physiologica*, 191(3), 229-236.

Tokuno, C. D., Garland, S. J., Carpenter, M. G., Thorstensson, A., and Cresswell, A. G. (2008). Sway-dependent modulation of the triceps surae H-reflex during standing. *Journal of Applied Physiology*, 104(5), 1359-1365.

Trimble, M. H., Du, P., Brunt, D., and Thompson, F. J. (2000). Modulation of triceps surae H-reflexes as a function of the reflex activation history during standing and stepping. *Brain Research.,* 858(2), 274-283.

Trimble, M. H., and Koceja, D. M. (1994). Modulation of the triceps surae H-reflex with training. *The International Journal of Neuroscience,* 76(3-4), 293-303.

Trimble, M. H., and Koceja, D. M. (2001). Effect of a reduced base of support in standing and balance training on the soleus H-reflex. *The International Journal of Neuroscience,* 106(1-2), 1-20.

Tsang, W. W., and Hui-Chan, C. W. (2003). Effects of tai chi on joint proprioception and stability limits in elderly subjects. *Medicine and Science in Sports and Exercise*, 35(12), 1962-1971.

Tsang, W. W., and Hui-Chan, C. W. (2004). Effects of exercise on joint sense and balance in elderly men: Tai Chi versus golf. *Medicine and Science in Sports and Exercise*, 36(4), 658-667.

Tsang, W. W., and Hui-Chan, C. W. (2006). Standing balance after vestibular stimulation in Tai Chi-practicing and nonpracticing healthy older adults. *Archives of Physical Medicine and Rehabilitation,* 87(4), 546-553.

Tsang, W. W., Wong, V. S., Fu, S. N., and Hui-Chan, C. W. (2004). Tai Chi improves standing balance control under reduced or conflicting sensory conditions. *Archives of Physical Medicine and Rehabilitation*, 85(1), 129-137.

Tucker, K. J., Tuncer, M., and Turker, K. S. (2005). A review of the H-reflex and M-wave in the human triceps surae. *Human Movement Science*, 24(5-6), 667-688.

Tucker, K. J., and Turker, K. S. (2007). Triceps surae stretch and voluntary contraction alters maximal M-wave magnitude. *Journal of Electromyography and Kinesiology*, 17(2), 203-211.

Verhagen, A. P., Immink, M., van der Meulen, A., and Bierma-Zeinstra, S. M. (2004). The efficacy of Tai Chi Chuan in older adults: a systematic review. *Family Practice,* 21(1), 107-113.

Versino, M., Candeloro, E., Tavazzi, E., Moglia, A., Sandrini, G., and Alfonsi, E. (2007). The H reflex from the abductor brevis hallucis muscle in healthy subjects. *Muscle and Nerve,* 36(1), 39-46.

Voerman, G. E., Gregoric, M., and Hermens, H. J. (2005). Neurophysiological methods for the assessment of spasticity: the Hoffmann reflex, the tendon reflex, and the stretch reflex. *Disability and Rehabilitation,* 27(1-2), 33-68.

Wolpaw, J. R. (2007). Spinal cord plasticity in acquisition and maintenance of motor skills. *Acta Physiologica*, 189(2), 155-169.

Wolpaw, J. R., and Carp, J. S. (2006). Plasticity from muscle to brain. *Progress in Neurobiology*, 78(3-5), 233-263.

Zehr, P. (2002). Considerations for use of the Hoffmann reflex in exercise studies. *European Journal of Applied Physiology,* 86(6), 455-468.

In: Posture: Types, Assessment and Control
Editors: A. Wright and S. Rothenberg, pp. 175-189
ISBN 978-1-61324-107-3
© 2011 Nova Science Publishers, Inc.

*Chapter 7*

# BODY SUPPORT AND DRIVING OPERATION OF A VEHICLE FOR WHEELCHAIR USERS

## *Hiroshi Ikeda[1] and Akihiro Mihoshi[2]*

[1]Holistic Prosthetics Research Center, Kyoto Institute of Technology,
[2.]Faculty of Civil Engineering, Kinki University

### ABSTRACT

Driving a vehicle is an important means to realizing participation in society for disabled people who want to become independent, however, the maintenance of laws in Japan concerning the driving environment is insufficiently established when compared to the support and welfare for disabled drivers in other advanced countries. A better and safer driving environment will be created if public opinion is taken into account positively, in a similar way to stations and other public areas. In this chapter, in order to determine the driving safety of wheelchair drivers, both a questionnaire survey and an experiment to measure the steering angle and acceleration-velocity during driving were conducted. As a result, it is shown that the driving environment for wheelchair drivers does not grant enough modifications for safe driving, and there are differences between physically unimpaired drivers and wheelchair drivers in the tendency for hazardous driving behavior. When driving at faster speeds, the methods of keeping body balance are shown to be different on right and left curves, and also a difficulty in maintaining a stable position during operation of the vehicle is indicated. Especially at the end of a curve, where there is greater acceleration velocity, the body balance is easily disrupted in terms of driving posture, and a reduction of both stability and usability of driving operation of the steering wheel and the acceleration lever is shown.

### 1. INTRODUCTION

In Japan, the number of physically impaired people with a driver's license has been increasing by 4,000 drivers every year, and it reached a total of 252,257 in 2011. The National Police Agency [1] reports about these drivers, 208,362 are limited to driving vehicles specially designed for disabled people, 39,374 people are permitted to drive provided they use hearing aids, and 4,112 wear a prosthetic limb and/or foot for driving a vehicle. In Japan, the provisional acquisition of a driving license by disabled people was legalized under Article 88 of the Road Traffic Law in 1960 [2]. In addition, the acquisition of a driver's license by disabled people with impediments to both upper limbs was legalized in 1982.

Recently, in order to support the independence of elderly and disabled people, the development of barrier-free environments in facilities and on roads has come under closer scrutiny as a social issue. In November 2000, the Barrier-free Transportation Law was implemented. This law involves the promotion of smoother transportation for elderly and disabled people in the public-transportation system. Also, the development of road networks has increased for the use of physically impaired people as a means to expand their positive contributions to society. However, roads are still designed on the premise of travel by physically unimpaired people. Therefore, in order to assure disabled people's needs, comfort and safety when they are actively involved with society as well as when they travel, there is a demand for further development of an ergonomic driving environment. [3, 4].

According to Ikeda et al. [5] and Dols et al. [6], the operational procedures and environmental set-up for physically impaired people are unsatisfactory, and almost no ergonomic considerations, which assure their safety and comfort during driving, are taken into account. Also, it was shown by Ikeda et al. [7] that it is difficult to maintain a correct course when driving on curves because of the necessity of controlling speed and steering at the same time. If these problems are solved and a stable environment for driving is developed, not only the improvement of safety and risk management but also the reduction of physical load for disabled drivers will be realized. Therefore, it is important to study various fields of driving environment for wheelchair drivers systematically. Concerning previous research of unimpaired drivers, Salvucci and Liu [8], Imsland et al. [9], and Kitahama and Sakai [10] used acceleration-velocity and steering angles as evaluation matrix in order to understand the traveling conditions of vehicles.

Development of the automobile environment is essential for physically impaired people to participate in society. However, so far, only small numbers of ergonomic studies on their driving conditions have been conducted. In this chapter, in order to focus on the situation of driving on curves, a questionnaire, acceleration-velocity, and steering angles were studied and the driving load for physically impaired people is discussed from the view of ergonomics.

## 2. QUESTIONNAIRE SURVEY

### 2.1. Method

#### *2.1.1. Subjects*

The subjects of the questionnaire included both people who require a wheelchair in their daily life and use driving support equipment when they drive a vehicle by themselves and also a group of unimpaired drivers. The questionnaire was distributed directly by hand, and after completion, it was collected by post mail. Wheelchair drivers returned 61 copies and unimpaired drivers returned 100 copies and the total percentage of return was 61.6 % for wheelchair drivers and 95.2 % for unimpaired drivers.

**Table 1. Characteristics of the subjects**

| Group | Wheelchair driver | Unimpaired driver |
|---|---|---|
| Sex | Male: 85.5 %<br>Female: 14.5 % | Male: 84.4 %<br>Female: 15.6 % |
| Age | 20-29: 27.3 %<br>30-39: 32.7 %<br>40-49: 23.6 %<br>50-59: 7.3 %<br>Over 60: 5.5 % | 20-29: 20.9 %<br>30-39: 18.7 %<br>40-49: 15.4 %<br>50-59: 20.9 %<br>Over 60: 24.2 % |
| Level of disability | First grade: 85.5 %<br>Second grade: 14.5 % | N/A |
| Driving experience | Under 1 year: 0.0 %<br>2-5 years: 18.9 %<br>6-10 years: 5.7 %<br>Over 10 years: 75.5 % | Under 1 year: 1.1 %<br>2-5 years: 11.1 %<br>6-10 years: 11.1 %<br>Over 10 years: 76.7 % |

The number of valid responses, fully completed, was 55 copies for wheelchair drivers and 96 copies for unimpaired drivers. Table 1 shows the characteristics of the subjects.

Figure 1 shows examples of remodeling to vehicles used by wheelchair drivers. The left picture shows an example of support equipment for subjects with impairments in lower limbs, and the right picture is an enlarged view of part of the accelerator and brake lever.

*2.1.2. Questionnaire items*

The questionnaire was concerned with the following three points; (1) necessity of driving equipment, (2) criteria for deciding seat position, and (3) driving behavior on various types of curves. In addition, this research is based on results from the use of right-hand side drive vehicles.

## 2.2. Results and Discussion

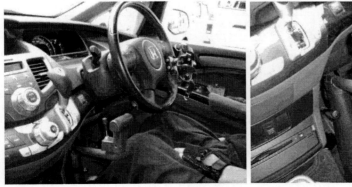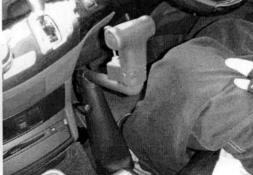

Figure 1. Example of support equipment for lower limb impairment.

## 2.2.1. Remodeling and Financial Grant Status

When asked about the necessity of remodeling driving equipment, except for the acceleration and brake lever (later called speed control lever), the group of wheelchair drivers responded that "steering wheel" was the highest at 57 %. The next was "indicator lever" at 41 % and then "headlight switch" at 15 %, as shown in Figure 2. This indicates the necessity for many modifications of the operation system.

Next as shown in Figure 3, the wheelchair drivers were asked about the method of keeping body posture during driving. 85 % of drivers do not use special support equipment, but use a normal seatbelt with 3 points. Then, when asked about their requirements for body support, about half, 49 % responded that they require more support in a "right-left direction" and 24 % in a "front-back direction". The response "not necessary" was 16 %.

Concerning the driving support equipment of vehicle remodeling in Figure 2, when the group of wheelchair drivers was asked whether they receive or do not receive a financial grant for modification, 85 % responded "yes".

Then, the subjects were asked about the total amount of the grant for driving support equipment. As shown in Figure 4, 35 % of subjects paid "50 %" of the total cost and 27 % of subjects paid "60 %". Therefore, over 70 % of wheelchair drivers paid over half of the total cost by themselves.

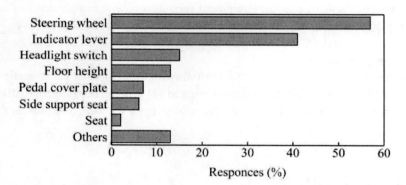

Figure 2. Situation of remodeling.

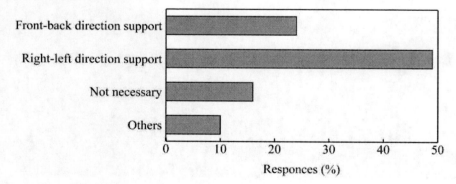

Figure 3. Requirement of body support.

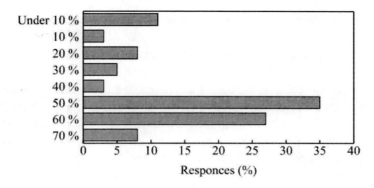

Figure 4. Rate of payments by self.

The main points of remodeling of driving support equipment, except for the speed control lever, were the steering wheel and the indicator lever, which are essential for driving. However, even though it is not enough to meet their special requirements, wheelchair drivers used a normal driving seat and seat belt which are important factors in keeping body balance. The reason is that although almost all wheelchair drivers received financial support for remodeling, about 70 % of drivers must pay by themselves for more than half the total cost, therefore, it can be said that the high cost of total remodeling is an important factor in terms of deciding the necessity of driving support equipment.

Financial grants for driving support equipment cost have a fixed maximum amount, therefore, the payment by self will be higher for people who have severe impairments and need many kinds of support equipment. Therefore, they can only pay for the basic support equipment necessary for driving, however, this does not cover enough support to improve safety and create a comfortable environment. Even though they have special requirements, they have to use the current driving operation environment.

### 2.2.2. Driving Seat and Seat Position

As shown in Figure 5, when the subjects were asked about their experience of posture sliding or tilting forward on the seat, the response of "often" was just 1 % for wheelchair drivers, "sometimes" was 17 %, "seldom" was 34 %, and "never" was 48 %. A low frequency, but about 20 %, of wheelchair drivers responded that they experience unnatural posture and they have problems with the driving seat.

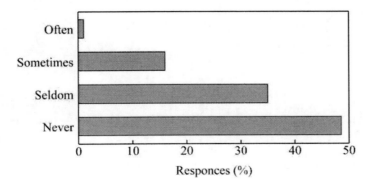

Figure 5. Changes of seating posture when driving.

Next, the subjects were asked if they had ever experienced a dangerous situation caused by an unnatural sitting posture while driving. The wheelchair drivers response was 2 % "often" and 22 % "sometimes", therefore, about a quarter of the drivers had experienced such a situation (see Figure 6).

Then, the subjects were asked about the criteria for determining the position of the driver's seat. As shown in Figure 7, for the wheelchair drivers, 23 % responded that the "acceleration and brake" is the most important criteria, 35 % for the "steering wheel", and 38 % for "both". On the other hand, for the unimpaired drivers, 47 % responded "acceleration pedal", 9 % "steering wheel", and 43 % "both". Between the groups, there were significant differences ($\chi^2 = 19.06$, $p < 0.01$), therefore, it can be thought that for wheelchair drivers the criteria of the operation of the steering wheel when adjusting the position of the driver's seat is greater than for unimpaired drivers.

Vehicles which are used by wheelchair drivers have been designed based on the standards of unimpaired drivers. Therefore, there is only limited space for attaching a remodeled speed control lever. If the position of the driver's seat is adjusted for the priority of the operation of the steering wheel, operation of the speed control lever would become more difficult. Also, if the priority is for the speed control lever, operation of the steering wheel would become more difficult.

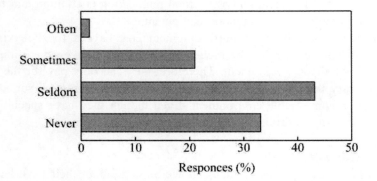

Figure 6. Hazard caused by unnatural sitting posture.

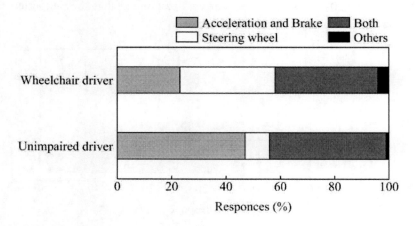

Figure 7. Standard seating position.

Therefore, this effects seating posture and the driver's posture becomes unstable. There is a tendency for the seating posture to be disrupted, and, although not often, some drivers feel this causes trouble during driving.

## *2.2.3. Experience of Risk Behavior*

The subjects were asked if they had ever had a problem with driving operation when driving at high speed on curves because of the centrifugal force that makes the driver's body lean to the side. As shown in Figure 8, the response of wheelchair drivers was 9 % "often" and 50 % "sometimes", therefore, about 60 % of the wheelchair drivers answered that they had experienced a problem. For the group of wheelchair drivers, it can be said that there is a stronger possibility of a problem with driving operation occurring compared to the unimpaired drivers.

Next, when the subjects were asked about the problem of driving operation with centrifugal force on several traffic conditions, the response of the wheelchair drivers was higher than the unimpaired drivers for all conditions, as shown in Figure 9. The most noticeable difference was on a "left curve" ($\chi^2 = 16.52$, $p < 0.01$), the response of wheelchair drivers was 38 % and unimpaired drivers was only 10 %. The next was on a "left corner" ($\chi^2 = 15.02$, $p < 0.01$), the response of wheelchair drivers was 28 % and unimpaired drivers was only 5 %. Especially, the "left curve" and "left corner" conditions showed a high response, and the common point is that when centrifugal force makes the body lean to the right side, the drivers experience some problem with driving operation.

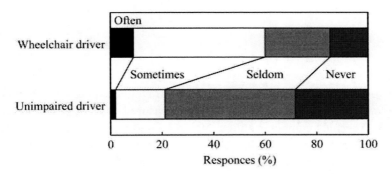

Figure 8. Frequency of problems with driving operation on curves.

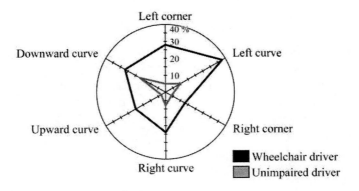

Figure 9. Problems caused by centrifugal force.

Concerning the effect of centrifugal force when driving on curves, about 60 % of the wheelchair drivers responded that they experience problems. Wheelchair drivers, who have lower-body impairments, have to keep body balance during driving with only their upper body. Therefore, it is easy to receive the effects of centrifugal force, and so the frequency of problems becomes higher. Also, there is a tendency for a higher rate of responses for "curves" and "corners" traveling in a left direction. Therefore, this may be the reason for the alternative methods of keeping driving posture when experiencing the effects of centrifugal force.

## 3. DRIVING MEASUREMENT

Drivers sense vibrations and the centrifugal force of traveling in vehicles both consciously and unconsciously, and the driver's feedback concerning this information can be used to support safe driving. The change of acceleration-velocity in traveling and its effect on the vehicle reflects the driving conditions. These are important indicators for evaluating the safety of driving. Acceleration and deceleration of vehicles are shown as acceleration-velocity in a front-back direction, while the information on centrifugal force created by steering operation on curves is indicated as acceleration-velocity in a right-left direction. Using these indicators, the situation of driving on curves was clarified and the environment, which is designed based on the driving style of unimpaired people, was examined to determine if it is satisfactory for wheelchair users.

### 3.1. Method

#### 3.1.1. Procedure for Measurement

In order to examine the driving operation and traveling conditions of vehicles, both the steering angle and acceleration-velocity were measured. All of the measured data was recorded onto a personal computer online. Video images were also used in order to examine driving performance. Figure 10 shows a schematic diagram of the measurement system.

Examiners explained to the subjects of this study about the purpose, method and possible risks of the experiment. A sensor was attached and the conditions for measurement were checked. Measuring equipment was set inside the vehicle, and the personal computer was turned on by the power source in the vehicle. The experiment was conducted with the subject's consent.

#### 3.1.2. Measuring Steering Angle

The steering angle is one of the indicators to evaluate driving techniques. Video images of the subjects driving on roads were shown on the computer screen, and the steering angles were measured from selected curves according to the frame numbers. The time required for driving on a curve was divided into 10 segments, and the starting point of the curve was set. The relationship between the size of steering angles and the time required on 11 points were compared.

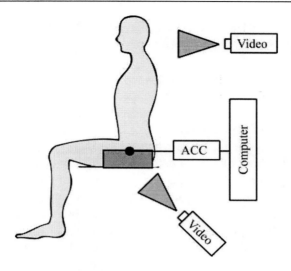

Figure 10. Schematic diagram of the measurement system.

### 3.1.3. Measuring Acceleration-Velocity

Driving conditions were evaluated by right-left and front-back acceleration-velocity indicators. Gauges for measuring acceleration-velocity were set in different places inside the vehicles since the vehicles used for the measurement, owned by each subject, were different. In order to obtain the best information about the influence on the drivers, the acceleration sensors were set around the most stable place near the driver's seat. The gauge for measuring acceleration-velocity was a tri-axial acceleration gauge MA3-04HD of Microstone. The sampling speed was 100 Hz. The detection range was 0-4 G.

### 3.1.4. Characteristics of the Subjects

Five physically impaired people and three physically unimpaired people participated in this experiment. All of them were volunteers and all of the vehicles used for this experiment were personally owned by them. The average age of the physically impaired subjects was 39.0 years old (27-58 years old). Three of them obtained a driving license after becoming disabled. Their average period of driving experience was 16.6 years (8-35 years). All of them belong to the first grade of disability. They had damage in their cervical and thoracic spine regions. When they were outside, they used manual wheelchairs as an aid. The engine capacity of two vehicles was 2,500 cc, another two were 2,400 cc and one was 2,200 cc. All vehicles had modified steering in order to assist driving; the accelerators and brakes of all vehicles had been remodeled, and the alterations were due to impairment in upper and lower limbs. Table 2 shows the characteristics of the subjects including the three physically unimpaired drivers.

### 3.1.5. Characteristics of the Course

In order to understand the driving conditions of physically impaired people, data analysis was conducted on curves because information that was gained from previous interviews showed that driving load is greater on curves. The selected curves are shown in Figure 11 as right and left curves. Each curve zone was divided into 5 sections. Section 1 and 5 are the start and end of the course, Section 2 and 4 are the start and end of the curve, and Section 3 is the middle of the curve.

## 3.2. Results and Discussion

### 3.2.1. Steering Control Performance

Figure 12 shows the steering angle when the starting point of a curve is set as 0° and the end part as 100 %. On both of the curves, and with a slow driving speed, after changing the steering angle through the middle of the curve, the angle of the steering wheel was corrected once, and then changed again for both disabled and unimpaired drivers. However, as the speed conditions became faster, the operation of correcting the steering wheel was not at the middle of the curve. The steering wheel angle was constant from the beginning to the end of the curve. When the speed condition becomes faster, the locus tends to change from M-shaped to a smooth shape, therefore, it would be difficult to keep a correct course. Especially, on the section from the end of the curve to becoming straight, the steering wheel was turned back quickly on the right curve more than left curve.

**Table 2. Characteristics of the subjects**

| Group | Age | Level of disability | Spinal cord injury | Driving experience | Vehicle capacity |
|---|---|---|---|---|---|
| Wheelchair driver | 27 | First grade | C6 | 9 years | 2,500 cc |
| | 42 | First grade | C6 | 16 years | 2,500 cc |
| | 58 | First grade | C6 | 35 years | 2,400 cc |
| | 31 | First grade | C6 | 8 years | 2,200 cc |
| | 37 | First grade | C6 | 15 years | 2,400 cc |
| Unimpaired driver | 41 | N/A | N/A | 20 years | 2,500 cc |
| | 37 | N/A | N/A | 19 years | 2,500 cc |
| | 24 | N/A | N/A | 4 years | 2,500 cc |

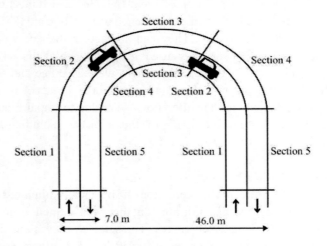

Figure 11. Experiment course.

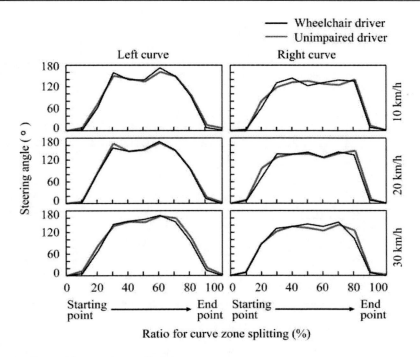

Figure 12. Comparison of the steering angle on a curve.

When the speed condition becomes faster, the locus tends to change from M-shaped to a smooth shape because of a reduced degree of correcting the steering wheel. In other words, when the steering angle of the curve remains constant, driving can not be commensurate with the course. This procedure affects the steering and speed in order to maintain posture, and seems to be too heavy an impact on driver performance. Especially, on the section of leaving the right curve, both groups turned the steering wheel back more quickly than on the left curve, however, this might be because of different ways of controlling body posture when experiencing centrifugal force. The trunk and appendicular muscles of upper and lower body impaired people are not the same as unimpaired people, so it is easy for them to lose body balance and difficult to stabilize usability of the steering and/or speed control lever when driving.

### 3.2.2. Changes of Acceleration-Velocity

In order to compare the acceleration-velocity of different conditions for both groups, the driving time on the selected zones was divided into 100 time-units, and the acceleration-velocity of the vehicle in right-left and front-back directions was compared. An average time was used for this data. Figure 13 shows the directions and size of the acceleration-velocity on right and left curves. The waveform noise of the velocity was smoothed, and the average velocity was calculated in time units.

In a comparison of the average acceleration between each speed condition, the acceleration of front-back directions did not show such a significant difference, however, right-left directions showed changes at the section between leaving the curve to becoming straight. When the driving speed was over 30 km/h, there were greater effects on driving operation due to centrifugal force.

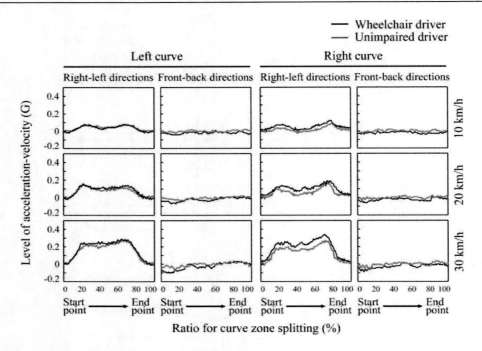

Figure 13. Comparison of the acceleration-velocity on a curve.

Next, the driving load was studied by examining the acceleration-velocity at five sections of the course shown in Figure 11. This evaluation of acceleration-velocity was conducted by a different method from the indicators in Figure 13. An absolute figure was calculated after the measured waveform was equalized, and a comparison was made by using the figure as an index of the size of the acceleration-velocity. The driving time at curves was divided into 100 time-units and the average acceleration during each 1 % was calculated. The borderlines of the curve zones were identified, and the average acceleration-velocity at each zone was calculated. Figure 14 shows a comparison of the acceleration-velocity at five different sections.

A comparison of the acceleration of right-left direction for both groups on the sections 1-5 showed a tendency to increase the difference between sections 1 and 2, and also 4 and 5 when the speed became faster. Sections 1-2 are from a straight to the curve approach, and sections 4-5 are a straight line after exiting the curve. These are the sections which are most influenced by centrifugal force through operation of the steering wheel. When leaving the right curve, the difference of the acceleration-velocity for right-left direction was 0.22 G, which showed the strongest influence. On this section, drivers feel tension in order to keep their posture and the upper half of the body leans as a backlash on Section 5 where the direction of acceleration-velocity changes, and then the upper limbs are under strain from the effort of keeping body balance and controlling the vehicle. Thus, it is possible that more severe muscle tension is triggered and this will put more driving load onto the driver than under normal driving conditions. In the driving research with the use of an electromyogram by Ikeda et al. [11], it was shown that the muscle load on the left curve was basically higher than on the right curve, however, on the section of leaving the curve on the right curve, the use of the trapezius muscle, which is used for steering operation, was greater.

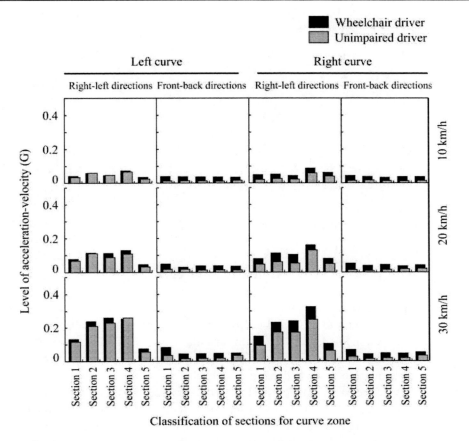

Figure 14. Comparison of the acceleration-velocity on each section of curve.

On this section, the driver received the effects of centrifugal force in a right-left direction when leaving the curve, therefore, it can be said that such a section is a typical case of difficult driving for wheelchair drivers.

As shown in Figures 13 and 14, significant differences were found in the acceleration velocity on the right-left direction in accordance with the increase of speed on both the right and left curves. Especially, the influence of centrifugal force showed a remarkable increase of velocity for disabled drivers when leaving the right curve. Also, when correcting the angle of the steering wheel at the immediate end of the curve at section 4-5, a tendency of a "severe swerve of the vehicle" was observed.

The wheelchair driver does not maintain body balance by using the legs as unimpaired people do on a curve with centrifugal force, upper body posture is kept by the arm being straight and the shoulder and back pushing against the seat on the right curve, as shown in Figure 15 (b). Also, it can be assumed that on the left curve, the driver keeps his right arm straight to press on the steering wheel, and the body trunk is fixed and centered around the left shoulder, Figure 15 (a). However, on leaving the curve, it seems that there is a disruption of the balance due to correcting the steering angle and pushing the upper body against the seat for support, possibly causing the vehicle to swerve strongly. It was shown that on this section, the body balance was easily disrupted, and the operation of steering wheel and speed control lever was unstable which shows a decrease in the level of driving control environment.

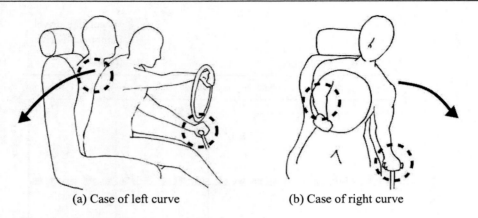

(a) Case of left curve     (b) Case of right curve

Figure 15. Image of driving style for wheelchair user.

## CONCLUSION

In this chapter, it was found that levels of driving load were different depending on speed, and also it is difficult to drive and keep a safe posture on some conditions.

As for the reduction of driving load, the installation of support equipment to vehicles built basically for the movements of unimpaired people and the alternation of driving methods are not enough to support driving by wheelchair drivers. With an understanding of this situation, it is necessary to acknowledge the driving situation scientifically and to understand driving load. When wheelchair users are driving vehicles, one hand is mainly used for the steering wheel and the other hand is used for controlling acceleration and braking. They cannot control the steering wheel with both hands; thus their posture is unstable when they are driving. In this view, for safe driving, the following are required: (1) driver's seats which can stabilize the driver's posture even on curves; (2) development of a human interface system of controls for wheelchair drivers, especially when driving on curves.

If a driving-seat to support posture, which would decrease muscle tension, is developed, unimpaired people will also find it comfortable for driving. The road conditions created for unimpaired people will only increase the driving load for wheelchair drivers.

As a future task, it is important to clarify dangerous areas from the viewpoint of wheelchair drivers. It is also necessary to evaluate conditions when people drive on curves, and this should happen not only for people with both upper and lower body impairments, but also in comparison to people with only lower body impairments and also physically unimpaired people.

## REFERENCES

[1] National Police Agency. (2011). Driver's license statistics.
[2] National Rehabilitation Center for Persons with Disabilities. (1994). Physically handicapped people/senior citizens and driving: Historic process and present conditions. Tokyo, Chuohoki Publishers.

[3] Ikeda, H., Mihoshi, A., and Kimura, N. (2007). Problems of driving vehicles for disabled people, *Journal of Human Environmental Studies*, Vol. 5, No. 1, pp. 27-33.

[4] National Rehabilitation Center for Persons with Disabilities. (1990). Driving guidance handbook for physically handicapped people. Tokyo, Chuohoki Publishers.

[5] Ikeda, H., Mihoshi, A., Ikeda, H., and Hisari, Y. (2007). Physical load related to highway-driving among disabled people, *IATSS Research*, Vol. 31, No. 1, pp. 100-109.

[6] Dols, J. F., Garcia, M., and Sotos, J. J. (1996). Procedure for improving the ergonomic design of driving positions adapted for handicapped people, *Boletín Factores Humanos*, No. 12-13, pp. 7-17.

[7] Ikeda, H., Mihoshi, A., Kimura, N., and Amemiya, K. (2008). Driving behaviour on curves for wheelchair users, *Journal of Traffic Science Society of Osaka*, Vol. 39, No. 1, pp. 60-65.

[8] Salvucci, D. D., and Liu, A. (2002). The time course of a lane change: Driver control and eye-movement behavior, *Transportation Research*, Part F, Vol. 5, No. 2, pp. 123-132.

[9] Imsland, L., Johansen, T. A., Fossen, T. I., Grip, H. F., Kalkkuhl, J. C., and Suissa, A. (2006). Vehicle velocity estimation using nonlinear observers, *Automatica*, Vol. 42, No. 12, pp. 2091-2103.

[10] Kitahama, K., and Sakai, H. (2000). Measurement method of normalized cornering stiffness, *JSAE Review*, Vol. 21, No. 2, pp. 213-217.

[11] Ikeda, H., Hirose, H., and Mihoshi, A. (2010). Study of movements of the head and muscle load of the shoulders and lower arms in driving for wheelchair drivers, *Journal of Human Environmental Studies*, Vol. 8, No. 1, pp. 75-79.

# INDEX

## A

accelerator, 177
ACL, 15
action potential, 20, 156, 157, 160
active feedback, 106
activity level, 5, 14
adaptation, xi, 23, 25, 56, 58, 67, 77, 79, 81, 94, 155, 166, 167, 168
adaptations, vii, ix, 1, 12, 25, 46, 61, 63, 64, 67, 75, 80, 81, 92, 141, 166, 172, 173
adiposity, 30
adjustment, 35, 37, 133, 136, 143, 150, 151, 159, 162, 163, 164
adolescents, 77, 78, 82, 87, 93
adults, 8, 9, 10, 11, 12, 14, 16, 17, 18, 19, 20, 23, 24, 25, 26, 27, 28, 29, 31, 32, 54, 55, 61, 74, 75, 76, 93, 132, 152, 162, 167, 168, 174
aerobic capacity, 18
age, vii, x, 2, 6, 8, 10, 11, 12, 13, 15, 16, 17, 19, 20, 21, 24, 26, 27, 28, 29, 30, 31, 43, 63, 65, 67, 71, 72, 74, 75, 76, 81, 87, 90, 91, 95, 134, 135, 145, 149, 162, 168, 183
age-related decline in postural control, vii, 2, 21
aggregation, 128
agonist, 15, 17, 162, 165
akinesia, 44
alters, 28, 174
amplitude, xi, 5, 9, 36, 40, 42, 47, 48, 142, 144, 155, 156, 159, 160, 161, 162, 163, 164, 165, 169
anatomy, 37, 43
ankles, 8, 16, 42, 47, 120
anthropometric characteristics, 97
APA, 37
appropriate motor responses, vii, 1, 6, 21
arthritis, 147
artificial intelligence, 51

assessment, vii, x, 2, 21, 27, 29, 90, 101, 131, 132, 134, 138, 151, 160, 165, 170, 174
assessment techniques, 21
asymmetry, 27
asymptomatic, 93
ataxia, 132
athletes, ix, x, 15, 29, 61, 63, 64, 67, 68, 69, 71, 73, 76, 78, 79, 80, 82, 83, 88, 90, 91, 94, 96, 146, 151
atrophy, 8
attachment, 88
avoidance, 21
awareness, 53, 83
axons, 156, 157

## B

back pain, x, 63, 67, 69, 72, 79, 83, 91, 92, 93, 95, 96, 97
backlash, 186
basal ganglia, vii, 1, 6, 56
base, vii, 1, 2, 4, 17, 27, 28, 35, 36, 41, 65, 86, 100, 101, 106, 129, 134, 173
behavioral change, 47
behaviors, 55
bending, 67, 69, 85, 89, 91, 92, 93, 95, 144, 153
beneficial effect, vii, 1, 19, 21, 27, 82, 167
benefits, 18, 84
bias, 171
biceps femoris, 87
biofeedback, 24, 126, 128
biomechanics, 5, 6, 60, 61, 100, 101, 131, 133, 134, 139, 149
bipedal, 2, 14, 31, 54
blindness, 44
blood, 128
body composition, 83
body image, 44, 68, 83

body mass index, 140, 149
body schema, 36, 37, 41, 43
body shape, 37
body size, 152
body weight, 21, 163
bone, 23, 77, 79, 138, 147, 148, 151
bone mass, 23
bones, 11, 139, 145
boxing, 145
brain, 6, 8, 17, 44, 51, 56, 128, 172, 174
brainstem, 6
breathing, 41, 93, 103, 112, 120, 128
brevis, 161, 174

# C

calibration, 52, 55
canals, 44
capsule, 3
cardiac activity, 103, 120
cardiac muscle, 31
cardiac output, 128
cardiovascular risk, 30
caricature, 43
cartilage, 139
case studies, 39
case study, 97
cataract, 10, 22
cauda equina, 170
central nervous system, vii, 1, 11, 36, 43, 44, 61, 100, 130, 139
centre-of-pressure (COP), vii, 1, 10
cerebellum, vii, 1, 6, 11, 51
cerebral cortex, 60
chaos, 134
Chicago, 57
childhood, 91, 97
children, 44, 54, 59, 71, 78, 87, 91, 93, 95, 96
citizens, 188
clarity, 89
classes, 83
climate, 78
clinical application, 149
closure, 9
CNS, 6, 9, 10, 11, 16
coefficient of variation, 14
cognitive performance, 61
cognitive perspective, viii, 33
cognitive process, 44, 51
cognitive research, 43
cognitive science, 53
cognitive tasks, 17, 28
cognitive theory, 38, 50, 51

coherence, 43, 44, 52
collagen, x, 64
combined effect, 127
community, 19, 21, 25, 28, 32, 51, 52
compensation, 26, 35, 36, 149
competition, ix, 52, 63, 67, 71, 81
competitive sport, 67
complement, 141
complexity, viii, ix, x, 34, 45, 48, 51, 53, 99, 102, 128, 130, 131
compliance, 150, 152
complications, 15
comprehension, x, 138
compression, 65, 67, 77, 79
computation, 23, 51, 52
computer, 133, 182
computing, 3, 5, 55
conception, 36
conceptual model, 58, 134
concordance, 82
conditioning, 83, 128, 158, 159, 160
conference, viii, 22, 34
configuration, ix, 36, 63, 76, 78, 79, 95, 160
congress, 150
Congress, 22, 23
consensus, 38
consent, 182
construction, 37
consumption, 146
contact time, 143, 146
contour, 10
contradiction, 36, 46, 50
contrast sensitivity, 10, 27
control group, x, 63, 70, 72, 75, 78, 81, 82, 91, 168
conviction, 52
coordination, viii, ix, 10, 30, 33, 34, 37, 41, 45, 48, 49, 54, 55, 57, 58, 59, 61, 83, 133, 135
correlation, 5, 14, 31, 90, 152, 160, 173
correlation coefficient, 90, 160
correlations, 14, 15
cortex, vii, 1, 6, 10, 43, 44, 54, 158, 159
cost, 18, 20, 21, 35, 41, 42, 43, 50, 142, 178, 179
counterbalance, 3
creep, x, 64, 78, 81
criticism, 41, 48, 50, 141
cues, 57
cycles, 67
cycling, 70, 78, 79, 80, 92, 95, 145

# D

daily living, 96
damping, 152, 153

dance, 68, 70, 83
dancers, ix, 61, 63, 91, 95
danger, 43, 130
data analysis, 183
data set, 97
decrease of neuromuscular capacities, vii, 1
deep brain stimulation, 56
deficiencies, 90
deficit, 37, 43
deformation, x, 45, 64, 78, 81, 139
degenerate, 44
degradation, 8
dependent variable, 46
depression, 162, 164, 166
depth, 9, 10, 15, 52, 107, 131
depth perception, 10
destiny, 58
detectable, 90
detection, 12, 38, 183
determinism, 47, 60
deviation, 6, 40, 47, 65
diabetes, 131
diabetic neuropathy, 135
differential equations, 113, 114, 116, 126, 128
diffusion, vii, 1, 3, 5, 6, 29
digestion, 130
disability, 26, 65, 177, 183, 184
discomfort, 91
discs, 64, 66, 95
disorder, 44
displacement, vii, 1, 3, 4, 5, 6, 35, 38, 39, 42, 47, 49, 100, 105, 152, 167
distribution, 35, 38, 46, 64, 100, 103, 120, 128, 130, 132, 165
dominance, 47
dopaminergic, 44
drawing, 56
DSC, 135
dual task, 22
dynamical systems, 49, 59

# E

education, 87
elaboration, 60
elastic deformation, 144
elderly population, 27, 28
electrodes, 40, 160
electromagnetic, 92
electromyograph, 156
elementary school, 96
e-mail, 99
embryogenesis, 39

EMG, x, 20, 23, 24, 152, 155, 156, 160, 161, 163
empirical studies, 49
EMS, 20
endurance, 32, 146, 151
energy, x, 35, 41, 42, 50, 61, 106, 112, 118, 126, 130, 134, 137, 138, 139, 142, 144, 145, 146, 148, 153
energy consumption, 144
energy expenditure, x, 61, 118, 130, 137, 138, 142
engineering, 55
environment, viii, ix, xi, 3, 9, 25, 34, 35, 38, 40, 46, 58, 59, 61, 64, 77, 175, 176, 179, 182, 187
environmental change, 160
environmental factors, 64
epiphysis, 77
epithelia, 30
equilibrium, 2, 5, 10, 16, 19, 53, 56, 58, 65, 99, 100, 103, 104, 110, 113, 114, 115, 118, 120, 123, 124, 129, 131, 132, 170
equipment, 21, 176, 177, 178, 179, 182, 188
ergonomics, 176
error detection, 37, 39, 41, 43
evidence, xi, 13, 18, 21, 23, 28, 48, 155, 160, 166
evoked potential, 156, 158
evolution, 90, 91
excitability, 157, 158, 159, 160, 161, 163, 164, 165, 170, 171, 173
excitation, 156, 157, 159, 170, 172
excitatory postsynaptic potentials, 156
execution, viii, 33, 160, 161
executive function, 44, 51
executive functions, 44
exercise, vii, viii, xi, 1, 2, 8, 18, 19, 20, 21, 22, 23, 26, 27, 29, 30, 32, 68, 74, 75, 76, 79, 85, 86, 87, 89, 94, 144, 151, 153, 155, 166, 167, 173, 174
exercise programs, 20, 21
exertion, 36
experimental condition, 163
exposure, x, 63, 67, 78, 90
extensor, 20, 28, 31, 32, 161
extensor carpi radialis longus, 161
external environment, 9
exteroceptive feedback, ix, 34
extraction, 5

# F

families, 102
fat, 22
fiber, 27
financial, 178, 179
financial support, 179
Finland, 150

fitness, 20, 21, 25, 83, 84, 86
flex, 86
flexibility, 20, 21, 25, 64, 83, 88, 91, 92, 93, 96, 97, 122, 142, 151, 153
flexion movements, 90
flexor, 3, 7, 13, 14, 15, 22, 24, 27, 141, 148, 149, 150, 151, 161
flexor carpi radialis, 161
flight, 42, 166
fluctuations, 14, 28, 31, 49, 60
fluid, 19
football, 25, 71, 78, 88, 97
force, ix, 2, 3, 4, 11, 12, 13, 14, 16, 18, 22, 23, 24, 25, 26, 31, 34, 38, 40, 52, 60, 91, 95, 100, 101, 118, 120, 129, 130, 132, 135, 139, 140, 142, 143, 144, 145, 146, 147, 148, 151, 168, 169, 181, 182, 185, 186, 187
formula, 90
foundations, viii, 34, 132
France, 33, 58, 60, 129
freedom, 16, 47, 102, 105, 106, 107, 108, 113, 122, 128, 139
friction, 45
functional approach, 38
fusion, 59

## G

gait, 12, 22, 44, 50, 56, 62, 129, 133, 140, 142, 144, 149, 150, 153
gastrocnemius, 2, 7, 23, 39, 41, 144, 152, 153, 161, 165, 169, 170, 171
gender differences, 142
Generalized Motor Program (GMP), ix, 34
geometry, 36, 109, 120, 129, 130, 131, 142, 144
gestures, 37
grants, 179
graph, 46
gravitational force, 36, 45
gravitational pull, 35
gravity, vii, 1, 2, 3, 7, 10, 35, 36, 37, 40, 42, 45, 56, 133, 135, 150, 164
grouping, 8
growth, x, 51, 63, 64, 67, 77, 82, 88, 90, 92
growth factor, 64
growth spurt, 67
guidance, 52, 55, 189
gymnastics, 68, 71, 78, 83
gymnasts, ix, 63, 69, 72, 78, 83, 91, 93, 97
gyms, 87

## H

hair, 11
hair cells, 11
hamstring, 15, 25, 28, 31, 80, 82, 83, 87, 88, 89, 91, 92, 93, 94, 95, 96, 97, 142, 150
handicapped people, 188, 189
health, 18, 19, 27, 29, 65, 84, 86, 158
health status, 65
height, 42, 68, 100, 146, 148, 166, 171
hemisphere, 44
heterogeneity, 8
hip joint, vii, 1, 2, 3, 16, 107, 120, 131
history, 13, 29, 92, 163, 173
Hoffmann reflex (H-reflex), x, 155
homogeneity, 49
horses, 50, 57, 142, 150, 151
H-reflex modulation, xi, 155, 156, 158, 160, 162, 163, 164, 165, 166, 167
human body, 21, 41, 64, 108, 118, 120, 139, 143, 148
human development, 166
human subjects, 25, 146, 169, 171
Hunter, 103, 133, 140, 151
hybrid, 4, 51
hybridization, 52
hypothesis, 3, 6, 10, 16, 17, 36, 42, 43, 44, 49, 51, 53, 103, 105
hysteresis, 49

## I

ICC, 90, 160, 161
ideal, 19, 93, 139
idiopathic, 95
illusion, 39, 40
illusions, 10
images, 182
immersion, 45
impairments, 177, 179, 182, 188
improvements, 18, 19, 89, 128
impulses, 7, 11, 129, 171
in transition, 50
in vivo, 95, 97, 140, 149, 150, 152, 169
inattention, 57
incidence, 65, 70, 79, 87, 93, 96
independence, 46, 176
individuals, 8, 9, 11, 12, 13, 14, 15, 16, 17, 18, 19, 20, 37, 38, 39, 44, 57, 79, 81, 82, 90, 95, 96, 128, 153
inertia, 51, 55, 103, 122, 141
inertial effects, 108

information processing, ix, 34, 35, 37, 40, 44, 57
information-processing system, viii, ix, 34, 41, 43
inhibition, 36, 158, 162, 164, 169, 170, 171, 172
initiation, ix, 34
injuries, 15, 21, 22, 25, 82, 83, 84, 87, 93, 95, 96, 100, 131, 138, 140, 147, 148, 166
injury, x, 15, 20, 31, 63, 67, 82, 83, 84, 85, 87, 137, 138, 146, 147, 148, 149, 184
injury prevention, 83
inner ear, 10
integration, ix, 6, 26, 35, 37, 39, 40, 57, 134
intentionality, 46
interface, 151, 188
internal consistency, 90
interneuron, 158
interneurons, 159, 160
intervention, x, xi, 20, 21, 46, 138, 155, 166, 167
intervertebral disc, ix, x, 63, 66, 92, 93, 95, 97
invariants, ix, 34, 46
inverted pendulum, x, 16, 23, 36, 42, 48, 99, 102, 104, 105, 107, 108, 109, 111, 112, 113, 126, 129, 130, 133, 134, 141
ipsilateral, 53
Islam, 32
issues, ix, 34, 51, 101, 128, 141, 147
Italy, 99, 129, 134

## J

Japan, xi, 175
joint damage, 131
joints, 2, 7, 9, 11, 16, 19, 20, 31, 32, 49, 100, 103, 105, 107, 108, 109, 110, 111, 114, 120, 122, 124, 125, 126, 128, 129, 139, 153
jumping, 30, 148, 170
justification, 43

## K

kinetics, 59, 60, 106, 148
knees, 36, 42, 48, 77, 80, 88, 120
kyphosis, 64, 65, 66, 67, 68, 69, 70, 71, 72, 73, 74, 75, 77, 78, 79, 82, 83, 84, 85, 86, 87, 91, 92, 95, 96

## L

landings, 171
landscapes, 59
latency, 156, 158, 161, 163, 167, 169
latissimus dorsi, 85, 86, 94
laws, xi, 67, 175

lead, ix, 13, 18, 40, 63, 67, 79, 81, 82, 84, 140
learning, 48, 51, 53, 55, 60, 166
legs, 16, 35, 108, 116, 117, 120, 144, 187
lens, 10
lesions, 39, 41, 44, 54, 56
ligament, 12, 28
light, 10, 37, 41, 52, 62
light transmission, 10
load balance, ix, x, 63
locus, 184, 185
logical reasoning, 38
longitudinal study, 22, 24, 97
lordosis, 64, 65, 66, 67, 68, 69, 70, 71, 72, 74, 75, 76, 78, 81, 82, 83, 84, 85, 87, 91, 93, 94
lumbar spinal curvatures, x, 64, 81
lumbar spine, 81, 82, 83, 84, 86, 87, 92, 95, 97
lying, 61, 161, 169

## M

macular degeneration, 10
magnetic field, 158
magnetic resonance, 31, 140, 147, 148, 150, 151
magnetic resonance imaging, 31
magnitude, 2, 12, 14, 67, 78, 100, 106, 130, 142, 174
majority, 4, 19, 67, 82, 163
man, 53, 60, 132, 135, 136, 151, 169, 170, 171, 172
management, 96, 97
martial art, 19, 167
Maryland, 133
mass, vii, 35, 42, 48, 58, 65, 99, 102, 103, 117, 120, 124, 128, 130, 139, 141, 142, 143, 144, 150, 152
mastoid, 40
matrix, 117, 176
mean square COP displacement, vii, 1, 4, 5
measurement, 3, 4, 90, 96, 100, 101, 131, 132, 139, 149, 151, 152, 160, 162, 163, 182, 183
measurements, 4, 67, 90, 96, 97, 100, 149, 150, 153, 160, 161, 172
mechanical loadings, x, 63
mechanical properties, ix, 63, 64, 120, 128, 142, 152, 153
medicine, 51, 172
medulla, 11
MEG, 44
membership, 21
memory, ix, 34, 52
messages, 25, 36, 41
meta-analysis, 20, 29, 30
Metabolic, 61
metaphor, 52
metatarsal, 160
methodology, 20, 38, 40, 46, 160

MHC, 27
mice, 150
microgravity, 35, 36, 39, 56, 58
military, 93
modelling, 149
models, vii, x, 44, 49, 51, 54, 97, 99, 100, 101, 102, 103, 106, 107, 108, 112, 113, 117, 118, 120, 122, 128, 129, 130, 131, 133, 135, 140
modifications, xi, 13, 22, 35, 50, 79, 92, 175, 178
modules, 35, 41
modulus, 148
Moon, 18, 23
morbidity, vii, 1, 101
morphology, 25, 93
mortality, 101
mortality rate, 101
motion sickness, 40
motivation, 8
motor activity, 61
motor behavior, viii, 34, 44, 48, 51, 52, 53, 60
motor control, viii, 33, 34, 37, 53, 135, 140, 172
motor neurons, 43
motor skills, 166, 174
motor system, 6, 7, 9, 44, 138, 143, 147, 148, 169
motor task, xi, 14, 140, 147, 155, 160, 161, 165
MRI, 95
multiple sclerosis, 131
muscle mass, 142
muscle strain, 31, 166
muscle strength, vii, 1, 7, 10, 13, 15, 19, 27, 29, 32, 68, 87, 167
muscles, x, 2, 3, 5, 6, 7, 9, 11, 12, 13, 15, 16, 17, 18, 19, 23, 26, 27, 29, 31, 38, 41, 53, 64, 66, 67, 80, 83, 85, 87, 88, 89, 91, 92, 95, 100, 106, 122, 127, 128, 139, 140, 143, 144, 145, 147, 148, 150, 151, 152, 156, 159, 161, 162, 165, 169, 172, 185
musculoskeletal system, viii, x, 10, 34, 137, 138, 145

## N

neglect, 44, 130
nerve, x, 11, 38, 155, 156, 158, 160, 161, 169
nervous system, vii, 1, 8, 9, 11, 16, 30, 31, 37, 41, 43, 44, 128, 171
neuromotor, 140, 147
neurons, 8, 11, 158
neuropathy, 40
neurophysiology, 100, 171
neuropsychology, 51
neurotransmitters, 156, 159
neutral, 15, 65, 66, 77, 80, 82, 83, 84, 86, 89, 161, 164
New Zealand, 22

NMR, 153
normal development, 64, 77
Norway, 22
nuclei, 11, 43
nucleus, 43
null, 140
nystagmus, 11

## O

obesity, 141
oculomotor, 39
old age, 24, 132
opacity, 10
operations, 51
optimal performance, 144
organ, 7, 164
organize, 40
organs, 7, 10, 11, 130
oscillation, 48, 49, 102, 106, 112, 113, 140, 142
osteoarthritis, 147
overweight, 23
overweight adults, 23
oxygen, 146
oxygen consumption, 146

## P

pain, 65, 67, 83, 84, 93, 97
parallel, 16, 37, 139, 164
participants, 21, 69, 82, 162, 163, 169
patella, 153
pathology, 41, 43, 44, 96, 101, 130
pathways, 16, 37, 38, 43, 44, 136, 158, 159, 162, 167, 171, 173
pedal, 180
pelvis, 3, 64, 65, 79, 87, 88, 89, 90, 92
penetrability, 61
perceptual learning, 55
performers, 83
peripheral neuropathy, 55
permission, 157, 158, 159
permit, 46
PET, 44
phase transitions, 49
Philadelphia, 22
physical activity, 18, 22, 26
physical education, 96
physical fitness, 23
physicians, 87
physics, 139, 141

Physiological, 8, 21, 25, 27, 28, 30, 31, 55, 58, 60, 97, 170
physiological factors, 9, 27
physiology, 27, 43, 44, 102
plantar fasciitis, 147
plantar flexion, 14
plasticity, 166, 174
platform, 2, 3, 4, 12, 35, 40, 42, 55, 101, 118, 119, 132, 133, 135, 146, 163
playing, 70, 88, 97
PM, 95
poor performance, 13
population, 8, 15, 18, 20, 27, 32, 72, 77, 81, 82, 89, 95, 101, 159
population group, 101
Portugal, 1, 137
position effect, 93
positive correlation, 14, 64
positive relationship, 142
positivism, 53
post-hoc analysis, 87
postural control, vii, viii, ix, xi, 1, 2, 3, 4, 5, 6, 7, 8, 9, 10, 11, 12, 13, 14, 15, 16, 17, 18, 19, 20, 21, 22, 23, 24, 25, 26, 27, 28, 29, 30, 31, 33, 35, 36, 37, 38, 39, 43, 45, 47, 48, 50, 51, 54, 56, 57, 58, 59, 61, 100, 101, 103, 107, 130, 132, 134, 135, 155, 162, 167, 169, 171, 173
Postural control, vii, 1, 6, 29, 36, 45, 58
postural loading, ix, x, 63
postural sway, vii, 1, 8, 14, 17, 20, 24, 27, 32, 39, 41, 44, 46, 53, 54, 57, 60, 61, 62, 100, 101, 133, 134, 156, 171, 173
prevention, 15, 18, 19, 20, 23, 27, 30, 31, 95, 161
primacy, 42
primary school, 70
principles, viii, 33, 87
programming, 54, 56
project, 53
propagation, 144
proprioceptive modalities, vii, 1
protection, 130
psychology, 48, 51
public opinion, xi, 175

## Q

quadriceps, 3, 7, 13, 15, 18, 22, 23, 29, 31, 41, 151, 169
quality of life, 17
quantification, 60
questionnaire, xi, 175, 176, 177

## R

racing, 97
radiation, 90
radius, 46
ramp, 160
random walk, 5
reaction time, 8, 10, 167
reactions, 8, 36, 39, 41, 43, 53
reading, 45
reality, 3, 101, 106, 112, 130, 152
recall, viii, ix, 33, 34
reception, 39
receptors, ix, 6, 7, 11, 12, 34, 35, 38, 40, 45, 156, 160, 164
recognition, ix, 34, 52
reconciliation, 51
recovery, 22, 29, 61, 138, 143
recreation, 84
recreational, 70, 75, 84, 85, 87, 94, 96
recurrence, 46
redistribution, 143
redundancy, 40
reference frame, 41
reference system, 11
reflex action, 166
reflexes, 8, 11, 128, 160, 164, 169, 171, 173
regression, 17
rehabilitation, x, 20, 26, 39, 95, 131, 137
reinforcement, ix, 34
rejection, 50
relaxation, ix, 34, 49, 95, 96, 150
relaxation properties, 150
relevance, 43, 45, 140, 173
reliability, 88, 90, 101, 131, 132, 160, 161, 165, 168, 169, 170, 172, 173
remodelling, 30
repetitions, 101
requirements, 43, 78, 178, 179
researchers, x, 3, 44, 51, 52, 102, 137, 139
resistance, 18, 19, 21, 23, 24, 45, 64, 138, 140, 168
resolution, 10, 128
resources, 43
respiration, 130
response, x, 7, 9, 11, 24, 41, 42, 46, 47, 51, 56, 67, 95, 96, 140, 141, 142, 149, 150, 151, 155, 156, 157, 160, 162, 163, 164, 165, 166, 167, 178, 179, 180, 181
restoration, 12
retina, 10
retinitis, 44
retinitis pigmentosa, 44
rhythm, 87, 88

rhythmic gymnasts, ix, 63, 72, 83, 91, 93
right hemisphere, 44
risk, vii, x, 1, 13, 14, 18, 19, 21, 28, 31, 52, 78, 83, 84, 87, 90, 93, 101, 137, 138, 147, 148, 176, 182
risk factors, 31
risk management, 176
robotics, 51
root, 4, 9, 10, 14
root-mean-square, 4
rotational matrix, 124
rotations, 105, 120, 122, 134
routines, 8, 83
rowing, 68, 72, 82
Royal Society, 150
rugby, 69
rules, ix, 34, 38

## S

safety, xi, 92, 175, 176, 179, 182
Sagittal alignment, ix, x, 63, 97
Sagittal spinal curvatures, ix, 63, 81, 94
sarcopenia, 24
scaling, 5, 17
scapula, 82
schema, ix, 34, 36, 37, 42, 51, 60
school, 52, 93
science, viii, 33, 52, 58
scoliosis, 95
self-organization, ix, 34
semicircular canals, 164
semimembranosus, 87
sensation, 7, 10, 11, 12, 19, 27, 30, 38, 58
sensations, 7, 160
senses, 10, 38, 45, 61
sensitivity, 10
sensors, 92, 100, 183
sensory modalities, 11, 21, 132
sensory systems, viii, 34, 38, 40
sex, 141, 148, 153
sex differences, 141
shape, 64, 65, 67, 92, 139, 184, 185
shear, x, 63, 65, 67, 84, 85, 105
shock, 64, 146, 147
showing, 140
signals, 16, 26, 32, 47, 57, 58, 101, 156, 158, 164
simulation, 10, 22, 26, 120, 126, 131
simulations, 106, 128
skeletal muscle, 60, 152, 153, 168
skeleton, 31, 77, 145
skin, 7, 39, 92, 100
soccer, ix, 28, 63, 69, 70, 71, 97
society, xi, 175, 176

software, 120
soleus, xi, 2, 3, 12, 153, 155, 156, 168, 169, 170, 171, 172, 173
soleus (SOL) H-reflex, xi, 155, 156
solution, 51, 52, 59, 113
South Africa, 137
Spain, 63, 95
spasticity, 174
spatial processing, 57
specialists, 87
spinal cord, 7, 8, 11, 43, 100, 156, 157, 160, 161, 162, 172
spinal stenosis, 162, 170
spinal tissues, ix, 63, 81
spindle, 7, 31, 32, 60, 162, 169
spine, ix, x, 63, 64, 65, 66, 67, 68, 72, 76, 77, 78, 79, 83, 84, 85, 86, 87, 91, 92, 93, 94, 95, 96, 97, 103, 128, 134, 148, 183
Spring, 152
stability, vii, x, xi, 5, 7, 8, 9, 10, 11, 12, 13, 15, 16, 18, 19, 20, 22, 23, 24, 27, 28, 29, 31, 32, 36, 40, 42, 45, 48, 49, 54, 55, 58, 99, 100, 101, 106, 118, 126, 128, 130, 132, 133, 134, 135, 137, 138, 140, 141, 147, 148, 149, 151, 152, 156, 162, 167, 173, 175
stabilization, 36, 56, 60, 61, 106, 126, 130, 132, 170
stabilogram diffusion analysis, vii, 1, 3, 29
stable states, 49
state, 5, 6, 45, 49, 61, 143, 144, 159, 164
statistics, 3, 9, 188
stimulus, 20, 50, 60
storage, 138, 143, 144
strategy use, 105, 120, 129
strength training, 18, 25, 28, 153, 166, 172
stress, 64, 77, 82, 132, 142, 147, 150
stress fracture, 147, 150
stretching, 39, 77, 88, 89, 93, 95, 96, 170
striatum, 43
stroke, 80, 81, 82, 163, 171
structural changes, 8, 10
structure, x, 27, 46, 61, 64, 100, 120, 128, 142, 149
style, ix, 23, 63, 73, 78, 95, 182, 188
subjectivity, 53
succession, 35
Sun, 23, 149
supervision, 51
suppression, 160, 170
surface properties, 58
surplus, 40
susceptibility, 17
symmetry, 29
symptoms, 44
synapse, 11

# Index

synaptic transmission, 156
synchronization, 37
syndrome, 44
synthesis, 29, 59

## T

Tai Chi, vii, 2, 18, 19, 21, 23, 24, 25, 27, 31, 32, 166, 167, 168, 170, 171, 173, 174
target, 38, 45, 47, 48, 49, 156, 157
task demands, 58
task performance, 46
team members, 70
techniques, 22, 83, 87, 100, 120, 169, 182
tendon, vii, x, 7, 11, 12, 37, 38, 55, 60, 106, 137, 138, 139, 141, 143, 144, 145, 148, 150, 151, 152, 153, 174
tendons, 7, 11, 100, 139, 140, 143, 145, 147, 152
tension, 3, 7, 11, 78, 87, 88, 151, 186, 188
terminals, 164
testing, 14, 21, 93, 101, 161, 162
test-retest reliability, 160, 161
thalamus, 43
thorax, 120, 122
thoughts, 14
three-dimensional multi-link models, x, 99
threshold level, 157
tibia, 3
tibialis anterior, 7, 12, 18, 24, 160, 170, 172
time series, 4, 5
tissue, 82, 96, 138, 144, 147, 148
tonic, 100
trade, 130
trainees, 93
training, vii, ix, x, xi, 1, 15, 18, 19, 20, 21, 22, 23, 24, 25, 26, 27, 28, 29, 30, 31, 32, 63, 64, 67, 68, 69, 71, 72, 73, 74, 75, 76, 77, 78, 79, 80, 81, 82, 83, 84, 85, 87, 88, 89, 90, 91, 92, 93, 95, 96, 97, 153, 155, 156, 166, 167, 168, 169, 170, 171, 172, 173
training programs, 21, 83
trajectory, 2, 135
transformation, 58
translation, 2, 54, 110, 123
transmission, 131, 145, 146, 157, 171
transport, 21
transportation, 176
trapezius, 186
treatment, 96
trial, 28, 31, 82, 117, 120
triceps, 18, 74, 76, 85, 87, 94, 141, 148, 149, 152, 169, 173, 174
trochanter, 3

Turkey, 23
type 2 diabetes, 23

## U

ultrasound, 140, 147
uniform, 46

## V

validation, 51, 97, 128, 129
variables, vii, 1, 3, 18, 38, 47, 54, 82, 92, 106
variations, 9, 24, 35, 42, 64, 101
vastus medialis, 161, 169
vector, 4, 13, 100
vehicles, 78, 175, 176, 177, 182, 183, 188, 189
velocity, xi, 4, 9, 14, 27, 29, 61, 106, 128, 139, 141, 145, 147, 148, 152, 163, 164, 165, 170, 175, 176, 182, 183, 185, 186, 187, 189
ventilation, 93
vertebrae, 64, 77, 83, 86, 94
vertigo, 11
vestibular system, ix, 11, 34, 35, 39, 44, 45, 101, 164
vibration, 12, 27, 37, 38, 55, 56, 60, 62, 140
viscoelastic properties, 148
viscosity, 111, 114, 124, 125, 126, 139
vision, ix, 7, 10, 11, 27, 34, 37, 39, 40, 43, 44, 46, 54, 59, 60
visual acuity, 10
visual environment, 9, 28, 46
visual field, 9, 10
visual system, 7, 10, 37, 38
volleyball, 68, 70, 71, 74, 78, 88, 92

## W

walking, 18, 19, 25, 28, 31, 50, 51, 54, 135, 144, 150, 152, 156, 166, 169, 171, 172
water, 80, 82
weakness, 13
wear, 176
weight loss, 23
welfare, xi, 175
withdrawal, 166
wrestling, 68, 71, 73, 78
wrists, 120

## Y

young adults, 9, 10, 14, 16, 17, 23, 30, 94, 162, 169
young women, 26, 83